Men's Cancers

◆ ◆ ◆

"The distinguishing quality of this lay reader's guide to men's cancers is that it is written by nurses who recognize the need for medical expertise with an emphasis on patient education in a clear, plainly written text. Recommended as a complete guide to survivorship strategies."

— *Library Journal*

Praise for *Women's Cancers*

"They take pains to make the content as easy to understand as possible, including a glossary of technical terms highlighted in the text, illustrating procedures and findings with clear line drawings, and listing questions to ask physicians about each disorder or therapy. Their guide is also significant for its encouragement of women's self-empowerment, advice on pursuing a healthy life-style, and advocacy for women's health funding and research."

— *Booklist*

"Readers will find all the answers to questions either patients are afraid to ask their doctors or that doctors don't know how to answer themselves."

— *The Richmond Review*

"Discussions of exactly what happens during surgery or while getting chemotherapy are excellent . . . and so are explanations of how different cancers develop. The authors suggest reasonable explanations for why people get cancer—the mix of cancer-causing factors in each woman's life will be unique—thereby downplaying fear-mongering news reports that say the cause of cancer is this chemical or that bad habit.

"WOMEN'S CANCERS will benefit women and their families, and should help some beat their disease."

— *Natural Health*

DEDICATION

To my dad, who fought a gallant but losing battle with lung cancer, and my mom, who was his advocate and caregiver;

To Don, Glenn, Jim, Gene, Boris . . . and the men whose lives are touched by cancer;

And especially to my twelve nursing colleagues who so generously gave time to prepare their contributions and share their wisdom in these pages, and to the thousands of our nursing colleagues who provide care and compassion on a daily basis to men—and their loved ones—who face cancer.

Other books in the Hunter House Cancer & Health series

Breast Implants—Everything You Need to Know (Bruning)
Cancer Doesn't Have to Hurt (Haylock & Curtiss)
Cancer—Increasing Your Odds for Survival (Bognar)
The Feisty Woman's Breast Cancer Book (Ratner)
How Women Can Finally Stop Smoking (Klesges & DeBon)
Lymphedema (Burt & White)
Recovering from Breast Surgery (Stumm)
Women's Cancers (McGinn & Haylock)

Ordering

Trade bookstores in the U.S. and Canada, please contact:

Publishers Group West
1700 Fourth Street, Berkeley CA 94710
Phone: (800) 788-3123   Fax: (510) 528-3444

Hunter House books are available at bulk discounts for textbook course adoptions; to qualifying community, health care, and government organizations; and for special promotions and fund-raising. For details please contact:

Special Sales Department
Hunter House Inc., PO Box 2914, Alameda CA 94501-0914
Phone: (510) 865-5282   Fax: (510) 865-4295
E-mail: ordering@hunterhouse.com

Individuals can order our books from most bookstores or by calling toll-free:
(800) 266-5592

Men's Cancers

How to Prevent Them,
How to Treat Them,
How to Beat Them

◆ ◆ ◆

Edited by
Pamela J. Haylock, R.N., M.A.

Hunter House
PUBLISHERS

Hunter House Inc., Publishers
PO Box 2914
Alameda CA 94501-0914

Library of Congress Cataloging-in-Publication Data

Haylock, Pamela J.
Men's Cancers: how to prevent them, how to treat, how to beat them / edited P. J. Haylock.
p.cm.
Includes bibliographical references and index
ISBN 0-89793-267-6 (cloth) — ISBN 0-89793-266-8 (paper)
1. Cancer in men—Popular works. I Title

RC281.M4 H395 2000

616.99'4'0081—dc21   00-063111

Project credits

Cover Design: Jil Weil Graphic Design
Book Production: Keri Northcott, Hunter House
Developmental and Copy Editor: Lydia Bird
Proofreader: Lee Rappold
Indexer: Kathy Talley-Jones
Graphics Coordinator: Ariel Parker
Acquisitions Editor: Jeanne Brondino
Associate Editor: Alexandra Mummery
Editorial & Production Assistant: Melissa Millar
Publicity Manager: Sarah Frederick
Sale & Marketing Assistant: Earlita Chenault
Customer Service Manager: Christina Sverdrup
Order Fulfillment: Joel Irons

Publisher: Kiran S. Rana

Printed and Bound by Publishers Press, Salt Lake City, Utah

Manufactured in the United States of America

9 8 7 6 5 4 3 2 1   First Edition   00 01 02 03 04

Table of Contents

List of Tables ix

List of Figures xi

List of Contributors xii

Important Note xiv

Introduction 1

Men and Cancer — Men and Communication — Regaining Power and
Control — The Premise—and Promise—of This Book — Expert Nurse
Contributors — Power, Control, and Survivorship — Cancer Victim,
Cancer Patient, or Cancer Survivor?

**Part I: Diagnosis and Beyond: Understanding Cancer
and Cancer Treatment** **7**

Chapter 1: About Cancer 8

What Is Cancer? — Causes of Cancer — Cancer Prevention — Cancer
Risk Analysis, Genetic Testing, and Genetic Counseling

Chapter 2: Finding Cancer 23

A Complex Process — Signs and Symptoms of Cancer —The First
Doctor's Appointment — Diagnosis — Staging of Cancer

Chapter 3: Your Cancer Care Team 34

The Idea of Self-Advocacy — Joining Your Treatment Team —
Choosing the Right Doctor — Second Opinions — Other Team
Members — Information Sources — Final Thoughts

Part II: Different Types of Cancers 51

Chapter 4: Prostate Cancer 52
Issues and Concerns — The Normal Prostate — Risk Factors,
Prevention, and Detection — Diagnosis and Workup — Treatment —
Follow-Up — Recurrence — Future

Chapter 5: Lung Cancer 84
Causes of Lung Cancer — Lung Cancer Prevention — Early Detection
— Types of Lung Cancer — Diagnosis and Workup — Treatment —
Symptom Management — Survivorship Issues — Future Directions

Chapter 6: Colorectal Cancer 100
Anatomy and Physiology — Risk Factors and Protective Factors —
Screening and Early Detection — Diagnosis and Workup — Treatment
— Questions to Ask When the Diagnosis Is Colorectal Cancer —
Follow-Up — Resources for You and Your Family

Chapter 7: Testicular Cancer 118
Normal Structure and Function of the Testicles — Statistics and Risk
Factors — Early Detection — Diagnosis and Workup — Treatment —
"What Does the Future Hold?"

Chapter 8: Penile Cancer 130
Risk Factors — Prevention and Early Detection — Diagnosis and
Workup — Treatment — Future

Chapter 9: Male Breast Cancer 136
About Breast Cancer in Men — Diagnosis — Treatment and Prognosis
— Support

Chapter 10: The Boy with Cancer 141
Types of Cancers That Affect Children — Cancers That Occur More
Frequently in Boys — Cancers Specific to Childhood — The Challenges
of Childhood Cancer — Resources for Children with Cancer and Their
Families

Part III: Treatment and Management of Cancer 155

Chapter 11: An Overview of Cancer Treatment 156
Goals of Cancer Treatment — Sequence of Cancer Therapy — Making
Treatment Decisions — Where Treatment Occurs — Finding Resources

Chapter 12: Surgery 164

Before Surgery — The Surgery Experience — The Postoperative Period
Going Home — Postoperative Healing

Chapter 13: Radiation Therapy 178

How Radiation Works Against Cancer — Radiation Therapy
Techniques — General Side Effects of Radiation and Self-Care —
The Future

Chapter 14: Systemic Therapy: Chemotherapy and Biotherapy 193

Chemotherapy — Biotherapy — Future Directions in Systemic
Therapy

Chapter 15: Clinical Trials 209

Types of Clinical Trials — Participating in a Clinical Trial — Finding
Information — Making a Decision — The Future of NCI-Sponsored
Clinical Trials — Final Thoughts

Chapter 16: Complementary and Alternative Therapies for Cancer 220

Defining and Differentiating Conventional, Alternative, and
Complementary Therapies — Complementary Practices and Cancer —
Known Alternative Practices — Less Known Alternative Practices —
Evaluating Complementary and Alternative Therapies

Part IV: Quality of Life Issues 247

Chapter 17: Taking Control of Cancer Pain 248

Sources of Pain — Barriers to Appropriate Pain Management — Pain
Assessment — Pain Management — Dispelling Myths about Pain
Medicines — Final Thoughts

Chapter 18: Cancer, Sexuality, and Sex 260

The Sexual Response — Sexuality and Fertility — Sexual Function —
Sexuality and Intimacy — Changes in Sexuality Related to Cancer —
Sexually Transmitted Diseases — Final Thoughts

Chapter 19: End-of-Life and Palliative Care 279

End-of-Life Concerns — Maintaining Control in Life's Concluding
Chapter — Crucial Questions and Decisions — Hospice and Palliative
Care — Paying for End-of-Life Care — Final Thoughts

Chapter 20: Survivorship 296

> Needs of Cancer Survivors — Cancer Victim, Cancer Patient, and
> Cancer Survivor — Survivorship Skills — You Are Your Own Best
> Advocate — The Politics of Cancer — What Does It All Mean?

Bibliography 317

Resources 322

Index 339

List of Tables

2.1: Cancer Definitions 30

2.2: Benign and Malignant Cell Traits 31

2.3: Common Sites of Metastasis from Primary Tumors 32

4.1: Diagnostic Tests for Prostate Cancer 61

4.2: The TNM Classification System for Prostate Cancer 64

4.3: The AJCC Staging System for Prostate Cancer 64

4.4: Treatment Options for Prostate Cancer 66

4.5: Treatment Options for Recurrent Prostate Cancer 81

5.1: AJCC TNM Staging System for NSCLC 90

5.2: Stage 0–4 Staging System for NSCLC 90

5.3: Comparison of Staging for Non-Small-Cell Lung Cancer 91

6.1: Nonmalignant Growths That Occur in the Colon 104

6.2: Routine Screening Tests for Colorectal Cancer 107

6.3: TNM Classification System 111

6.4: Comparison of Staging Systems 111

6.5: Treatment Options 112

8.1: TNM Staging System for Squamous Cell Carcinoma
of the Penis 133

13.1: Types of External Beam Radiation Equipment
and their Clinical Uses 180

13.2: Radioactive Materials Used in Brachytherapy 184

13.3: Skin Care During External Beam Radiation Therapy 187

13.4: Radiation Side Effects and Self-Care Interventions 189

14.1: Cytotoxic Chemotherapy, Mechanisms of Action,
      and Common Uses 195

14.2: Common Chemotherapy Side Effects 199

15.1: Typical Eligibility and Ineligibility Criteria 213

16.1: Herbs Used in Cancer Treatment 235

17.1: Medicines for Treating Severe Cancer Pain 255

19.1: Suggested Interventions for Symptoms Common
      at the End of Life 286

20.1: Financial Assistance Programs 312

List of Figures

1.1: Cell Cycle 10

1.2: USDA Food Guide Pyramid 17

1.3: Summary of the ONS Position on Genetic Testing 21

4.1: Normal Male Genitourinary Anatomy 54

4.2: Transperineal Approach and Technique for Radioactive
     Seed Implants in the Prostate 73

6.1: Anatomy of the Colon and Rectum 101

6.2: Structural Layers of the Colon 103

6.3: Polyp Arising from the Bowel Mucosa 103

7.1: Normal Male Anatomy 119

7.2: How to Do TSE 122

15.1: ONS Position on Cancer Research and Cancer Clinical Trials .. 210

19.1: ONS and AOSW Joint Position on End-of-Life Care 281

19.2: *Five Wishes*™ 284

20.1: Decision-Making Model 302

20.2: ONS Position on Patient's Bill of Rights for Quality Care 305

20.3: Self-Advocacy Strategies in Cancer Care 306

List of Contributors

LYNN M. COLLINS, R.N., M.N., A.O.C.N.
Oncology Clinical Nurse Specialist
Dallas, Texas

CAROL P. CURTISS, R.N., M.S.N.
Curtiss Consulting
Greenfield, Massachusetts

FRED FANCHALY, R.N.
Senior Systems Analyst
Information Technology and Services
Catholic Hospitals West
San Francisco, California

PAMELA J. HAYLOCK, R.N., M.A.
Oncology Consultant
Medina, Texas

JEROME KOSS, R.N., O.C.N.
Staff Nurse
Fox Chase Cancer Center
Philadelphia, Pennsylvania

PATRICIA J. KROFT, R.N., B.S.N.
Operating Room Nurse
Millbrae, California

JEAN LYNN, R.N., B.S.N., O.C.N.
Breast Health Nurse
George Washington University Hospitals
Washington, D.C.

KERRY A. MCGINN, R.N., M.A., N.P.
Nurse Practitioner
Kaiser Permanente Medical Center
South San Francisco, California

JAMIE S. MYERS, R.N., M.N., A.O.C.N.
Oncology Clinical Nurse Specialist
Research Medical Center
Kansas City, Missouri

JODY PELUSI, R.N., F.N.P., A.O.C.N., Ph.D.
Nurse Practitioner
Cancer Outreach and Wellness Program Coordinator
Maryvale Hospital
Phoenix, Arizona

MARCIA ROSTAD, R.N., M.S.
Pediatric Oncology Clinical Nurse Specialist
Tucson, Arizona

CYNTHIA J. SIMONSON, R.N., M.S., C.S., A.O.C.N.
Oncology Clinical Nurse Specialist
Massey Cancer Center
Virginia Commonwealth University
Richmond, Virginia

DEBRA THALER-DEMERS, B.S.N., R.N., O.C.N.
Staff Nurse
Good Samaritan Hospital
San Jose, California
Vice President, National Coalition for Cancer Survivorship

Important Note

The material in this book is intended to provide a review of information regarding the cancers that affect men. Every effort has been made to provide accurate and dependable information, and the contents of this book have been compiled through professional research and in consultation with medical professionals. However, other professionals may have differing opinions and advances in medical and scientific research are made very quickly, so some of the information may become outdated.

Therefore, the publisher, authors, editors, and professionals quoted in the book cannot be held responsible for any error, omission, or dated material. The authors and publisher assume no responsibility for any outcome of applying the information in this book in a program of self-care or under the care of a licensed practitioner. If you have questions concerning your nutrition or diet, or about the application of the information described in this book, consult a qualified health care professional.

◆ ◆ ◆

Introduction

A known set of skills can help people with cancer cope most effectively. These skills include finding information and making decisions. *Men's Cancers* was written to provide cancer survivors and anyone concerned about cancer with good, solid information about cancer and cancer treatment that can, in turn, help them make the crucial decisions that will impact the remainder of their lives. Each contributor has sought out important resources that readers can access, and questions that can provide the basis for a man's conversations with his doctor and other members of the cancer care team. The man who has information about what to expect throughout the cancer experience will make more effective plans about treatment, activities of daily living, and safe and effective self-care strategies.

Men and Cancer

Why a book on men's cancers? At the start of the twenty-first century, at least in the United States and many other Western countries, one in two men will eventually be diagnosed with some form of cancer. Of the approximately 1.2 million Americans diagnosed every year with cancer, just over half will be males.

Some kinds of cancers only affect men, or only affect women, by virtue of our distinctive anatomies. Other forms of cancer affect the two genders differently. For example, both men and women get breast cancer, but breast cancer affects men much less often, probably because of the differences in physiological function.

Some forms of cancer occur more often in one sex than another as a result of behaviors and environmental exposures. Men have historically worked in occupations where exposure to substances such as asbestos and other chemicals increased the risk of certain forms of cancer. At least for the moment, more men smoke cigarettes and cigars than do women, and more men than women are diagnosed with lung cancer. Sadly, women are "catching up" with men—both in the numbers of women who smoke and in the number of women who develop lung cancer—and new evidence suggests that women are actually more susceptible to the cancer-causing effects of tobacco. On the positive side—and "Hooray for the guys"—men have successfully stopped smoking in greater numbers than have women.

Men and Communication

It comes as no surprise that a good many men—and women, too—have difficulty with communication. When it comes to taking care of health needs, and talking about health-related problems, most experts agree that men are more than a step behind women. Many men—certainly not all, to be fair—just find it difficult to talk about a topic such as cancer that evokes fear, particularly when it might be perceived as a physical weakness. The woman has historically been the family member who takes care of the health-related problems of the rest of the family, and it has been primarily women who aggressively seek out health-related information. Ultimately, women are often responsible for making health care decisions.

When men do make valid attempts to talk about health-related concerns—with a doctor, for example—they run into systematic barriers that make successful communications difficult to achieve. A Louis Harris Survey conducted in 1995 revealed critical unmet communication needs of men facing cancer. In this study, almost all physicians surveyed reported that they discuss treatment options with their male patients with cancer, yet one in six men surveyed recalled no such discussions, and older men were even less likely to have these important patient-physician talks. Every doctor surveyed also reported that he discussed quality-of-life factors with his patients, but about a third of the male patients said their doctors did not talk with them about how treatments would affect their quality of life. The point? It is clear that men have informational needs, and it is also clear that some real communication problems occur between men and their doctors.

What we have is a situation in which people who are already less than comfortable talking about serious threats to their health are placed in what could only be referred to as a minefield. To further complicate the picture, physicians and other health care professionals unwittingly contribute to communication problems, resulting in inadequate information being provided to the man facing a possible cancer diagnosis. Ultimately, the lack of information can leave the man feeling inadequately prepared to face the challenges ahead.

Regaining Power and Control

A common reaction to the diagnosis of cancer is a feeling of powerlessness—a lack of control over one's life—and helplessness. A person who feels helpless is more likely to assume a passive role in his health care, and a person who is passive quite often does not fare as well as his counterpart who takes an assertive, active role. Doesn't it make sense to give one's fight against cancer the best shot possible? This book is about doing just that.

Timely, accurate information is the true source of power and control. Advances in technology, including the introduction of the Internet, have created an explosion of available information. So much so that it can be hard to sort out the good information from the bad. This book is intended to be a primer—a basic starting place—in the search for good, reliable information about many of the cancer problems that concern men, as well as the other people in these men's lives.

The Premise—and Promise—of This Book

Nurses have always been on the front lines with people facing cancer. Throughout any cancer journey, the experienced nurse who specializes in cancer care—the oncology nurse—is in my opinion the lifeline. The nurse has the most personal of interactions with people in his or her care. He or she is likely to be the one who responds to unscheduled telephone calls and questions that arise through the course of events, and who provides comfort and caring on a day-to-day basis. What many people fail to realize is that these nurses also possess incredible amounts of knowledge about the disease entity and its treatment—the core of their professional practice—and the wisdom that accompanies years of experience. Their knowledge is likely to be quite different than that of the physician. Nurses often characterize their unique set of skills and knowledge this way: "Doctors are primarily concerned with curing the problem. Nurses provide the care." Obviously, to provide adequate and optimal care, the nurse must also possess knowledge about the set of problems that needs to be addressed. Nurses can be—and should be—a primary source of information, advice, and support for people who face cancer. This is the premise behind the creation of the book.

Expert Nurse Contributors

Each chapter in this book was written by a nurse who has special expertise in the topic being presented. The contributors were selected specifically because of their cancer nursing knowledge and experience, and also because they have skills in writing and providing information to the patients with whom they interact on a daily basis. In creating his or her chapter, the nurse-authors were asked to write "as if you are sitting down with a man and/or his family member to talk about this cancer-related topic." The individual style of each author contributes, I think, to a more interesting and varied book.

The expert nurses represented in *Men's Cancers* work in varied cancer care settings ranging from rural and office-based settings to large university comprehensive cancer centers. Some of them are young, while others have been members of the nursing profession for two or more decades. Together, they represent well over a century of cancer nursing experience. Regardless of their identities, their areas of expertise, or their practice settings, these nurse-authors share a common goal: that of making vital information available to people facing the difficult challenges imposed by cancer and cancer treatment.

Power, Control, and Survivorship

We are committed to the belief that information is the source of power and that people facing cancer need to retain or regain a sense of power over their lives despite the cancer diagnosis. Some people refer to this as *empowerment*—assisting others to develop and use power in ways that help them cope with life's challenges more effectively.

Many health care professionals—especially nurses—have been trained to try to "do it all" for the patients in their care. This was probably never a realistic goal, but in the modern health care environment it is truly impossible. More and more, people facing a serious illness—and those around them, such as family members and friends—will find it necessary to pitch in. Most cancer care will occur in ambulatory care settings, doctors' offices, and, increasingly, in the home, with everyone—including the man with cancer—playing a role, perhaps confirming that medicines are taken correctly, or managing surgical wounds and other postoperative care, or overseeing nutritional support and symptom management. Learning and using self-care and caregiving skills is critical to both physical and emotional wellness.

Cancer Victim, Cancer Patient, or Cancer Survivor?

The emergence of the idea of empowerment has given rise to a social movement referred to as *advocacy:* standing up for one's rights. For years, people with cancer struggled to find and use good information that would allow them to take more active roles in making their own health care decisions. Many people worked on this independently. Eventually, as cancer treatment methods grew to be more successful, more and more people survived their cancers to the point that today between eight and ten million Americans are alive who have a cancer history. A good number of these people have banded together to promote the idea of *cancer survivorship*.

The word "survivor" is an important one. Consider the difference between the words "victim" and "survivor"—or even between "patient" and "survivor." The word "victim" denotes someone who is totally powerless and weak. The word "patient" would seem to refer to someone who is passive and waits, "patiently." Increasingly, people with cancer choose to reject powerlessness, or even passivity. Instead, they demand the right to play an active role in making decisions about their own care and in creating an environment that gives them the best chance to achieve an optimal level of health—despite the diagnosis of cancer. In other words, these cancer survivors are demanding that we help them do whatever it takes to be as well as they can be.

The National Coalition for Cancer Survivorship defines *cancer survivor* in this way: "From the time of its discovery and for the balance of life, an individual diagnosed with cancer is a survivor."

It is our intent that this book be a useful guide to successful survivorship strategies—just as the title implies: *Men's Cancers: How to Prevent Them, How to Treat Them, How to Beat Them.*

Pamela J. Haylock
October 2000

Part I

•••

Diagnosis and Beyond: Understanding Cancer and Cancer Treatment

1

◆ ◆ ◆

About Cancer

Pamela J. Haylock, R.N., M.A.

Most men, upon hearing the words, "You have cancer," will wonder, "What exactly does this mean?" and, "What does this diagnosis mean for me?"

Cancer means many things to many people. In addition to the physical aspects of having cancer, there are expected—and unexpected—emotional aspects as well. The more the person who is newly diagnosed can learn about cancer the better off he will be. He may find himself in the midst of people who seem to speak a different language—some even call it "medicalese." Learning the language can help a man quickly get on board and be part of the team. So let's start at the beginning and go through the basics, including an introduction to many of the unique words and phrases used in association with cancer.

What Is Cancer?

Cancer is not a new disease. Egyptian papyrus writings from 17 B.C. describe cancer, pointing out that there is no treatment. Over a thousand years later, Hippocrates—the Father of Medicine—said the same thing about treatment, advising physicians not to attempt to treat patients with cancer. It wasn't until the 1800s, with the development of anesthesia, that doctors made any real attempt to heal the disease.

The early Egyptians believed various gods caused cancer. Hippocrates' theories of disease, including cancer, involved the idea of an imbalance of critical bodily substances he called "humors." In the 1800s, cancers were often viewed as God's punishment, a cause for shame. Though people in developed societies in theory reject these ideas, myths and misunderstandings based on early beliefs still surround cancer even at the start of the twenty-first century.

Cancer is a common disease. By the end of their lives, half of all men and about a third of all women in the U.S. will develop some form of cancer. Despite its prevalence, and the progress that has been made in its treatment, cancer is still a major source of fear for most Americans. The good news is that statistics gathered between 1997 and 2000 reveal the first-ever sustained decline in cancer-related deaths in the U.S. As research evolves, there is every reason to hope that these positive trends will continue.

Cancer is not one disease. Rather, the term is used to describe common traits that cells in the body acquire. Cancer starts when cell functions go awry or get out of kilter. When many of these abnormal cells amass somewhere in the body—within organs, for example—they can interfere with normal tissue and organ functions, causing the signs and symptoms of cancer. The American Cancer Society offers this definition of cancer: "Cancer is a group of diseases characterized by uncontrolled growth and spread of abnormal cells. If the spread is not controlled, it can result in death."

Cell Cycle

To understand how cancer cells grow, divide, and spread, it is helpful to know a little about normal cells. The function of all cells is to take in food, use energy, and reproduce. The process of cell division, called the *cell cycle*, is the series of changes that a cell goes through from the time it is first formed until it divides—or splits—into two new *daughter cells* that are identical to their *parent cell*. The time it takes for a cell to complete this process is called *the generation time* or *doubling time*. Different kinds of cells have different generation or doubling times, but regardless of the doubling time, each cell goes through the same stages. A new cell is created at the end of the division part of the cell cycle, called *mitosis*. That particular cell ceases to exist when it goes into the mitosis phase itself and divides into two new daughter cells.

Cell cycle stages between mitosis phases are important: they prepare the cell to reproduce and create daughter cells. DNA, the basic genetic structure, controls the processes of cell division and differentiation—the process that determines the adult cell's actual function. Before a cell can start the process of mitosis, it has to create new DNA. DNA is made, or synthesized, during what is called the S phase (for synthesis). Between

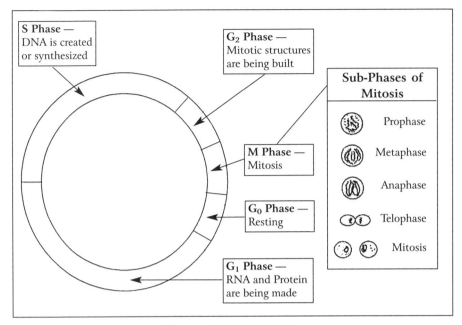

Figure 1.1: Cell Cycle

The cell cycle is the series of changes that the cell goes through from the time it is formed until it divides into two identical daughter cells. The cycle begins and ends with Mitosis—the "M" phase. Before a cell can enter the Mitosis phase, it makes new DNA during the S (for "synthesis") phase. There are gaps between the S and M phases—G_1 and G_2. G_0 is the "resting" or dormant phase.

mitosis—the M phase—and the start of the S phase, there is a gap phase—called G_1—during which the cell prepares itself to create DNA. After the S phase, there is second gap phase, this time called G_2, when the cell prepares for mitosis by making RNA and other special proteins. After mitosis, the daughter cell goes into a G_1 phase and stays there until it gets a message telling it to enter the S phase. Cells also have a third gap phase, called a resting phase, referred to as G_0. Figure 1 depicts the cell cycle.

During cell mitosis important activities take place that create the daughter cells. Mitosis is a continuous process with no clear breaks between stages, but cells' mitotic activities are separated into four phases called *prophase, metaphase, anaphase, and telophase.* It's important at least to know these phases exist because it is during these phases that cancer cells are most vulnerable to the various forms of cancer treatment. On the other hand, most cancer treatments cannot damage cells during the G_0 phase.

Most normal cells go through about fifty doublings before they are no longer able to reproduce. As normal cells die, they are replaced by new cells so that the organ or tissue made up by these cells achieves and maintains its normal size. Cancer cells can continue to divide beyond this number of doublings, giving cancer cells the property often called *immortality*—they don't die—and causing the abnormal growth or enlargement of organs or body parts usually associated with cancer.

Cancer Cells Versus Normal Cells

There are five basic differences between normal cells and cancer cells:

1. Cancer cells are immortal. They do not have a natural life span, but instead can continue to grow and divide indefinitely.

2. Cancer cells lose the property called *contact inhibition* or *density-dependent growth*. In normal tissues, cells stop growing when they touch each other. Cancer cells, on the other hand, don't seem to mind crowds; they pile on each other and form masses of cells.

3. Cancer cells have lower needs for the substances that stimulate cell growth. In other words, cancer cells can continue to grow and divide even when some of these substances are missing.

4. Cancer cells do not need a foundation or "anchor" on which to grow. Normal cells have a trait called *anchorage-dependent growth*— they need a surface on which to grow and survive.

5. Cancer cells cannot go into the resting phase, as normal cells can. Instead, cancer cells will continue to divide even when nutrients needed by the normal cells are missing.

It is the combination of these five characteristics of cancer cells that leads to the most significant differences between normal and cancer cells: The cancer cells can continue to grow, uncontrolled by any other body functions, and can spread—or *metastasize*—beyond the place where the cancer started, often called *the site of origin*.

The View under the Microscope

Under the microscope, cancer cells can look different than normal cells. This microscopic picture can say a lot about what to expect from a certain form of cancer. Normal cells usually look well organized, and cells of the same type are generally the same shape and size. You might liken this to a football team standing in formation just before kick-off: everyone is in a defined place, ready to do a defined job. Staining chemicals help the pathologist analyze the cell's parts; normal cells and cancer cells often react differently to these stains, allowing the pathologist to see the cell parts more clearly.

Sometimes, however, clumps of normal cells or benign cells will look the same as—or at least very similar to—cancer cells. When this occurs, the pathologist needs to assess the behavior of the cells—whether the cells resemble mature cells that would be expected in the tissue and how quickly they are dividing to produce new cells. Cells from different organs normally have different characteristics of division and growth.

Mature normal cells have very clear functions to perform. Think of it as the evolution of an infant to an adult. The infant's function in life is to survive, grow to adulthood, and perform some useful role in society. The new daughter cell can be likened to that infant. The mature cell, like an adult, takes on a very specialized function in life—in cellular terms, this is called *differentiation,* or *specialization*. As the cell takes on its special function, it also assumes a very characteristic structure or appearance. The process of differentiation involves some other chemicals that are created by other kinds of cells or parts of cells. The *growth factors* used to stimulate growth of different cell types are examples of these helpful chemicals.

Cancer cells tend to be less differentiated than cells from the normal tissue surrounding the cancer. The degree of differentiation is an important trait that conveys the speed of growth and/or destructive nature of cancer cells: poorly differentiated cells least resemble surrounding normal cells and are generally very destructive and fast growing forms of cancer. Well-differentiated cells, on the other hand, closely resemble surrounding normal tissues and are less aggressive and less destructive forms of cancer.

Causes of Cancer

Cancer occurs as a result of a defect in the control of the cell cycle that allows the cell cycle to go on over and over again and a second defect that prevents these abnormal cells from dying. In some forms of cancer, various defects causing just these changes have been found to exist on specific genes. Many experts predict that eventually all cancers will be related to specific genetic changes.

The Process of Carcinogenesis

Cancer develops as a result of the stepwise process called *carcinogenesis,* in which, over time, a cell changes from normal to abnormal, and finally becomes a cancer cell. *Carcinogens* are factors that produce cell changes that *can* lead to cancer through carcinogenesis. Carcinogens include external factors—factors that come from outside the body—such as radiation, chemicals, and viruses, and internal factors such as hormones, changes in the immune system, and familial or genetic traits. It is believed that more than one type of exposure or *initiating event* is common.

The first exposure to a carcinogen is called *initiation*. Not every exposure to a carcinogen results in the development of cancer; in fact, most do not. For cancer to occur, another series of events, referred to as *promotion*, must take place. Promotion occurs after initiation and helps—promotes—the development of cancer. The targets of carcinogens are the "on" and "off" switches for cell growth—cell genetic components called *oncogenes* and *cancer-suppressor genes*. These genes can spur other genes into action or turn them off—actions that, depending on the normal function of the targeted gene, allow cancer to develop. More often than not, ten or more years pass between an initiating event and the development of detectable cancer.

Chemical Carcinogenesis Chemical carcinogens are cancer-causing substances a person is exposed to in the course of his lifetime. Their existence has been recognized since tobacco was first identified as a carcinogen in 1761. Soot was identified as a cause of scrotal cancers among chimney sweeps in 1775. Man-made chemicals such as the aniline dyes used in tanning leather and aromatic amines used in drug manufacturing increase the risk of bladder cancer. Many other chemicals have been found to cause cancer in animals, but not many have been clearly identified as carcinogenic for humans. Dioxin from chemical plant emissions, industrial waste disposal, and pesticide residues in food products are suspected, but unproven, carcinogens. The plot of *A Civil Action*—the novel and movie starring John Travolta—broached this issue. Even though there is some evidence of carcinogenesis as a result of industrial chemical exposure, fewer than 5 percent of all cancer deaths in the U.S. can be related to on-the-job exposure.

Convincing evidence links both obesity and a high-fat, low-fiber diet to cancers of the colon. Food additives used in food processing common to industrialized countries may also be associated with the eventual development of cancer. These dietary factors could very likely be considered chemical carcinogens, as ingested chemicals as well as end-products of the digestive process could be carcinogenic. It is possible that carcinogenic chemicals are produced in the digestive system as dietary fats are broken down in the digestive process. Diets that are low in fiber content increase the gut transit time—the time it takes food to move through the digestive processes in the colon and be eliminated during normal bowel movements. This places potentially damaging chemicals formed during the digestive process in contact with the lining of the bowel for a longer period, increasing the chances of damaging the colon's cells.

Familial Carcinogenesis Familial carcinogenesis is based on a group of protective genes—*cancer suppressor genes*—that prevent cancer when they function normally. When these genes are changed or mutated, do not function normally, or are missing, a cancer is likely to develop. For example, the mutated gene *BRCA-1* is linked to breast and ovarian cancers and the *BRCA-2* gene is associated with breast cancer in women. A malfunction of a tumor-suppressor gene is associated with the condition called familial adenomatous polyposis that is responsible for a certain kind of colon cancer. Though only a few such mutated genes have been identified, many researchers suspect that mutations are, in fact, linked to the eventual development of many forms of cancer.

Physical Carcinogenesis Much of what causes mutations in cells falls into the category of *physical carcinogens*, which includes the fiber asbestos and ultraviolet and ionizing forms of radiation. *Ultraviolet radiation* (UVR) comes from sunlight and causes changes in DNA. If a cell is unable to repair the damage to DNA, it can undergo changes—called *malignant transformation*—that turn it from a normal cell into a cancer cell. Basal cell and squamous cell skin cancers and malignant melanoma are examples of cancers linked to UVR. Ultraviolet B (UVB) is the most carcinogenic of the UVR wavelengths.

Radiation breaks parts of exposed cells into smaller pieces—an effect called *ionization*. Ionizing radiation occurs in our environment naturally, and much of our exposure to it cannot be avoided. The radioactive gas *radon*, a decay product of radium and uranium, occurs in nearly all soil and rock, although there is quite a lot of geographic variation and the level of exposure depends on where you live. The jury is still out with regard to the actual effects of radon exposure. It is believed that radon can be a factor in the development of some forms of lung cancer, but only an estimated 5 percent of all cancer deaths are due to exposure to naturally occurring radiation.

Asbestos is a fiber that has been used in many industries, including construction and shipping. It is believed that the continuous irritation caused by inhalation of asbestos fibers, over time, results in the development of cancer, especially cancers affecting the lungs. Exposure to asbestos in combination with tobacco smoke produces a sort of double whammy: a smoker exposed to asbestos has a much greater chance of developing cancer than he would have with exposure to either tobacco smoke or asbestos alone. Asbestos exposure is especially linked to the development of a deadly form of lung cancer called *mesothelioma*.

Viral Carcinogenesis Although the numbers of viruses clearly known to cause cancer are few, some viruses have strong links to the development of cancer. The two viruses with the strongest identified links are the hepatitis B virus (HBV), associated with cancer of the liver, and the human T-cell leukemia virus type 1 (HTLV-1), linked to T-cell lymphoma. HBV is very common in Asia and Africa and accounts for the high numbers of liver cancers among people who live in or migrate from these countries.

The Epstein-Barr virus (EBV) is linked to another form of lymphoma, Burkitt's lymphoma, especially if the infected person's immune system is already weakened. The ability that viruses have to damage DNA is the most likely reason that some kinds of lymphoma are common in persons with weakened immune systems—most often referred to as *immunosuppressed* or *immunodeficient*—as a result of infection with the HIV virus, the cause of AIDS. The EBV is also highly associated with the development of cancers of the head and neck—*nasopharyngeal carcinoma*—among people of Chinese descent.

There are many strains of the human papillomavirus (HPV). One strain causes common warts as well as genital warts. There is mounting evidence that some strains of HPV relate to the development of cancers of the penis and prostate.

Bacterial Carcinogenesis So far, there is little evidence that bacteria cause cancer. One exception that has been a source of excitement among cancer researchers is the discovery that a bacteria called *Helicobacter pylori* is not only a cause of stomach and duodenal (small bowel) ulcers, but also seems to be involved in the development of a certain kind of lymphoma and some cancers affecting the stomach. The reason for the excitement is that this bacteria can actually be destroyed by treatment with antibiotics, resulting in reversal of the cancer-causing mechanisms and the prevention of these forms of cancer.

Cancer Prevention

Only as causes of various forms of cancer are identified does it become possible, in a scientific way, to prevent these diseases. As scientists close in on the actual carcinogenic mechanisms, it is increasingly possible to interfere with the processes that result in cancer.

Primary Versus Secondary Prevention

Most of the preventive actions mentioned here are called *primary* prevention—the avoidance of exposure to known cancer-causing agents or carcinogens. In secondary prevention, people who have known risk factors are followed more closely to check continuously and frequently for precancerous (or premalignant) conditions and early cancers.

These days, it can seem like everything causes cancer. If it's not smoking or something in our environment, then it's something we eat. And if it's diet, it seems like the newest study says that our favorite food or dietary additive—things like saccharine—may cause cancer.

This is where the element of choice—informed choice—enters the picture. We all need to make informed choices about which risks we are willing to assume and which we make concerted efforts to avoid. Some risks only affect the risk taker, such as decisions about diet and exercise. Other choices, such as smoking cigarettes and cigars, often increase another person's risk as well. This involuntary exposure to carcinogens is the source of a great deal of conflict among families, communities, and even in policy-making circles.

For now, we can focus on the primary prevention of several of the most common forms of cancer. The ACS says that "behavioral factors such as tobacco use, dietary choices, and physical activity modify the risk of cancer at all stages of its development." Behavioral factors or lifestyle choices are key in making a personal commitment to cancer risk reduction.

Reduce Exposure to Carcinogens in Tobacco Products It is estimated that as much as 90 percent of all cancers of the respiratory system (including the larynx, lung, and bronchus) are caused by exposure to carcinogens in tobacco smoke and tobacco products. While everyone knows someone who "has smoked every day of his life, is now in his eighties, and is still very healthy," most of us know *more* people who *were* smokers and have succumbed to lung cancer. In addition, there is mounting evidence that spouses of smokers have higher rates of lung cancer than spouses of nonsmokers. Clearly, the elimination of exposure to tobacco products and tobacco smoke goes a long way toward reducing a person's chances of developing this deadly form of cancer.

Modify Diet to Reduce Exposure to Carcinogens It is estimated that about one-third of all cancers—especially cancers of the colon and breast—might be related to diet. Dietary fat and subsequent obesity are the most likely suspects. Combining a balance of calories and physical activity with a diet that is high in plant foods such as fruits, vegetables, grains, and beans, and limited in amounts of meat, dairy, and other high-fat foods reduces the risk of cancer. The ACS issued an update of its nutrition guidelines in 1999, making them consistent with the U.S. Department of Agriculture (USDA) Food Guide Pyramid and dietary recommendations of other agencies that promote health (see Figure 1.2). The ACS rec-

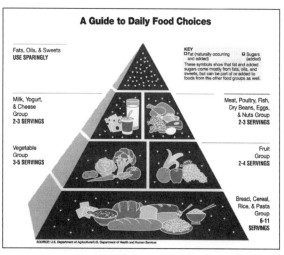

Figure 1.2: USDA Food Guide Pyramid

Reprinted courtesy of the United States Department of Agriculture

ommendations include these general suggestions:

- Choose most of your foods from plant sources.

- Limit intake of high-fat foods, especially those that come from animal sources.

- Be physically active and achieve and maintain a healthy weight.

- Limit intake of alcoholic beverages.

Limit Environmental Exposure to Carcinogens As Much As Possible

The American Cancer Society estimates that about 75 percent of all cancer cases in the U.S. are caused by environmental factors, including exposure to tobacco products, diet, and infectious diseases. There are undeniable risks associated with exposure to pollutants in food, air, and water. The degree of risk depends on the amount of exposure (concentration), the amount of time or duration of that exposure, and how intense the exposure is (high levels of exposure over short periods of time). The chemicals benzene, asbestos, vinyl chloride, arsenic, and aflatoxin are thought to cause cancer. Other chemicals, including chloroform, DDT, formaldehyde, polychlorinated biphenyls (PCBs), and polycyclic aromatic hydrocarbons, might cause cancer, but the evidence on these is not yet conclusive.

Limiting exposure to ionizing and ultraviolet forms of radiation is a sure way to reduce one's chances of developing basal and squamous cell skin cancers and malignant melanoma, the most common forms of skin cancer. Ways to avoid exposure to ultraviolet radiation include avoiding direct sunlight as much as possible and the routine use of sunblocks that block UVB radiation. X-rays used in medical and dental examinations—including mammograms—use the lowest dose levels possible while still maintaining the quality of the X-ray image.

With the exception of avoiding or at least limiting radon exposure, there is little chance of totally avoiding environmental exposure to ionizing radiation. The U.S. Environmental Protection Agency (EPA) estimates that nearly one of three houses in the U.S. has high radon levels. In 1988, the U.S. Public Health Service urged that houses be tested for radon. Information about radon testing is available from EPA offices.

People who have had radiation treatment for a previous cancer have an increased risk of developing second cancers in the area exposed previously.

Physical Activity The evidence linking cancer to low physical activity levels is, as Perry Mason would say, circumstantial. But there does seem to be quite a clear relationship between obesity, diet, physical activity, and some forms of cancer. Physical activity is known to stimulate the bowel and, in doing so, speeds up the transit time. The risk of breast cancer in physically active women is also reduced. Possible links between physical activity and development of specific men's cancers have not been thoroughly explored.

Chemoprevention Chemoprevention—the use of natural or man-made chemicals or medications to prevent precancerous conditions from becoming cancer—is a relatively new idea that has provoked great interest. Evidence exists that the regular use of small doses of aspirin, even as little as one baby aspirin per day, might help prevent the development of colon cancer. A major study is underway to test usefulness of the drug finasteride, usually used to treat benign prostate enlargement, to prevent the development of prostate cancer. It seems clear that the study of additional chemicals that offer protection against cancer is attractive to many scientists.

Cancer Risk Analysis, Genetic Testing, and Genetic Counseling

As more is learned about the role of genetics in the development of cancer, it will be increasingly possible to identify persons who are at higher risk for developing cancer. Awareness of increased risk allows the individual to take advantage of screening programs that increase the chances of discovering and treating a precancerous condition (such as a colon polyp) before it becomes cancer, or detecting a cancer in its earliest, most curable stage. Even though these technological advances offer great hope, they also open a Pandora's box: Legal, ethical, financial, and emotional issues tied to the use of genetic technology have yet to be addressed.

Cancer Risk Analysis

Cancer risk analysis is a process that allows a person to determine fairly accurately his chances of developing cancer. While many community cancer care programs are beginning to offer cancer risk analysis, only health care professionals with special education and training—medical doctors, advanced practice nurses, and medical geneticists—are truly qualified to offer this service. During a full analysis, an individual's risk is determined through assessment of many pieces of information. A full analysis explores options as well as determining risks and may include the following:

- detailed personal and family history—a "pedigree"—going back at least three generations and taking into account

  — personal risk factors

  — medical risk factors

  — environmental risk factors

  — family risk factors

- physical examination and assessment

- multidisciplinary evaluation resulting in development of a plan to minimize or control risk

- assessment of the man's and his family's informational needs

- development of a program of care that focuses on the man's identifiable risk factors

- genetic counseling that provides support and the information needed to make health care decisions

- information about access to clinical trials that relate to the man's particular risks

- possible genetic testing

Genetic Testing

Identification of an individual or family at high risk for developing cancer due to an inherited gene is made possible through *genetic testing*. (Genetic testing is also used for other health problems.) This process examines DNA for indications that the development of cancer is likely. So far, it has been useful in identifying people at risk for colon cancer and in diagnostic settings where different types of leukemia can be identified through DNA traits. A recent advance in the use of genetic tests involves the development of antibodies that can block a gene product that stimulates the growth of breast cancer, offering a new and exciting form of breast cancer treatment.

Predictive gene testing helps identify people at risk of getting a disease *before* symptoms appear. Since it is generally agreed that "all cancer is genetic," research and the manipulation of genes as a form of treatment can only be expected to grow in importance as time goes on. The National Institutes of Health and National Cancer Institute's illustrated booklet *Understanding Gene Testing* (NIH Publication No. 96-3905) provides a useful overview of gene testing. The booklet is available though the Cancer Information Service or via the NCI website.

During genetic testing, a sample of a person's DNA is taken from cells in his blood, other body fluids, or tissues. The DNA is tested for an anomaly or *glitch* in the makeup of the DNA, which is indicative of an actual or potential health problem.

Genetic Counseling and Other Issues

Genetic testing opens a Pandora's box of dilemmas. Emotional and behavioral consequences may be expected when a person learns his likelihood of developing cancer. If family members, such as children, are also at higher risk for cancer due to their genetic makeup, the emotional issues are compounded. For these reasons, an important service that must be included in any genetic testing program is genetic counseling—access to a skilled and knowledgeable genetic counselor who can help an individual and his family understand what the test results mean and use the information in responsible ways.

Another major issue is this: Who has access to a person's genetic information? Should an employer have the right to this information? What about an insurance provider or an HMO? There is growing concern that the issues of privacy and protection from genetic discrimination have not been fully explored, and many policy makers believe that legislation is needed to provide protection.

The issues abound. Who should get genetic testing and counseling? Who pays? Complete cancer risk analysis with genetic testing and counseling can cost over six thousand dollars, and most insurance plans do not cover these services.

What qualifications or credentials should be required of professionals who perform genetic testing and counseling? There are still no nationally accepted standards or guidelines for credentialing either facilities or personnel. When these techniques were first being offered, many providers thought genetic testing would create opportunities to reap a huge financial windfall. People with less than adequate training were sometimes—though certainly not always—set up in small cancer risk services that lacked the full range of services required to provide adequate information and support. The Oncology Nursing Society (ONS) recommends that nurses who provide cancer genetic counseling must be advanced practice oncology nurses with specialized education in genetics.

Since there are no standards for genetic testing, how do you know if a genetic testing service is one of the good ones? The Oncology Nursing Society offers these suggestions for assessing the quality of genetic testing services:

Figure 1.3: Summary of the ONS Position on Genetic Testing

Genetic testing services should:

1. Include informed consent and pre- and posttest counseling by qualified individuals (certified genetic counselors, advanced practice nurses with specialized education in genetics)

2. Be based in ethical practices that guide the development and use of genetic counseling

3. Offer counseling services that are consistent with the individual's cultural beliefs

4. Have educational resources available to help the individual and his family understand the implications of his genetic makeup

From the Oncology Nursing Society Position: Cancer Genetic Testing and Risk Assessment Counseling, 1997

Cancer risk analysis and genetic testing can help a man and his family look at their cancer risk profile. Does the risk affect only the man? Does it extend to family members? From this information, the man—and sometimes his family members—can determine which risk factors can be altered to reduce the chance of developing cancer. Risk factors that cannot be changed, such as genetic flaws, provide clues to help the man design a plan of action that assures that precancerous conditions will be monitored and that cancer will be discovered early, while it is most curable.

In the end, information is still the greatest weapon against cancer. Information allows us to make wise decisions. Knowing about and understanding cancer risks can help every person balance the risks of developing cancer with his own priorities and his own lifestyle.

2

◆ ◆ ◆

Finding Cancer

Pamela J. Haylock, R.N., M.A.

A natural response to hearing "You've got cancer" is denial. "It can't be true." "The test is wrong." "They've made a mistake." "How are the doctors so sure that they've got the right diagnosis?" With recent press about medical mistakes, who wouldn't ask these questions? The person with a possible cancer diagnosis must be confident that his diagnosis is accurate and understand the rationale for each step of the diagnostic process. Let's start at the beginning.

A Complex Process

The fact is, the diagnosis of cancer is most often made after not one but several different kinds of medical examinations and tests. The initial detection occurs when a man or his health care professional—doctor or nurse—notices a change in a body function or appearance. Sometimes a pain that won't go away or is not easily ignored brings a man to the doctor's office. Detection can also occur as a result of screening tests or by comparing results of a current test with those of an earlier, similar test. Suspicions lead to further tests, and eventually a conclusive diagnosis is made. After it is determined that a cancer is present, further testing determines the extent, or stage, of disease.

Usually, the conclusive test to diagnose cancer is one in which cells from the suspicious area are examined under a microscope by the pathologist.

Most of the symptoms that point to a possible cancer can also indicate health problems that are *not* cancer-related. So, except when a cancer diagnosis is very obvious, it is reasonable to go through a medical *workup* process that rules out other causes for the sign(s) or symptom(s) a person is experiencing.

Routine physical and screening exams are not covered by the majority of insurance plans; as a result, many people do not routinely take advantage of these potentially lifesaving procedures. The low-cost blood tests offered at community-based screening programs often include the option for prostate-specific antigen (PSA) testing. Increasingly, men use this convenient service to check on prostate health. Some clinics or doctors offer fecal occult blood tests (FOBT), a simple and inexpensive way to check for bleeding in the colon and rectum. But it remains a problem that most people—especially men—wait until they have a symptom they can't ignore before making an appointment to see the doctor.

Signs and Symptoms of Cancer

It is the change in function caused by cancer that results in the most common symptoms of cancer. Of course, these symptoms will differ depending on where the cancer is located and how much a body system or organ's function is altered. It is usually one of these changes that encourages a man to make an appointment to visit his doctor.

The American Cancer Society (ACS) has identified the seven most common warning signs of cancer. These have been listed in an order that makes them easy to remember, spelling out "CAUTION" with the first letter of each warning signal:

<u>C</u>hange in bowel or bladder habits

<u>A</u> sore that does not heal

<u>U</u>nusual bleeding or discharge

<u>T</u>hickening or lump in the breast or elsewhere

<u>I</u>ndigestion or difficulty in swallowing

<u>O</u>bvious change in a wart or mole

<u>N</u>agging cough or hoarseness

The ACS recommends that if a person has any one of these warning signs, he should see his doctor or other health care professional.

The First Doctor's Appointment

The first time a man seeks a medical opinion about any symptom, the doctor, nurse, or physician's assistant will take a detailed medical history that will include questions about the symptom—or symptoms—the man has:

- How long it has been present?
- Has it gotten worse over time?
- How does it interfere with the man's daily activities?
- What, exactly, does it feel like?
- Are there things the man can do to make the problem go away, at least for a while?
- Are there things the man does that make the problem seem to worsen?
- Are there any similar problems in other family members?

After a thorough medical history is taken, the doctor, nurse (perhaps a nurse practitioner or clinical nurse specialist), or physician assistant will do a complete physical examination, paying special attention to what appears to be the source of the man's symptom. In medical terms, this symptom is often called the *chief complaint*. Some people find this term offensive: no one likes to be accused of complaining!

In most settings, any suspicious findings will be discussed with a doctor. He or she will recommend what tests need to be done next and follow up on information gathered during the history and physical. Objective signs—things that the man may not be aware of but are noticed during the physical exam—will be factored into the doctor's decision-making process.

What comes next depends on the problem, the symptoms, and the body part that seems to be affected. The diagnostic process specific to each kind of cancer is described in detail in the chapter covering that cancer. The following is a brief overview of a general diagnostic workup.

Diagnosis

The diagnostic process follows a fairly common course, going from the safest, easiest, and least costly to perform and advancing to more complex—and sometimes more risky—procedures in order to arrive at an accurate diagnosis.

Laboratory Tests

The chemical composition of body fluids such as blood and urine provides important information about body functions. Samples of body fluids are examined in a laboratory equipped with the appropriate instruments for performing these tests. Some doctors' offices have laboratory facilities in which some necessary analyses can be done. More often, blood and urine samples will be tested in hospital or other commercial laboratories. The sample might be collected in the doctor's office or clinic and then sent out—sometimes physically hand-delivered and sometimes mailed—to the laboratory. Or the man might go in person to the laboratory to provide the needed sample. Determining which laboratory will provide the analysis may depend on the man's insurance coverage—it makes sense to choose a facility covered by the plan. Sometimes a needed test might be available only in certain laboratories. The doctor or nurse ordering the laboratory test can usually help direct the man to the right laboratory facility, but it might also be left to the man to make sure his insurance pays for the test being ordered, or for the laboratory that is selected.

The chemical composition of blood and urine can reveal changes occurring in the body that *could* be the result of a suspected cancer. However, these chemical changes could also be related to a noncancerous condition. When changes in the makeup of blood or urine are found, they are pieces in a complex puzzle. The doctor uses his or her knowledge of the symptoms and the potential causes to guide decisions about which laboratory tests are most likely to provide answers and complete the puzzle. For example, a man who has symptoms the doctor believes might be related to a prostate problem is likely to have his prostate-specific antigen (PSA) level tested. If symptoms seem to originate in the colon or digestive tract, the doctor might include a carcinoembryonic antigen (CEA) level in the laboratory analyses. The PSA and CEA are examples of chemicals called *tumor markers*, measurements of proteins found in the blood that often, but not always, indicate the presence of cancer. In complex situations, or cases in which the test results lead to more questions, the *pathologist*—the doctor who specializes in laboratory analyses—may be asked to review the test results. In general, the laboratory results are reported back to the referring doctor, who is responsible for sharing the test results with the patient.

Imaging Techniques

In general, some sort of imaging study will be done at the same time as laboratory studies. Findings from a laboratory test will lead the doctor to ask for a specific imaging study or, conversely, the image may provide evidence of the need for a particular laboratory test. Imaging studies include the routine chest X-ray, computerized axial tomographic (CT or CAT) or magnetic resonance imaging (MRI) scans, bronchoscopy, gastroscopy, colonoscopy, ultrasound, and nuclear scans—techniques that allow doctors to get an actual picture of what is going on inside the man's body.

X-rays are used to assess bones and certain tissues and can show differences between normal and abnormal areas. For example, abnormal growth is a denser or lighter area (X-rays are black and white) on the X-ray film. CT and MRI scans show cross-sectional images of body parts. MRI scans use a magnetic field to direct radio waves through the body to create images. For X-rays and CT scanning, a *contrast medium* can be given orally, injected intravenously, or administered in an enema. The contrast helps to outline certain organs and show abnormalities more clearly.

Generally, an *X-ray technician* (or X-ray tech) is the person who "takes the picture." The technician helps position the man correctly for the desired imaging study and handles the equipment used in the procedure. The technician is like a photographer, taking the pictures using the correct procedures and techniques and processing the film. The technician usually will have the film checked by a *radiologist* (a doctor who specializes in diagnostic radiology) to make sure the image is accurate and clear. If the image is not clear, the radiologist might ask that the procedure be repeated. Once it is determined that a clear image is available, the man can leave the radiology department. The image or images created during the study are reviewed by one or more radiologists. Their findings are reported back to the referring doctor, and the referring doctor is generally responsible for talking to the patient about what the imaging study reveals.

Some imaging studies are conducted in a *nuclear medicine* department, usually a separate hospital-based laboratory where radioactive tracing chemicals are used to highlight changes in organs and tissues. Studies done using nuclear medicine techniques are the positive emission tomography (PET) scan, single-photon emission computed tomography (SPECT), Gallium scan, and other scans of the bone, liver, spleen, brain, thyroid, and kidneys, as well as studies that use radio-labeled monoclonal antibodies. Again, the results are reported to the referring doctor who, in turn, will discuss the test results with the patient.

Imaging studies have many uses and play important roles in the initial diagnostic phase as well as in the ongoing monitoring process during and after cancer treatment. Their use can also be controversial. One issue is the cost of these studies; most insurance plans do whatever possible to avoid paying for expensive, unnecessary tests. While routine chest X-rays are not particularly expensive, a hospital X-ray department charges, on the average, around $4,000 for a CT scan that takes about one hour!

It is always reasonable to make sure that any test—a laboratory analysis or imaging study—actually answers a question that needs to be asked. The most important question is, "Will the results of this test affect the treatment recommendation?" If the test request goes forward, the man's insurance plan may have contractual agreements with designated imaging facilities, as it does with laboratory facilities, meaning that the man will be encouraged to use the facility that accepts payment from that health insurance plan, negotiate acceptance of his plan's payment to the facility, or be prepared to pay the facility out of his own pocket.

If the information gathered through all of the laboratory tests and imaging studies supports the suspicion of cancer, the final step in making the cancer diagnosis is for cells from the suspicious area to be examined by a pathologist under a microscope.

Tissue Diagnosis

The microscopic identification of cancer cells—tissue diagnosis—is the best way to determine the presence of cancer and the only way to confirm the cancer diagnosis with 100 percent accuracy. A small sample of tissue must be taken from the suspicious area and examined under a microscope by the pathologist, who is knowledgeable about the look and behavior of cancer cells. This proof of cancer and the details it provides are critical for making appropriate treatment decisions. The skill of the doctor responsible for obtaining the tissue sample is key to assuring the accuracy of the diagnosis; if he or she misses the cancer cells, the pathologist will not have the information needed to assess the tissue thoroughly.

Getting this tissue sample usually requires some sort of *invasive* procedure, so called because it "invades" the body in some way, ranging from a relatively simple biopsy to a full surgical procedure. Prior to any invasive procedure the patient must provide his *informed consent*, which acknowledges that he has been fully informed about the purposes and benefits of the proposed procedure and any risks involved. More complete discussions on informed consent are included in Chapter 12, "Surgery," and Chapter 15, "Clinical Trials."

Biopsy is the process of removing a small piece of tissue for microscopic examination. If the area under suspicion is clearly visible—for example, on the skin surface—the doctor can snip or scrape a small piece of that tissue. For less accessible areas such as the colon, throat, or lung, procedures are used that require a scope to visualize inside the body and special tools to grab or snip a piece of tissue. Sometimes a needle is inserted through the skin to withdraw cells, tissue, or fluid. In other cases the tissue sample will not be available until after surgery is performed; the pathologist then examines all of the organ or tissue that was removed during surgery. Information about obtaining tissue samples for different forms of cancer is provided in the chapters covering the specific cancers.

Understanding the Pathology Report

The pathologist's report exemplifies how important it is to understand the language of cancer. This report provides the data that identifies the kind of cancer, the extent of the cancer, and its particular behavior. Along with the man's own physical and emotional status, the pathology report is the final piece of crucial information to be considered in deciding potential plans for treatment.

The pathology report generally begins with a review of the tissue sample the pathologist received. For example, the report will describe the size and overall appearance of the sample and reveal whether or not the edges of the sample contain cancer cells. The pathologist will use a phrase such as "margins are clear" (no cancer cells) or "margins are not clear" (all of the tumor has not been removed). For some diagnoses, the distance—measured in millimeters or a fraction of a centimeter—of clear margins is also important.

The report describes the cells of the tissue being examined. The most important distinguishing characteristics determine which cells are cancer and which are benign. Some terms are used interchangeably and incorrectly. For example, the word *neoplasia* is often used instead of the word "cancer." In fact, neoplasia simply means "new growth," and does not necessarily indicate that the new growth is cancer. Sometimes the word *benign* is used incorrectly as well. In general conversation, this word often describes something completely harmless. In medical terms, a neoplastic growth can technically be benign and still be dangerous. For example, a benign tumor inside the skull will not spread to other parts of the body. This tumor type is technically benign, yet it can still grow larger and larger within the skull's limited space. The growing tumor, even though noncancerous, creates serious symptoms linked to the increasing pressure inside the skull. Table 2.1 provides a short glossary of terms that describe cell traits—called *histological* traits—that are commonly found in biopsy reports. Table 2.2 provides a quick look at the differences between benign and malignant cells that the pathologist will assess.

The pathology report identifies the kind of cancer, using terms that indicate the tissue where the cancer is likely to have started. Each and every

Table 2.1: Cancer Definitions

Term	Definition
Neoplasia	*Neo* = "new" and *plasia* = "growth." *Neoplasia* simply means "new growth."
Anaplasia	The loss of structural organization and useful function of a cell.
Dysplasia	Disturbance in the size, shape, and organization of cells and tissues.
Hyperplasia	An increase in the number of cells in a tissue or organ causing an increase in bulk.
Hypertrophy	An increase in the size of individual cells.
Benign	Lacks the ability to spread to distant sites but can grow and cause problems locally. Benign neoplasia is usually designated by the suffix "oma" attached to the name of the cell composing the tumor.
Malignant	Has the properties of local invasion, destructive growth, and spread or metastasis beyond the site of origin. The word is derived from a Latin term that means "wicked."

part of the human body is derived from one of the following four basic tissues:

1. Epithelial tissue: Tissues that cover and line the body and organs and tissues that make up glands. Skin, membranes that line the mouth and stomach, and the prostate gland are examples of epithelial tissues.

2. Connective tissue: Tissues that connect all other tissues together and to the skeleton and support other tissues. Bone and bone-forming cells, cartilage, fat, and blood and blood-forming cells are all connective tissues.

3. Muscular tissue: Tissues that line blood vessels and intestines, attach to the skeleton, and are responsible for moving bones. The heart is made mostly of muscular tissue.

4. Nervous tissue: The brain, spinal cord, nerves, and parts of sensory organs (such as the eye and ear) are all made up of nervous tissue.

Cancer can arise from any of these four major tissue groups and is often named according to the *tissue of origin*. Most forms of cancer start in epithelial cells—the cells on the body's surface or lining internal organs and passageways—and are called *carcinoma*. The cancer type called *sarcoma* starts in connective tissues—muscles, bones, tendons, or blood vessels. Other cancers are named according to the specific cell type in which the cancer is

Table 2.2: Benign and Malignant Cell Traits

Benign	Malignant
Lacks the ability to spread to distant sites.	Can spread to distant sites through the lymph and blood circulation systems.
Is encapsulated—covered by a capsule.	Does not have a capsule of tissue that holds the tumor cells together.
Cells closely resemble normal cells.	Cells bear little resemblance to normal cells.
Neoplastic growth is slow.	Cells grow in an unrestrained manner.
Generally less dangerous.	If spread is not controlled, death can result.

growing. For example, *leukemia* arises from white blood cells, and *lymphoma* arises from lymph cells. *Glioblastoma* and *astrocytoma* are nerve cell cancers that arise from glial cells and astrocytes, both specific types of nerve cells. A few other forms of cancer—such as *myeloma* (arising from the plasma cells of the blood) and *melanoma* (a skin cancer that starts in the melanin cells that produce skin pigment)—don't fit into the usual way cancers are named.

Cancer cells usually keep some traits that help identify the precise organ system in which the cancer started. For example, cells from a prostate carcinoma will look very much like normal prostate cells, even though they are discovered in an area outside of the prostate gland. When lung cancer spreads to the bone or brain, those cancer cells will still resemble cells from the lung. Ultimately, the cancer will be named using the type of cancer and the primary site. For example, lung cancer might more accurately be called "lung carcinoma," or colon cancer "colon carcinoma." Knowing the site of origin is important in the diagnostic workup process and is crucial in determining the appropriate form of treatment. In rare cases, a cancer defies attempts to identify its source and is termed "cancer of unknown origin." In this type of situation, treatment will proceed based on the experts' "best guess" about the cancer's origin.

In addition to assessing the general appearance of cells, the pathologist performs tests on the cells that provide clues to how the cancer behaves and the man's prognosis. These tests include *flow cytometry* to measure the DNA characteristics and growth potential of the cells in question. The behavior of the cells—how quickly they are dividing and how closely they resemble normal cells from the site of origin—is reflected in what is referred to as the tumor's *grade*.

Staging of Cancer

Just knowing that a cancer is present is not enough. In order to determine the best form of treatment, the extent of a man's cancer—its *stage*—must be determined.

After biopsy results confirm the presence of a particular kind of cancer and describe the cancer's characteristics, the *staging workup* determines to what extent the cancer has spread beyond the site of origin. The staging workup is based on the scientific study of cancers, called *oncology*, and the anatomical structures affected by the cancer. By studying the way different forms of cancer behave when they are untreated—their *natural histories*—doctors can make a fairly educated guess about where a cancer might spread first. With this information, and through imaging and laboratory studies, doctors can then assess the stage of the cancer. Table 2.3 provides a brief overview of common sites of metastasis from primary cancers.

For many of the various forms of cancer, staging terms or staging systems are used to provide doctors with a common language and common understanding of the cancer being evaluated. For example, unique staging systems for both colon and prostate cancers are still in use in many cancer treatment centers. Over the years, however, variations in staging terms created a source of confusion, and the *TNM system* was devised as a way of standardizing staging terminology. Simply explained, the T refers to the size of the primary tumor, the N denotes the presence or absence of spread of cancer to the lymph nodes surrounding the primary tumor, and the M refers to the presence or absence of spread, or metastases, of the cancer to other organs. A number between 0 and 4 is attached to each of these letters, denoting size or extent of spread. For example, a T1 tumor will be much smaller than a tumor that is designated T3. N0 denotes that spread to the local lymph nodes was not

Table 2.3: Common Sites of Metastasis from Primary Tumors

Primary Tumor	Sites of Metastasis
Head and neck	Lymph nodes
Colon, pancreas, stomach	Liver, lung, bone
Breast	Lymph nodes, lung, bone, liver, skin, chest wall
Lung	Brain, liver, lymph nodes, bone
Bone, kidney, testicle	Lung
Melanoma	Liver, lung

found, whereas N1 indicates that cancer has spread to the local lymph nodes. The TNM system is used for most forms of cancer. Other staging systems for specific cancers are described in the chapter that describes that particular cancer.

The doctor uses stage and grading information, along with factors specific to each patient such as his general health and his own wishes, to determine treatment options that offer the best chance of cure or control of the cancer. Cancers that are small and contained within a limited space of an organ can often be treated with a *local therapy* such as surgery or radiation therapy. Cancers that have spread to other organs are more likely to require a *systemic* form of therapy that can reach all parts of the body, such as chemotherapy or biotherapy. The standard treatment methods are reviewed in chapters 11–14.

3

♦ ♦ ♦

Your Cancer Care Team

Kerry A. McGinn, R.N., M.A., N.P.

Cancer is too big a battle to fight alone. It takes a team effort. The most effective health care team includes:

- you at the center of the team, with a strong voice about what happens to *your* body

- the best doctors you can find: competent, knowledgeable, and the kind of people you can work with

- plenty of other very important players: health care providers other than doctors; family, friends, and coworkers; people who have been through a similar cancer as mentors or a support group

Each member of your cancer care team can contribute something special. Together, you can choose and carry through the best possible treatment plan for you.

The Idea of Self-Advocacy

Fighting cancer can be, quite literally, the challenge of a lifetime. As in any worthwhile endeavor, a person usually needs to develop and use new skills in order to achieve success. For example, a weekend jogger would need some training and conditioning before entering the Boston Marathon. Taking on the battle against cancer requires special skills as well.

There is literature to suggest that a defined set of skills will help people with cancer cope more effectively with the disease and its treatment. Six crucial skills are as follows:

1. Communication: Cancer survivors need to feel comfortable in bringing up and discussing concerns and questions and to talk openly about goals of planned treatments, reasonable expectations, and risks and benefits of suggested interventions.

2. Finding information: Knowledge, skills, and access to accurate, timely, and diagnosis-specific information will be key to making good decisions throughout the cancer experience.

3. Decision making: Every man with a cancer diagnosis needs to be able to make sound, informed decisions about treatment options and symptom management.

4. Negotiation: Cancer survivors and their family members will more than likely need, at least on occasion, to negotiate or make "deals" such as requesting time off from work, changes in work assignments, and changes in normal family roles.

5. Problem Solving: While moving through the stages of the cancer experience, a man and his loved ones will face many new situations and problems. Anticipation of and satisfactory resolution of problems will smooth out the rough parts in the road.

6. Self-Advocacy: Every person with cancer, as well as his family and loved ones, should expect that quality cancer care services include a level of respect for and attention to the man and his unique set of needs. Sometimes, getting the desired services or the desired level of care will require the man himself or a friend or family member to assertively make his needs known.

These skills can be learned and honed in many ways. Members of the treatment team, friends, family, Internet websites, and other kinds of publications can be valuable sources of information. Many cancer centers and clinic settings offer cancer resources centers—some even specific to certain kinds of cancer—that are open to the public. The American Cancer Society–sponsored *I Can Cope* program offers a structured educational program to help people understand the cancer experience. *The Cancer Survival Toolbox*, a collaborative project of the National Coalition for Cancer Survivorship, the Oncology Nursing Society, and the Association of Oncology Social Workers uses the six skills listed above in a program that helps a person learn to be an effective self-advocate. The consistent use of these skills increases a man's chances of getting the kind of care he needs, helps him regain or maintain a sense of control, and will be essential in giving him the best chance to develop a successful, working partnership with his treatment team.

The U.S. health care system is far from simple. Most other developed countries' systems are complicated as well, but in ways that differ from the U.S. system. Regardless of the country or the health care system, a man is likely to face some difficulties as he goes through the diagnostic processes and cancer treatment. Most men discover that their outlook is more positive when they play active roles in planning and coordinating their care. A first step is getting the skills and information that allow a man to be a fully functioning member of his cancer care team.

Joining Your Treatment Team

Some men prefer to leave all the control and decision making about the cancer in their doctors' (or other primary health providers') hands. This is one legitimate way of coping, but "Yes, doctor"/"No, doctor" is simply not enough for many men. These men want more control over the situation. And, as much as they trust their doctors, they know that it is not their doctors who will have to live day after day with the choices that have been made.

Men who become active members of their treatment teams expect their doctors to present treatment *options*, including the option of *no* treatment. The doctor may argue strongly for a particular choice but must explain the pros and cons of each choice so that the man can understand them.

Without having to become a medical expert, a man can learn enough about his cancer and its treatments to participate in making intelligent decisions. Decisions that are made will be key to the man's (and his family's) short- and long-term satisfaction with his care. Nothing could be worse than regretting a decision that is made without being fully aware of the pros and cons, the ifs and buts of making one choice over another.

Choosing the Right Doctor

One of the man's most important decisions will be choosing his doctor. Choosing the best doctor from among several candidates may not be a problem for the man with adequate insurance who also lives in or near a city. However, the man without such access may need to travel or have his records sent to a cancer center for assessment, development of a treatment plan, or perhaps therapy.

If all doctors made the best possible use of cancer therapies available today, more men would survive cancer. This is too serious a disease, and the long-term relationship with the primary cancer doctor is too crucial, to settle for the wrong doctor. But how does a man find the right doctor?

No doctor is perfect, and no doctor can be expected to combine all the qualities a man wants all the time. To decide which doctor best suits his individual needs, a man might ask these three questions:

- What is essential in a doctor?

- What is important but negotiable?

- What can I do without if necessary?

Basic credentials are essential. The *Directory of Medical Specialists* and the *American Medical Dictionary*, available in many libraries, list such factors as a doctor's education and specialty preparation. For instance, is a specialist "board certified"? Is the doctor a member of appropriate professional organizations such as the American Society of Clinical Oncology (ASCO), the professional organization of physicians and other health care professionals—who can join as "associate members"—involved in cancer care?

What else is essential? For many men, the doctor's services must be covered by the man's insurance plan, and the doctor must have admitting privileges at a hospital included in that plan. The man with Medicare or Medicaid (Medi-Cal in California) coverage needs a doctor who agrees to accept this form of payment.

Competence and experience come next. The doctor must have the basic skills to take care of a patient with this type of cancer. With a rare form of cancer, the man might have to seek out a "super specialist" who has developed special expertise.

Beyond these essentials, if a man has a choice between two or more well-qualified doctors, he must weigh what other factors matter most to him. There is no "right" answer. Sometimes, the decision will come down to a personality match, making sure that the man and his doctor can indeed work together, that they are cognizant of and respect each other's needs. In the "old days," a doctor's so-called bedside manner—the trait that often boils down to communication skills—was often a deciding factor.

Does a warm bedside manner matter? Or is a brisk, no-nonsense presentation preferred? Will the man insist on access to cutting-edge clinical trials or will he favor a more conservative approach? Does he want a doctor who takes charge and makes most of the decisions or one who involves him in the decision-making process? Is this doctor known for no-holds-barred aggressive therapy or for a greater willingness to suggest comfort care if cure is unlikely? How clearly and honestly does the doctor communicate about diagnosis and the risks and benefits of proposed treatments? How carefully does he or she listen to the man and respect his input?

If there is a choice of doctors, any and all of these factors will be part of the man's overall satisfaction with his care. Health care is a product and patients are its consumers. While a man cannot expect perfection, he has a right to competent, considerate care. This includes reasonably knowledgeable, competent, helpful, and friendly office staff, appointments scheduled so he does not routinely have to wait long, and adequate telephone access in case of a problem.

Finding a Cancer Doctor

Generally, a surgical procedure is the first form of cancer treatment. For a good number of men, surgery might be the only form of treatment used. Sometimes, however, the surgeon will either know or suspect that some cancer cells have escaped from the local area and prefer to play it safe. This means that a man with cancer may have to deal with a combination of therapies: one or more local treatments, such as surgery or radiation, and one or more systemic treatments, such as chemotherapy, hormone therapy, or biological therapy. Combining two or more forms of cancer treatment requires a lot of effort to use these therapies wisely, so that the treatment achieves the desired outcome while avoiding undue side effects.

For some kinds of cancers, a medical oncologist may be the doctor who helps fit these pieces together. This doctor not only coordinates care, but also specializes in the systemic therapies for cancer. After completing training to become a doctor of internal medicine (internist), the medical oncologist has pursued advanced training in cancer therapy. (For prostate and some urinary tract cancers, the urologist may provide the systemic therapy as well as the surgery.)

Any of these specialists—or the man's primary care provider, such as his internist or family doctor—may assume the role of cancer therapy "chief." This individual prescribes and delivers therapy and/or coordinates treatment and sees the man frequently during treatment and at regular intervals afterward.

A man's internist or family doctor may suggest or make a referral to a particular doctor to treat the cancer. Many men today receive their health insurance through managed care in which the internist or other primary care provider acts as a "gatekeeper"—the person who decides when specialist care is needed and which specialists should provide it. If a man wants his insurance to pay all or most of the hefty costs of his cancer care, he may be limited to doctors who have agreed to work with his insurance or managed care plan, sometimes referred to as the plan's "network," although the network often includes a choice of physicians. The best advice is to check the health plan's network *before* beginning the decision-making process.

Recommendations may also come from a nearby medical school, the local medical society or the American Cancer Society unit, a nurse in the oncology unit or clinic at the local hospital, or friends. The Cancer Information Service of the National Cancer Institute which can be reached at (800) 4-CANCER provides a list of nearby cancer specialists.

The Patient-Doctor Relationship

Like other relationships, the patient-doctor relationship carries with it both rights and responsibilities. What does this mean for a man?

He listens to the doctor. Ideally, a few days after diagnosis, when he is past the initial shock, he brings a family member or friend with him, along with a small tape recorder or a pen and notebook with questions written beforehand. He and his companion then sit down with the doctor for a treatment planning session. The high stress after a cancer diagnosis affects any person's capacity to listen to and understand what is said; this is normal and does not indicate any deficiencies on the man's part. The doctor will need to repeat important points, but bringing someone along for any serious discussion, as a backup listener, saves missed information and misunderstanding. A tape recorder also lets the man replay the conversation later for himself and his family.

Many men complain that they do not understand what the doctor and other health professionals say—that the vocabulary is unfamiliar and the explanations too technical. But medical concepts can all be explained in ordinary words, and the right to clear explanations in words he understands must be a patient's right. It is always appropriate to ask, "Would you explain that again in simpler terms?" or "Could you rephrase that?" or "This is what I think you said—is that right?" Illustrations—either drawn by the health professional or printed—and books and pamphlets can be helpful. It also makes sense for a man to ask where he can get more information if he wishes (although some Internet enthusiasts may find far more information than they want or need!).

The man needs to think about what he wants and communicate it as clearly as possible. No matter how sensitive they may be, doctors cannot read minds. Unless the man answers questions honestly and raises issues that concern him, the doctor cannot know what is happening. That includes being frank about sensitive issues, including sex and alcohol and drug use. In particular, the man accepts responsibility for either following the treatment plan he and his doctor have devised or communicating any problems so that they can be resolved.

Many men feel they do not know what questions to ask or are reluctant to ask "silly" questions. Focusing on what is important to them is key to asking sensible questions. Cancer books and pamphlets often include lists of questions to ask the doctor, a useful way of jogging the memory. Many men find it helpful to keep a notebook handy so they can jot down questions when they arise and to review this list before the appointment.

It is common for *anyone* to feel a bit intimidated in this unfamiliar medical environment. Some men react by becoming silent, others by becoming very overbearing and demanding, often in an attempt to reassert control in a difficult situation. Neither response works very well. What works best is if the man expects and understands that this is a partnership of human beings, to which the doctor brings medical expertise and the man brings the equally valuable contributions of his intelligence, personality, ability to observe, and coping skills.

If he expects his doctor to treat him courteously, the man must return that consideration. He should take time before his appointments to collect his thoughts and questions, so that the doctor can meet his needs without having to change the whole day's appointment schedule. Courtesy also involves such basics as keeping appointments or informing the office otherwise, using advice phone calls reasonably, and not taking out his anger at the cancer itself on the medical staff.

Both the man and his doctor are human, and only human. Accepting each other as human beings, sharing each other's strengths, and acknowledging that both of them could, at times, do things in more effective ways are all part of forging the necessary bond between them.

An especially useful resource for a man (or his family) who wants to learn or strengthen skills to use in dealing with health care professionals is *The Cancer Survival Toolbox*, a self-learning audiotape program available free from the National Coalition for Cancer Survivorship [(877) 622-7937 or www.cansearch.org/programs/toolbox.htm]. The six modules cover the key skills of communicating, finding information, making decisions, solving problems, negotiating, and standing up for your rights.

Second Opinions

Cancer therapy changes all the time. What was state-of-the-art just last year may be outdated now. In many cases, doctors do not yet know the best way to treat particular cancers, and good doctors may legitimately disagree about what therapy to recommend. It often makes sense for a man to find out what different doctors think about the therapy options for his cancer.

This may mean consulting a medical and/or radiation oncologist after a biopsy, but before more surgery. If there are several acceptable ways to treat a particular cancer (as with prostate cancer), the surgeon or urologist may be more likely to look at surgical solutions, the radiation oncologist to recommend radiation, and the medical oncologist to propose systemic therapy. Seeking out their opinions tells a man that he has choices and helps him clarify what each might mean to him. In the long run, it may save him from having to repent at leisure a decision hastily made. In the short run, however, hearing all these different points of view may be confusing and distressing. In situations where there are several treatment options, the differences often lie in the effect on a man's quality of life. The choice of treatment then depends on factors that vary from one man to another.

Most doctors consider second opinions routine and welcome, a safety mechanism that protects both patient and physician. If at all possible, the second opinion should come from another doctor in the same specialty who is in no way connected to the one who provided the initial treatment recommendation—in other words, *not* the first doctor's business partner. It is possible to go overboard getting additional opinions. Visiting two surgeons makes sense; seeing six is usually too much.

Second opinions can also include a review of the biopsy microscope slides by a second pathologist with special expertise in his type of cancer. Slides and other medical records can be safely and quickly mailed for a prompt second look. The increasing use of technology in healthcare—or *telehealth technology*—provides ways in which pathology slides, imaging studies, and medical records can be transmitted to specialists in distant locations for review.

A man can get several opinions at one time if his case is reviewed by a *tumor board*, a group of health professionals from different cancer specialties who meet regularly. They listen to a presentation of the case and view visual evidence such as X-rays and other imaging films or biopsy slides, and then pool their expertise to recommend a course of treatment.

In the United States, a man may want to travel to one of the hospitals designated by the government's National Cancer Institute (NCI) as a Comprehensive Cancer Center, where new methods of cancer diagnosis and treatment are investigated. The NCI Cancer Centers program recognizes over twenty-five Comprehensive Cancer Centers that meet its criteria for large-scale, balanced programs of cancer research, patient care, and community outreach. Several other NCI-designated cancer centers fall into categories with a narrower research focus, but still offer potential resources for some men. Comprehensive Community Oncology Programs (CCOPs) and cooperative groups offer state-of-the-art cancer therapies in community-based settings. Other countries have similar programs. Information on NCI Cancer Centers is available from the NCI's Cancer Information Service at (800) 4-CANCER or its website, www.nci.gov. The Association of Community Cancer Centers (ACCC), a voluntary organization of community-based practices, also provides a nationwide listing of these cancer treatment settings (www.accc-cancer.org).

Traveling to a cancer center or having his case reviewed there before treatment makes sense especially for the man who has limited access to specialized cancer care in his community, has an uncommon cancer, or has a cancer with either no standard treatment protocols or many treatment options. Some men may be candidates for, and choose to participate in, a *clinical trial*, a study to evaluate a new therapy. Clinical trials are administered by cancer centers, or sometimes by oncologists in local communities. The experimental portion of the therapy (such as new drugs) may be given at reduced or no cost, although the man and/or his insurance often must pay for the cost of care associated with the treatment protocol. See chapter 15 for more information about clinical trials.

Doctors—and now patients—can access online computer databases to find out about up-to-date research and treatment protocols. *Physician Data Query* (PDQ) of the NCI is one popular resource. Some patient-advocate groups have compiled treatment protocol listings for patients with particular cancers. The better informed everyone is, the better care a man will get.

Other Team Members

There is much more to safe and effective management of cancer than prescribing and administering the actual treatment. In fact, most of cancer care involves the management of the physical and emotional side effects of the cancer itself and cancer treatment. Other health care professionals, family members, friends, and other people involved in resource and advocacy organizations can be critically important resources for a man and his family as they face cancer and cancer treatment.

Health Care Professionals

Depending on his type of cancer and its treatment, a man with cancer can come into contact with a bewildering array of health care providers besides his doctors. *Registered nurses*, whether in the doctor's office or the hospital, include general nurses, cancer specialist nurses such as oncology certified nurses (OCN), and advanced practice nurses.

Advanced practice nurses—nurses who have at least a master's degree in nursing—can be certified as advanced oncology certified nurses (AOCN). Certification is one way a man can tell if the nurses involved in his care have a high level of skill and knowledge about cancer, cancer treatment, and the needs of people facing cancer. Ask whether the nurses involved in your care are certified in oncology nursing. Knowing that they have the necessary knowledge and skills for the safe administration of chemotherapy and other forms of treatment will help you feel good about the quality of the care you are receiving. Because of their education and focus, registered nurses also teach patients and family members about cancer, its treatment, and quality-of-life issues such as dealing with symptoms or side effects.

Licensed vocational or practical nurses—LVNs or LPNs—have less formal education than registered nurses. Their titles differ from state to state. They often give much of the direct patient care in the hospital or doctor's office. Nursing assistants (sometimes *certified nursing assistants* or CNAs) or other patient care assistants have been taught to perform certain tasks such as taking blood pressure and giving baths. They should not, however, be charged with the responsibility of actually administering chemotherapy; in most states, such activities on the part of unlicensed personnel are illegal.

Technicians and *technologists* include personnel who draw blood samples, perform imaging studies such as X-rays and CT scans, or administer radiation treatments. A physical therapist can help a man regain strength; an occupational therapist can teach easier ways of performing everyday activities if cancer or its treatment have caused problems. A man might also be assisted by a dietician, respiratory therapist, social worker, volunteer, admission clerk, office staff, or hospital chaplain, according to his needs.

Your Cancer Care Team

Many men with cancer value the time spent with a psychotherapist, psychologist, or other *mental health professional*. Seeking help in coping emotionally with a cancer diagnosis does not mean a man is maladjusted or lacks control. It simply means he is making good use of resources to improve his life in a very difficult situation. Counseling can also be provided by a social worker, nurse, clergy, or other licensed counselor.

Family and Friends

Health professionals call them "significant others": spouses, family members, lovers, best friends. However strange the term is, it does reflect the fact that a special person makes a difference. Often, not-quite-so-significant others—friends, acquaintances, coworkers—can play major roles as well.

A diagnosis of cancer is difficult and distressing, not only for the man, but also for everyone around him. Serious illness changes roles and rules in relationships. Family members may have to face new responsibilities, often with little help or instruction. Family and friends may have to cope with their own feelings of fear, sadness, anger, and perhaps guilt.

Sometimes, people respond to the cancer diagnosis of a person close to them by being consistently loving, supportive, and helpful. However, cancer treatments may take a long time, and it is common for family and friends to react differently at different times. People may be supportive part of the time and run out of steam at others.

A man with cancer can encourage a helpful response from others by being frank about what is happening and about what he wants and needs. This gives cues to others so that they do not need to tiptoe around the subject. At the same time, if he can talk about other subjects as well and avoid concentrating completely on the cancer, he reminds them—and himself— that he is a person who just happens to have cancer, rather than a cancer that just happens to have a person attached.

Each man is an individual, with his own ways of coping with cancer. However, two tendencies occur commonly enough—and sometimes cause enough problems for a man and his family and friends—that they deserve comment. If a man comes to realize that he behaves in one of these ways, he may want to try some changes.

First, there is that old stereotype: the strong, silent type of man. He refuses to share his concerns with others and sometimes cannot even voice them to himself. He may prefer taking action, including making treatment choices quickly and independently, to taking time to talk over his feelings and options with others. He may feel that this way of dealing with the situation protects others from pain and worry. Unfortunately, his family members *are* involved in this man's cancer, treatment, and outcomes. If they do not know what is going on and are not part of the whole process, they often feel helpless, more afraid, and perhaps angry that they have been excluded from something so important in their lives. As always, communication—

with the man and his family exchanging honest information about what is happening and how each feels about it—works best. Sometimes, especially if the family has had trouble talking freely in the past, it helps to have the doctor, an oncology nurse, a member of the clergy, or a counselor ease the communication.

Second, many men have difficulty dealing with being sick. A psychotherapist I know comments that while women who become ill tend to try to protect those around them, men are more likely to sit back and let others take care of them. This happens often, even with the flu; in a stock comedy situation the woman, perhaps more ill, is fluffing up the pillows for her wretched spouse, who has no clue how to behave when he is sick and no longer has his accustomed control over the situation.

If this is how the individual man copes with illness, and he now has a cancer diagnosis, the problem gets much worse and lasts far longer. His partner may think, "Here I am, doing my job and his job, too—and he could be doing *something* to help, even if it's just folding the laundry."

Somewhere there must be a happy middle ground where a man (or a woman) neither takes on the whole burden nor leaves it all for others. Obviously, how much a man can do depends on the cancer and its treatment, but it makes sense to talk about this freely to be sure that resentment does not build up on either side. If his partner needs to take on some of the man's role, the man may be able to take on some of the partner's role. Negotiation—give and take—is key.

What if a man's behavior, such as heavy smoking or drinking, has probably played a key role in the development of cancer? This situation, most obvious in lung, head, and neck cancers, can add problems to an already difficult situation. The man may feel guilty and family members angry about this crisis that might have been avoided had he acted differently.

Tobacco or alcohol addiction is an illness itself, and distressing though addiction may be it is neither a measure of a man's moral worth nor a reasonable cause for guilt. Alas, no matter how well a man and his family may know this in theory, thcy may feel differently in the gut and may need help getting past this emotional roadblock. Blame—of self or of a family member—cannot change one whit what happened in the past and can cause a great deal of unnecessary unhappiness in the present. A therapist such as a psychologist or alcohol counselor can be especially useful in these situations.

What about the children when their father has cancer? It is crucial that children still at home be told very clearly (and repeatedly, if necessary) that they will be taken care of and that they are *in no way to blame* for the cancer. Most children are sensitive to undercurrents of emotion. They react better to a simple, reasonably hopeful explanation than to a wall of silence that leaves them imagining the worst. Of course, the explanation needs to be tailored to the situation and the age of the child. The father who is taking chemotherapy might tell his young child, "I got sick. I have to take strong medicine for a long time so I'll get well. The medicine makes me tired so I can't go for a walk with you today, but I still love you as much as always."

For many relationship issues, a useful booklet is *Taking Time: Support for People with Cancer and the People Who Care about Them*, available free from the Cancer Information Service (see the Resources section at the back of this book). *When Someone In Your Family Has Cancer*, also from the CIS, helps older children in this situation. Physician and cancer survivor Wendy Harpham's book *When A Parent Has Cancer* and its companion book *Becky and the Worry Cup* offer sensitive and realistic suggestions for parents who face cancer and their children.

Mentors and Support Groups

Men sometimes believe that they should be able to get through the cancer experience without help from support groups or mentors, that those are "a woman thing." Unfortunately, that often means a man must struggle harder and suffer more than if he were less reluctant to learn from those who have covered this ground before. Often, seemingly difficult problems turn out to have quite simple solutions.

A man who wants to talk to someone who has "been there" may already have a friend or coworker who has experienced the same kind of cancer. If not, his doctor or oncology nurse may be able to put him in contact with another man. This could be a mentor, someone who has already finished treatment successfully and can share successful techniques for getting through the experience. Or a man might want to be matched with someone undergoing treatment at the same time, so that they can support each other along the way. The Internet also provides several chat room or e-mail resources, geared either to general cancer or specific to a cancer type; some men find it easier and more convenient to ask for information or support online. Increasingly, application of technology—such as interactive telephone conferencing and radio and television talk-show formats—provides people with new ways to connect with others who can offer information, hope, and support.

Advantages of a good support group include access to information about treatment options and symptom relief. Group members can help a man explore his feelings—anger, sadness, helplessness, guilt—and learn how normal most of these feelings are and what others have done to cope with them. A support group gives a venue for practicing communication and for learning more effective ways of understanding others and making oneself understood; gives a sense of perspective, so that a man can see his own progress from diagnosis through treatment and beyond; allows a man to spend a short amount of time concentrating intensely on the cancer so that he can put it out of his mind at other times; provides a chance to help others by communicating his own experiences. Although studies so far have looked at women rather than men with cancer, researchers have been intrigued by early findings that women in support groups showed a marked survival edge over women not in groups.

Groups may be short-term (six to eight weeks, for instance, or a weekend retreat) or much longer; they can be composed of men getting treatment for the same disease or a mixture of men with varying diagnoses. Groups might be geared toward information, mutual support, or an equal mixture of the two. Some are limited to people with cancer while others welcome the involvement of family and friends. Some groups are open, allowing new participants to join in at any time; others are closed, allowing ongoing participation of only those who started the sessions together. A support group may have a particular focus, such as holistic treatment. Each group has a different personality, depending on its goals, members, and the facilitator or leader.

It helps a lot to have a group leader or facilitator who is experienced in guiding groups. That way, members can explore painful feelings safely and freely, because they know competent help is available to pull them out of any emotional quagmire. A skilled leader also helps keep group members from taking on the feelings and burdens of others. This means that the group becomes an enriching rather than a depleting experience.

Any type of group can be helpful and effective—or not. Some can be actively detrimental. It makes sense to promptly leave a group that induces strong guilt feelings in its members for having cancer or that advises them to use alternative therapies instead of standard treatments for potentially curable cancers.

Even the man who is ready and willing to join a support group could have difficulty finding one that meets his needs. Breast cancer groups abound for women, but men's information and support groups are much less common. Grassroots advocacy groups such as US TOO, a nonprofit prostate cancer advocacy organization, quite often form local support groups and educational programs. An oncology social worker, an oncology nurse, a member of the clergy, another counselor, or the local unit of the American Cancer Society (ACS) are good resources to help find support groups and other sources of emotional assistance. In many locations, ACS volunteers facilitate the *I Can Cope* program, a series of education and support seminars for cancer patients and their families. The *Cancer Survival Toolbox* programs offer an easy-to-adapt format for helping cancer survivors learn coping and self-advocacy skills. Sometimes the lack of an existing support group is an incentive for a man to form one, perhaps with the assistance of one of the grassroots advocacy organizations or members of his health care team.

Information Sources

In addition to receiving specific information about his case from health professionals and second opinion sources, a man can learn a great deal about his type of cancer and cancer in general from other resources. Trained personnel at the NCI's Cancer Information Service (CIS) answer general questions and will send free packets of information on almost any cancer topic. Physician Data Query (PDQ) of the NCI offers up-to-date treatment guidelines for anyone with access to a fax machine or the Internet. The ACS has units in most communities and can provide a wealth of information including booklets and computer reports.

Bookstores and libraries (including hospital, medical school, and health consumer libraries) offer an array of reading materials. As always, it is wise to examine the author's credentials and the reasonableness of the material presented. A number of worthwhile publications are listed in the Resources section at the back of this book.

Computers, the Internet, and e-mail have revolutionized the process of getting cancer information. The man who has access to a computer and a modem has at his fingertips information about state-of-the-art cancer thinking and therapy. Internet sites include cancer survivor accounts and encouragement. Accessing one Internet address usually opens the way to many more. For men without Internet skills or access, several community cancer organizations and local libraries offer help in getting started, including volunteer teachers and perhaps free access. A man may also wish to participate in a chat room, forum, or bulletin board where people communicate directly online or by way of e-mail. See the Resources section in the back of this book for helpful starting places.

One Internet caveat: Because *anyone*, with any—or no—credentials, can provide "information" online, including personal Web pages, it is especially important to double-check any treatment recommendations before following them.

Final Thoughts

Experienced oncology nurses generally share the opinion that a fully functioning cancer care team should be a priority of all cancer care health care professionals and all facilities that provide cancer care services. Although this idealistic picture occasionally becomes reality, in the real world the team often falls short of the ideal. Still, a man who is knowledgeable and aggressively advocates for his own needs can be instrumental in molding a team that will come through for him and his family. If the man is unable to mount this kind of effort himself, a family member or friend—or a health care professional willing to work in this kind of role—can help him achieve the same result.

Part II

◆◆◆

Different Types
of Cancers

4

Prostate Cancer

Pamela J. Haylock, R.N., M.A.

Most nurses have patients who leave a mark on their lives. For me, Boris was one of those. A Russian diplomat, Boris was one of my first patients and had advanced prostate cancer at the time he was diagnosed. I think he was typical of many men—stoic, private, and terribly embarrassed to ask questions of this young nurse. He had surgery to remove both testicles—the standard treatment for advanced prostate cancer at the time. When he was getting ready to leave the hospital, he showed me his discharge medication prescription for diethylstilbestrol (DES), the hormone treatment used in advanced prostate cancer. I'll never forget Boris's teary eyes when he asked me if the pharmacist would know what the surgeon had done to him just by seeing the prescription. I never saw Boris again. His story was very common in 1971. It's wonderful to know that thirty years after I met Boris, the vast majority of men like him would be diagnosed early, and would live long and productive lives after a prostate cancer diagnosis.

Issues and Concerns

The Most Common Men's Cancer

Prostate cancer is the most common cancer among American men. Every year, nearly 180,000 new cases of this cancer are diagnosed, and close to 37,000 American men die of it. For some unknown reason, prostate cancer is becoming more common. Men are increasingly concerned about their risks, as is clearly evidenced by the growing number of books on the bookstore shelves totally dedicated to prostate cancer topics.

In the past decade or so, prostate cancer has become a political issue, with prostate cancer advocacy groups demanding and increasingly winning attention and research dollars to support research into the cause and management of this common cancer.

Communication Between Men and Their Doctors

A Louis Harris Survey conducted in 1995 revealed critical problems for men facing prostate cancer. Almost all urologists surveyed reported that they discuss treatment options with their prostate cancer patients. Yet one in six patients said they *did not* discuss treatment options with their doctors, and older men were even less likely to have discussed options. Every doctor surveyed said he discussed quality of life factors, yet three of every ten men with prostate cancer say their doctors *did not* talk with them about how treatments would affect their quality of life.

US TOO International, Inc., a prostate cancer survivor support organization, stresses the importance of open lines of communication between the patient and doctor if men are to assume active roles in making informed treatment decisions. Prostate cancer presents many complex questions for the man and his family, and everyone involved must make concerted efforts to be completely honest and willing to discuss questions and concerns.

For a full report of the survey "Perspectives on Prostate Cancer Treatments: Awareness, Attitudes and Relationships—A Study of Patients and Urologists," contact US TOO (listed in the Resources section at the end of this book) or visit the US TOO website at www.ustoo.com.

Screening and Treatment Controversies

The uncertainty of the overall value of using the prostate-specific-antigen (PSA) as a screening test has recently created controversy. The PSA, like nearly all prostate cancer diagnostic tools, does not allow doctors to predict with any certainty whether the early cancers it picks up are the kinds that grow quickly or the kinds that grow slowly. This uncertainty, and a growing knowledge of how prostate cancers behave, fuels debate about what kind of treatment to offer or whether "no treatment" might be the best option. This might sound to some almost unethical: "What? Even though I know I have cancer I should forego any treatment at all?" Well, yes, this option might be right for some men. And all options will be reviewed a little later in this chapter.

Most prostate cancers grow very slowly and are discovered in older men. Even so, some prostate cancers grow quickly and spread to other parts of the body, causing symptoms and sometimes death. Treatment for men with these fast growing kinds of prostate cancer can help them live longer and prevent or relieve symptoms. One of the major problems in deciding on treatment for a man with prostate cancer is that it is not always possible to tell which man has a fast growing cancer and which has a slow growing kind. Clearly, not all men should get the same kind of treatment, and in some cases no treatment is considered the best option.

The Normal Prostate

The prostate, a male sex gland, is one of the few organs found only in men. It produces some of the seminal fluid that protects and nourishes sperm cells. The normal prostate gland is about the size of a walnut. When the man is standing, it is located in front of the rectum, behind the base of the penis, and under the bladder. It surrounds the upper urethra, the tube that carries urine from the bladder and semen from other sex glands out through the penis.

Testosterone, the sex hormone produced mainly in the testicles, affects normal and abnormal prostate growth. Therefore, eliminating testosterone is one way to treat prostate cancer.

Because the prostate is close to the rectum, the doctor or nurse practitioner can examine the prostate by inserting a finger into the rectum. This is called a *digital rectal examination* or DRE. Since the prostate surrounds the urethra, an enlarged

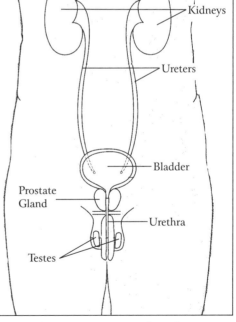

Figure 4.1: Normal Male Genitourinary Anatomy

Reprinted courtesy of the National Cancer Institute

or swollen prostate squeezes the urethra and can restrict flow of urine from the bladder to the penis.

Risk Factors, Prevention, and Detection

Prostate cancer results from the growth of abnormal prostate gland cells that multiply faster than normal prostate cells. The cancer usually begins on the outer area of the prostate and moves to the inner part. In later stages, the cancer can spread to other parts of the body.

Risk Factors

The causes of prostate cancer are as yet unknown. A noncancerous condition called benign prostatic hyperplasia (BPH), sometimes referred to as benign prostate enlargement, is not thought to be a risk factor for prostate cancer, though men can have both an enlarged prostate and prostate cancer. Factors that seem to increase the risk of a man developing prostate cancer include:

- age—older men have an increased risk
- family history
- African-American background
- diet high in fat and red meat
- sunlight exposure

Age is the single most important risk factor for prostate cancer. The older a man is, the more likely he is to develop the disease. As many as 30 percent of men over fifty may have early-stage prostate cancer. For men over eighty, the figure could be as high as 70 percent. Some experts believe that if a man lives long enough, he will eventually develop prostate cancer. Since just over 3 percent of all men die from prostate cancer, it is clear that the disease is not as life-threatening as other forms of cancer.

Prevention

An understanding of what seems to cause cancer, any kind of cancer, would logically lead to an understanding of how to prevent it. Although a few cancers, such as some forms of lung and skin cancers, are clearly linked to a specific cause, there is no clear link between any causative agent and the development of prostate cancer. Consequently, there is no clear directive about how to prevent the disease.

Nonetheless, some interesting observations have led to clinical trials studying the prevention of prostate cancer. The Prostate Cancer Prevention Trial (PCPT) involves nearly 20,000 men and will compare the incidence of prostate cancer in those who take the drug *finasteride* (a drug developed to treat benign prostatic hypertrophy) for seven years and those who take a placebo for the same length of time. The PCPT results should be known by 2004. Another study started in 1999 will, in a similar way, assess the value of combining selenium and vitamin E in the prevention of prostate cancer.

Early Detection

Since we can't select our family and have no control over family history, knowledge of a family history of prostate cancer does not really help prevent the disease. Family history is, however, important to include when talking about and deciding on screening for various kinds of cancer, including prostate cancer. Men with a family history of prostate cancer, meaning men whose father or brother has developed the disease, are thought to be more at risk. African-American men and men who are older are also more at risk for developing prostate cancer. Men who are more at risk and who use the screening methods available to them are more likely to find cancers at an early and more curable stage. This is the value of early detection.

Advances in early detection of prostate cancer have resulted in a dramatic change in the survival rate of men with this disease. Before the PSA and DRE tests became available around 1990, most men with prostate cancer were diagnosed with advanced or late-stage disease, and most died within a few years of diagnosis. Today, cancers found early are smaller and less likely to have spread to other parts of the body. Other early detection techniques include transrectal ultrasound and spring-loaded biopsy devices. Men with early-stage disease have almost a 100 percent chance of living at least another five years without physical symptoms and problems caused by their prostate cancer. Herein lies the crux of the debate about treatment for early-stage prostate cancer.

Although early diagnosis and treatment of prostate cancer can help some men live longer, it may not affect the life span of others. For a man with a life expectancy of less than ten years, many experts believe there is no need to make an early diagnosis. And, at least so far, there is no treatment for prostate cancer that does not have some risks that could affect a man's quality of life. At this time, there is no conclusive proof that early detection will affect the prostate cancer death rate. Studies are underway to prove that early detection in large groups of men will lower prostate cancer death rates, but the studies will not be completed and their results analyzed for several years. Until then, the decision to have tests for early prostate cancer detection is left up to each man—and perhaps each man and his health care provider.

Nevertheless, there are some organizations and experts who are more or less in charge of making recommendations for early detection policies. The U.S. Veterans Administration recently made it known that it would no longer routinely provide prostate cancer screening. Instead, veterans are encouraged to talk to their health care provider and, together, make decisions about going ahead with early-detection testing. The American Cancer Society (ACS) and the National Comprehensive Cancer Network (NCCN) recommend that PSA and DRE be done every year, starting at age fifty, for men who have at least a ten-year life expectancy, and for younger men who are at higher risk. These groups also recommend that men in high-risk groups, such as those who have two or more first-degree relatives (father and a brother, or two brothers) or African Americans, begin testing earlier, at forty-five years old.

The PSA Test

The PSA is a blood test; blood is drawn and sent to the laboratory for examination. The PSA level is measured in the unit *nagstrom per milliliter*, abbreviated ng/ml. In general, older men tend to have increased PSA levels. A normal PSA level for a man younger than fifty is considered to be 0-2.5 ng/ml, a level that does not indicate cancer. For men older than seventy, normal PSA can range from 0 to 6.5 ng/ml. Conditions other than cancer can cause a slight increase in the PSA level. The health care professional needs to have a clear understanding of a man's health history and habits in order to interpret the meaning of an increase in the man's PSA. For example, benign prostatic hypertrophy causes a slight increase in PSA level, as does inflammation of the prostate, called *prostatitis*. Still, when a PSA level is higher than 4 ng/ml, it is wise to look for an explanation, recheck the PSA level, and possibly go to the next level of diagnostic testing.

An important advance in prostate cancer diagnosis is the discovery that PSA exists in more than one form; it can be either linked or not linked with other molecules in the blood. Unlinked PSA is called *free PSA*; linked PSA is called *complexed PSA*. New tests that determine the amount of "free" compared with "total" PSA, called the "free-to-total" (or "free-to-complexed") PSA test, have been very helpful in increasing the accuracy of PSA in predicting the likelihood of prostate cancer. A lower level of free PSA (FPSA) compared to complexed PSA is more often associated with cancer. Conversely, a higher percentage of FPSA compared to complexed PSA is less often linked to prostate cancer.

A possible advance in prostate cancer screening is testing for the prostate-specific membrane antigen (PSMA), first reported in 1987. PSMA seems to be a type of protein that the body develops in response to increased prostate cell activity. PSMA is increased in benign prostate enlargement and is even higher when the cells are very active prostate cancer cells. PSMA is not currently used in screening, but could be in the future. In the meantime, it can help detect spread of prostate cancer even before there are signs and symptoms, and is believed to have the potential to help diagnose and monitor prostate cancer as a tumor marker. Human kallikrein 2, or hK2, first reported in 1997, is another molecule similar to PSMA. Researchers believe that hK2 could someday be an important prostate cancer tumor marker.

The PSA test is not 100 percent accurate in finding cancer. Some men with low PSA levels can still have cancer, while men with higher PSA levels may not. Generally, over half of all men with a PSA level of 10 ng/ml or higher—or a percent FPSA of 0 to 10 percent—have cancer.

There are some things every man can do to make PSA testing as accurate as possible. Ejaculation can cause a normal and temporary increase in blood PSA levels. Since it would be impossible to tell if the high level is caused by ejaculation or a cancer, it is recommended that men abstain from any sexual activity for two days before PSA testing.

Manipulation of the prostate through digital rectal examination (or other forms of rectal manipulation such as anal intercourse) also causes the PSA to rise. For this reason, it is important to have the blood levels drawn for PSA before having the digital rectal examination.

PSA levels tend to change over time. As already noted, PSA will increase slightly just because of normal aging. It is a good idea to keep track of PSA levels from year to year. From one year to the next, a man with a PSA that rises at a rate more than 0.75 ng/ml is at an increased risk of having prostate cancer.

If the total PSA level is over 10, a biopsy is recommended as the next step. A total PSA level of less than 10 must be considered along with two other types of PSA analyses, the PSA velocity and the percent of free PSA.

Signs and Symptoms

The PSA has allowed for the diagnosis of prostate cancer even before symptoms develop. While there is controversy about the value of early detection in the long-range management of prostate cancer, most experts still value early detection as the most reliable way to prevent premature deaths from this disease. Men should also be aware of the signs of prostate cancer and, even though the same signs could indicate other conditions, go to the doctor or nurse practitioner for a physical examination as soon as they experience symptoms.

The most common symptoms of prostate cancer are

- frequent urination (especially at night, called *nocturia*)

- inability to urinate

- trouble starting to urinate

- trouble holding back urination

- a weak or interrupted flow of urine

- pain or burning feeling during urination

- pain during ejaculation

- blood in the urine or semen

- frequent pain or stiffness in the lower back, hips, or upper thighs

Prostate cancers develop from cells of the prostate gland. The development of cancer starts with some cell changes in the prostate, when a few cells change from normal to abnormal. These abnormal cells have not yet developed into a cancer, do not cause symptoms, and cannot be felt during a physical examination. Eventually, these abnormal cells form a clump of cells or a tumor, usually developing in the outer part of the prostate. The tumor might not be in a place where it will put pressure on the urethra, though it could possibly be discovered by DRE. Even when the tumor cannot be felt by DRE, it may be detectable by PSA or some of the other early detection tests. When the tumor becomes large enough to squeeze the urethra, it will cause some of the problems with urination mentioned above.

As time goes on, the cancer cells continue to grow within the prostate and can spread outside of the prostate gland to the seminal vesicles, lymph nodes, and bones. Common sites of bone involvement with prostate cancer are the spinal column (vertebrae) and hip bones.

Lymph fluid is carried by lymphatic vessels to lymph nodes. Lymphatic vessels of the prostate lead to nodes in the pelvis. Cancer cells can enter lymph vessels and spread out along these vessels to reach lymph nodes, where they continue to grow or metastasize. If prostate cancer cells have spread to the pelvic lymph nodes, they are more likely to have spread to other organs, too.

Diagnosis and Workup

As with all forms of cancer, a full, complete examination or workup will take place after the first tests—in this case the PSA and DRE—indicate the possibility of cancer. For most men with prostate cancer, this full examination will be done by a doctor who specializes in problems in the urinary tract, the urologist. The urologist will need to learn about the man's past medical history and current state of health.

Additional diagnostic tests will be used to assess the man's cancer status (see Table 4.1). The man with suspected prostate cancer can expect to have a transrectal ultrasound of the prostate, a prostate biopsy, a bone scan, a CT or MRI scan, and cystoscopy.

As in all forms of cancer, determination of the cell type, grade, and stage of prostate cancer offers clues to prognosis and provides the basis for deciding which treatment option is most likely to offer hope for cure or control. A man's understanding of the grade and stage of his cancer is the key to his ability to make informed decisions.

Cell Type

Most prostate cancers—about 95 percent—are *adenocarcinomas*. The cell types of the remaining 5 percent of prostate cancers include *transitional cell carcinoma* and, even more rarely, *squamous cell carcinoma*. In addition to true cancers, there are two forms of abnormal prostatic cell growth: *atypical adenomatous hyperplasia* (sometimes referred to as *adenosis*) and *prostatic intraepithelial neoplasia,* or PIN. Both are considered precancerous.

Grade

The *tumor grade* indicates how quickly the cancer cells are growing and dividing, and offers a picture of how quickly the cancer itself is growing and its likelihood of spreading or metastasizing. The *Gleason score* is used specifically to describe the grade of prostate cancer cells and is determined in two steps. First, the pathologist determines what cell features are most common throughout the tumor and gives this pattern a number score ranging from 1 to 5. Lower numbers correspond to cell features that are most like normal prostate cells, while higher numbers suggest more bizarre cellular features that have little resemblance to normal cells. A second number that reflects the second most common cell features is added to the first. The sum of the two numbers is the *Gleason score,* or *Gleason grade*. A Gleason

Table 4.1: Diagnostic Tests for Prostate Cancer

Test	What It Shows	How It Is Done
Prostate Specific Antigen (PSA)	Higher than normal levels suggest prostate cancer. PSA is done as a screening test, can be helpful in predicting prognosis and assessing the effectiveness of treatment, and is also used to determine if prostate cancer has recurred after treatment. The PSA test should also include the percentage of free PSA. The PSA level normally increases as a man ages: the normal PSA for a man who is 40 to 49 years old is 0–2.0ng/ml; for a 70- to 79-year-old man, 0–5.5ng/ml.	Blood is drawn in the doctor's office, clinic, or laboratory and is sent for testing. Results are available within two to five days, depending upon the laboratory. The PSA should be routinely followed by the digital rectal exam.
Free PSA	How much PSA is circulating in the bloodstream in an unbound form, compared to how much PSA is bound with other proteins in the blood. When the routine PSA is at a borderline level, a low percentage of free PSA is more likely to occur with prostate cancer, and indicates the need for a biopsy of the prostate.	Same as routine PSA
PSA velocity	Measures how quickly the PSA level increases over time. By comparing annual PSA levels, PSA velocity provides a way to follow a man with borderline PSA levels.	Same as routine PSA
Digital Rectal Exam (DRE)	Enlargement and abnormal contours of the prostate gland, tumors in the rectum, and swelling that pushes the rectal walls. Stool collected during the exam can be used to do a fecal occult blood test (FOBT).	Can be performed in a doctor's office, a clinic, or the inpatient setting as a part of a complete physical examination. It may be performed by a nurse practitioner, physician's assistant, or a physician. It should not cause pain.
Transrectal ultrasound (TRUS)	Guides placement of the biopsy needle used to get a specimen of suspicious tissues or mass in the prostate.	In the X-ray department, a special probe is inserted into the patient's rectum. Sound waves are sent out by the probe, creating an image on a video screen so that the doctor can guide placement of the biopsy needle. Most men say this is mildly uncomfortable but not painful.

Table 4.1: Diagnostic Tests for Prostate Cancer (cont'd.)

Test	What It Shows	How It Is Done
Biopsy	Several small tissue samples—typically six to eighteen samples—of different areas of the prostate, including any suspicious mass, are needed to make an accurate diagnosis. The many samples provide a representative sample of the prostate and show how much of the prostate is involved by the cancer. The examination of the biopsy might include a DNA ploidy analysis.	Guided by the ultrasound video image, the doctor inserts a narrow needle through the rectum into the abnormal area of the prostate. The needle removes a small sample of tissue that will be examined under a microscope to find or rule out cancer. The microscopic exam will also determine the Gleason's score, an indicator of the cancer cells' variation from normal prostate cells.
Bone scan (radionuclide bone scan)	If cancer is discovered in the prostate, a bone scan will help determine if the cancer has spread to bones. These findings will help determine the plans for treatment.	Can be done during an outpatient visit or during an inpatient stay. After a dye is injected into a vein, a series of X-ray images are taken. Areas of the bone that are changed due to disease, as well as healed fractures and even arthritis, will be highlighted in the images. These highlighted areas will be examined further to determine if the changes are caused by the spread of cancer.
DNA ploidy analysis	Though its value has yet to be proven, some physicians include DNA ploidy in their treatment-related considerations. It should be used only in situations where its results would potentially alter a man's treatment options.	Tissue samples taken during the biopsy are tested to determine how quickly cancer cells are growing. Cancer cells classified as diploid grow slowly. Cells classified as aneuploid or tetraploid grow quickly. DNA ploidy analysis is done by the pathologist during the microscopic examination of biopsy samples using flow cytometry techniques. It assesses the DNA characteristics of the cancer cells.
Computerized axial tomographic (CAT or CT) scan	A CT scan is a sophisticated X-ray exam that uses computer techniques to obtain more detailed cross-sectional X-ray images of body structures than a routine X-ray offers. A CT scan can show enlarged lymph nodes in the pelvis and the spread of cancer to other internal organs.	CT scanning can be done with and without the addition of contrast dyes injected into the vein. The dye can be injected just before the CT scan starts. The IV needle and tubing are used only during the scan and can be removed as soon as it is completed. The patient lies on a table and is surrounded by a donut-shaped machine that snaps multiple X-rays. A CT scan generally takes less than one hour to complete although the doctor may order more than one scan to be done during one appointment. A CT scan is usually not used in early-stage prostate cancer.

Table 4.1: Diagnostic Tests for Prostate Cancer (cont'd.)

Test	What It Shows	How It Is Done
Magnetic resonance imaging (MRI)	MRI is an X-ray technique that uses magnetic fields to create very detailed cross-sectional images of the targeted body structures. It can picture abnormalities in lymph nodes or organs that may suggest spread of cancer.	MRI is done in an X-ray department, specially constructed MRI units, and even MRI mobile units—specially converted trailers that contain the MRI equipment. MRI is similar to a CT scan. MRI is usually not done in early-stage prostate cancer.
Blood tests	Complete blood count (CBC) counts the number of the various kinds of blood cells. Low white and red blood cell counts can be an indication of spread of cancer to the bone marrow.	Blood chemistry tests assess for chemical changes in the blood caused by alterations in the liver, kidney, or bone marrow function.
Prostatic acid phosphatase (PAP)	PAP was a very common blood test used to detect prostate cancer until the PSA was introduced. PAP is still used as an indicator that cancer has spread outside of the prostatic capsule, and to confirm recurrence of prostate cancer.	Blood is drawn in the doctor's office, clinic, or laboratory and is sent for testing.

score of 1 to 2 is indicative of a small, slow growing cancer. Scores of 5 or more generally indicate larger and faster-growing cancers.

Stage

Depending on where a man's cancer is diagnosed, one of two common staging systems will be used to describe the extent of prostate cancer. The American Urologic Association (AUA) System is an update of a staging system developed by Whitmore that was itself updated by Dr. Hugh Jewitt. You might hear this staging system called the AUA System or the Jewitt System. Increasingly, the tumor-node-metastasis classification system—the TNM—developed by the American Joint Committee on Cancer (AJCC) is used.

The Jewitt System, first described in 1975 and since modified, groups stages into four categories that range from A (indicating a clinically undetectable tumor confined to the prostate gland) to D (indicating advanced disease with distant metastases).

The TNM classification, which offers a more exact distinction within each staging category, is outlined in Table 4.2, and the AJCC system in Table 4.3. The AJCC system groups TNM classes into stages I–IV.

Table 4.2: The TNM Classification System for Prostate Cancer

T =	**Primary Tumor Characteristics**
TX	Primary tumor cannot be assessed
T0	No evidence of primary tumor
T1	**Tumor is not clinically visible by X-ray nor felt in examination**
T1a	Tumor is found while performing other type of surgery but involves less than 5 percent of the tissue removed
T1b	Same as T1a, but involves more than 5 percent of tissue removed
T1c	Tumor is discovered by needle biopsy after elevated PSA
T2	**Tumor is found only in the prostate**
T2a	Tumor involves one lobe of the prostate gland
T2b	Tumor involves both lobes of the prostate gland
T3	**Tumor extends through the prostate capsule**
T3a	Tumor extends to outside the capsule
T3b	Tumor has invaded one or both seminal vesicles
T4	**Tumor is attached to or invades organs or structures other than the seminal vesicles such as the bladder, sphincter, rectum, abdominal muscles, or pelvic wall**
N	**Involvement of Regional Lymph Nodes (N)**
NX	The regional lymph nodes cannot be assessed
N0	There is no evidence of regional lymph node involvement
N1	There are metastases in regional lymph node or nodes
M	**Distant Metastasis (M)**
MX	Distant metastasis cannot be assessed
M0	No distant metastasis
M1	Distant metastasis (when more than one site of metastasis is identified, the most advanced category—M1c—is used)
M1a	Nonregional lymph node(s)
M1b	Bone(s)
M1c	Other site(s)
G	**Histologic Grade (G)**
GX	Grade cannot be determined
G1	Well differentiated
G2	Moderately differentiated
G3–4	Poorly differentiated

Table 4.3: The AJCC Staging System for Prostate Cancer

Stage	Criteria
I	T1a, N0, M0, G1
II	T1a, N0, M0, G2, 3–4
III	T3, N0, M0, any G
IV	T4, N0, M0, any G
	Any T, N1, M0, any G
	Any T, any N, M1, any G

Treatment

Treatment options are determined based on several factors that make each man's condition unique:

- The man's age: Even without the cancer diagnosis, would this man be expected to live less than or more than five years?

- The man's general health status: Are there other conditions—called *co-morbidities*—that would rule out a particular form of treatment, or medical conditions that would interfere with a particular treatment protocol?

- The stage and grade of the man's cancer.

- Symptoms of cancer that the man may already have.

Active treatment for prostate cancer can involve surgery, radiation therapy, hormone treatment, and chemotherapy, in addition to new treatment modalities being explored such as monoclonal antibodies (MCAs) and vaccines. Any of these therapies might be used alone in *single modality* therapy, or used together in *combination* or *combined modality* therapy. Treatment options are outlined by stage of disease in Table 4.4.

Watchful Waiting

For some men, a viable but controversial option to active treatment is *watchful waiting*, which involves periodic observation without active treatment. Watchful waiting is considered a valid option for men with early stage-A or B1-prostate cancer, particularly men who are over seventy years old. It might also be used for men with a low Gleason score and low PSA. Periodic observation will include monitoring of the PSA level and physical examination every three to six months. Active treatment will be started if there are signs that the cancer has progressed.

Some physicians suggest watchful waiting because they recognize that most prostate cancers grow slowly and may never become life threatening. Since the advent of the PSA, very early, asymptomatic, and clinically undetectable prostate cancers are diagnosed more often. As a matter of fact, only about 3 percent of all men who develop cancer cells in their prostate will actually die of the disease. For men who have asymptomatic prostate cancer, the treatment and its short- and long-term effects can cause more problems than the cancer. Still, the idea of watchful waiting can be difficult for many men to accept; the idea of having any untreated cancer is almost foreign. The value of watchful waiting as an option has not yet been fully proven in

Table 4.4: Treatment Options for Prostate Cancer

Stage	Considerations	Treatment Options
Stage I	Is life expectancy more than or less than twenty years? General health status PSA level Gleason score	Watchful waiting/periodic evaluation External beam radiation therapy Radical prostatectomy with pelvic lymphadenectomy Brachytherapy/interstitial radioactive seed implants
Stage II	Is life expectancy more than or less than twenty years? General health status PSA level Gleason score	Watchful waiting/periodic observation External beam radiation Radical prostatectomy with pelvic lymphadenectomy Brachytherapy/interstitial radioactive seed implants Ultrasound-guided percutaneous cryosurgery is being studied
Stage III	Life expectancy General health status Symptoms	External beam irradiation with or without hormonal therapy Orchiectomy or hormonal manipulation (LHRH) Brachytherapy/interstitial seed implants Radical prostatectomy No treatment Symptom management and/or palliative surgery Ultrasound-guided percutaneous cryosurgery is being studied
Stage IV	Age Coexisting medical conditions Symptoms Presence of distant metastases	Symptom management—transurethral resection, radiation therapy Hormonal therapy Bilateral orchiectomy Chemotherapy is being studied
Recurrent prostate cancer	Prior treatment Site of recurrence Coexisting medical conditions Patient's needs and wishes Symptoms	Radiation to the site of recurrence Radical prostatectomy Hormonal therapy Cryosurgical ablation at the site of recurrence is being studied Palliative radiation therapy Radioactive isotopes for the management of bone metastases

prospective, randomized clinical trials, so controversy remains. Until trials demonstrate its value, men—particularly older men with disease—may be asked to consider watchful waiting as a valid alternative to more risky treatment, but will most likely be offered standard therapy as well.

Decision Making

For prostate cancer, more than any other kind of cancer that affects men, choosing from among available treatment options can be very confusing. The three crucial pieces of information men need to make good treatment decisions are:

- the baseline PSA

- the Gleason score

- the clinical stage of disease

US TOO International, a prostate cancer survivor support organization, advocates the "Medical Miranda for the Prostate Cancer Patient." The Miranda, as anyone who watches television dramas, reads crime novels, or simply reads the paper knows, is the warning an arresting police officer must give to a crime suspect: "You have the right to remain silent, you have the right to an attorney...."

US TOO suggests that the "Medical Miranda" reads like this:

You have the right to know your prognosis.

You have the right to understand principles of evaluation and treatment.

You have the right to be familiar with the pros and cons of available treatment options.

This idea of the Medical Miranda applies not just to men with prostate cancer, but to all people facing any cancer diagnosis. With respect to prostate cancer, US TOO advocates that men understand these concepts:

Organ-confined disease: Is the cancer limited to the prostate itself, or is there a high risk that the cancer has spread outside of the prostate? If the cancer has spread beyond the prostate, then local therapies such as prostatectomy, radiation therapy, or cryosurgery will not cure the disease.

Determination of extent of disease: Is the Gleason score determined and the stage of the disease fully explored?

Neoadjuvant hormone blockade (NHB): For some men, taking hormonal therapy before surgery or before radiation therapy helps to reduce the size of the tumor and, in some studies, has been shown to reduce the spread of cancer.

Pros and cons of different therapies: It is important that the man know the source of the numbers or statistics the surgeon is quoting to describe risks and benefits. Are they numbers that reflect the surgeon's own practice, the collective experience of a major medical center, or another community practice? What is the treating surgeon's own experience? US TOO recommends that a man ask the surgeon for the names and telephone numbers of his last five patients who had prostatectomy and that the man talk to these other men. US TOO also recommends that the man get a copy of the explanations of pros and cons that have been provided by the surgeon, as well as a copy of any consultant's report.

A good decision-making process is one in which the man fully understands what the treatment is designed to do, as well as the more common and less common risks and the expected benefits of any form of treatment. This is referred to as weighing the risks and benefits, or pros and cons. It has been demonstrated over and over again that the choice of treatment will affect the quality of the remainder of the man's life. Unfortunately, there is currently no cancer treatment that is completely without some risk of long-term, unpleasant, or adverse side effects. On the other hand, a man may decide that the potential adverse effect is something that is relatively unimportant, if the trade-off is the likelihood of curing or controlling the cancer. These are the issues that each man needs to consider as he goes through the process of selecting from among the treatment options available to him.

Surgery

Surgery is quite often the first treatment option presented once a diagnosis of prostate cancer is certain. Surgery is a viable, valuable, and generally accepted treatment. But, as the saying goes, "If the only tool you have is a hammer, everything looks like a nail." In other words, a surgical specialist is more likely to recommend surgery. This is not necessarily wrong; it's just that most specialists are true believers in the techniques they know best. There is a wide difference of opinion among the many specialists who play roles in the management of prostate cancer, resulting in the confusion that many men experience as they wade through the information about risks and benefits linked to the various forms of treatment.

The following discussion is designed to help a man with prostate cancer understand the treatment modality and create a baseline level of information, so he can then ask the right questions of his health care team, and evaluate the answers.

Transurethral Resection of the Prostate (TURP) Transurethral resection of the prostate (TURP) is used to treat blockage of urine caused by an obstruction in the bladder. It is not uncommon for a man to undergo a TURP for what he and the surgeon believe to be a noncancerous condition called benign prostatic hyperplasia (BPH), only to discover that the obstruction is actually caused by prostate cancer. In the TURP procedure, a scope is inserted through the penis into the urethra, and small pieces or chips of prostate tissue are removed through the scope. Bleeding is stemmed by cautery, burning the small blood vessels causing them to seal over.

During and immediately after the TURP procedure, the bladder is continuously flushed or *irrigated* with a saline solution via a three-way catheter inserted through the penis into the bladder. The continuous irrigation helps prevent the formation of blood clots that can cause bladder distention. The irrigation procedure is likely to continue for about twenty-four hours. When the bleeding has more or less ceased, generally by three to four days after the procedure, the catheter is removed. Bladder spasms and pain related to the procedure are expected, but should be relatively easy to manage with medicines such as belladonna and opium suppository, oxybutynin, or propantheline. After the catheter is removed, it will be important for the man to urinate frequently, as soon as he notices even the slightest urge. Waiting or holding urine can cause the bladder to distend or become too full, which can lead to urinary retention.

The man should expect to need and use pain medicines during the postoperative phase. Some of the medicines used to control bladder spasms can cause constipation; stool softeners and laxatives should be used to make sure that constipation does not occur. The man will be expected to drink large amounts of fluids, and can anticipate other routine postoperative procedures such as coughing, deep breathing, and walking.

Radical Prostatectomy After a biopsy-proven Stage I–II (A, B) prostate cancer is detected, the surgical procedure called *radical prostatectomy* is often posed as a curative method of treatment, particularly if the man can reasonably be expected to live at least another ten years. Sometimes this surgery is offered even for Stage III (C), although surgeons are generally less confident that they will be able to achieve a cure with surgery alone when treating Stage III prostate cancer. If a urologist is the only physician involved in the diagnostic and staging workup, it is more likely that he or she will recommend surgery. In late-stage prostate cancer, other types of surgery might be used to manage distressing symptoms, but surgery is not likely to result in a cure. In assessing the value of surgery, the man needs to consider many factors, including what the surgery and recovery will entail, and the expected short- and long-term effects.

The surgeon uses one of two approaches to do a prostatectomy. In what is called the *retropubic* approach, the surgeon makes the incision in the abdomen. In the *perineal* approach, the prostate gland is accessed through an incision in the perineal region. If the surgeon does a *radical prostatectomy*, he or she removes the prostate gland, the prostatic capsule that surrounds the gland, ejaculatory ducts, seminal vesicles, and sometimes the lymph nodes in the pelvis. In the past, this surgery resulted in permanent erectile dysfunction (impotence) and urinary incontinence (the inability to control urination, resulting in more or less continuous leaking or dribbling). Many surgeons have now become skilled in what is referred to as *nerve sparing* technique, which preserves erectile function and urinary control. Still, erectile dysfunction affects 30 to 40 percent of all men who undergo this surgery. There is a slightly lower risk for urinary problems; recent reports show that 90 percent of all men who undergo nerve sparing radical prostatectomy have complete urinary control. Of the remaining 10 percent, some have stress incontinence that requires them to wear a pad, and a small number have no control over the flow of urine at all and must use a diaper, drip collector, condom catheter, penile clamp, or even a small ostomy pouch to collect urine.

The immediate risks of surgery can include infection, pneumonia, unexpected bleeding, blood clots, difficulty urinating, and accidental puncture or tears of the bowel. During the first several days following surgery, it will be important to watch for early signs of infection such as fever or chills, and redness or drainage from the incision. An indwelling catheter (also called a *Foley* catheter) will be left in place for several days to ensure that urine drains well, and also to make monitoring of urine color and quantity easier. The nursing staff in the recovery room and the surgical unit will monitor the man while he remains in the hospital. Once he leaves the hospital, he or his caregiver will be expected to watch for any unexpected symptoms and to call the doctor as soon as urinary problems or signs of infection occur.

Later, another set of nurses can be help a man reach his highest possible level of recovery. Specialty nurses, sometimes called *enterostomal therapy* nurses or *wound, ostomy, and continence* nurses, have a thorough understanding of the anatomical and physiological causes of incontinence and impotence and understand the emotional impact these problems have on men.

Such a nurse can help a man select from any of the available devices to collect urine, and learn to manage the device in a way that is compatible with his lifestyle and his unique needs. This nurse also has the knowledge to teach men with urinary incontinence new skills, such as timed voiding techniques, Kegel exercises, and biofeedback, which may help them regain some if not total control over urinary flow.

There are also likely to be bodily changes that affect sexual activity following radical prostatectomy. When the prostate is removed, the amount of semen that is expelled at ejaculation will be reduced. Sometimes the ejaculate goes backward up into the bladder instead out through the penis, resulting in *dry ejaculation*. The urine might be cloudy because it contains sperm. Orgasm can still occur even without ejaculation; nevertheless, partial or complete erectile dysfunction or impotency—inability to have or maintain an erection—is a relatively common occurrence after radical prostatectomy. Men over seventy are less likely to regain erectile function. Men under fifty are likely to regain potency after the surgical wound heals and the swelling from surgery goes away, generally within six weeks to three months. Clearly, if impotency is one of the aftereffects of surgery, a full exploration of its cause should be done; some men may find ways to regain erectile function. When erectile function is absent, the man and his partner can explore other ways of expressing sexuality and intimacy. Chapter 18 deals more directly with sexuality and concerns surrounding sexual activity.

Cryosurgery *Cryosurgery* is a form of surgery in which liquid nitrogen probes are used to take targeted prostate tissue to temperatures low enough to kill tissue, including any cancerous tissue. The cryoprobes are guided by transrectal ultrasound. The use of cryosurgery is still new, and its long-term effectiveness is not yet known. Some serious potential side effects or problems are associated with cryosurgery, including injury to the bladder and rectum, urinary incontinence, and impotence.

External Beam Radiation Therapy

Radiation therapy is used in the management of prostate cancer in several ways. *External beam radiation therapy* (XRT) can be used alone to treat early stages (A2-, B1, B2) of prostate cancer, and is also useful in the management of problems such as bone metastases (spread to bones) and urinary obstruction that can occur in late-stage, advanced disease. In some treatment plans, radiation is used along with hormone therapy over a sixteen-week course of therapy. Sometimes, particularly when the spread of cancer is discovered during surgery, a treatment plan might be to apply radiation *after* surgery. Radiation might also be a preferred treatment for a man who has medical conditions that place him at higher risk for problems relating to surgery. The external beam radiation treatments are given five days a week over a period of five to seven weeks. The actual dose of radiation to be used, and the schedule, will depend on the stage of disease.

Some protocols involve a course of external beam radiation followed by the seed implant procedure. The combination of external beam radiation therapy and the brachytherapy technique described in the next section is called *Combined Precision Irradiation* or CPI. This approach has been recommended for men who have stage C (III) disease, when the cancer is located outside of the prostate gland itself. Usually, external beam radiation will be started about three weeks after the implant procedure.

Brachytherapy

There is renewed interest in the use of *brachytherapy* techniques in the treatment of prostate cancer. Its general application was first reported in 1917; during the 1970s, brachytherapy gained popularity in the management of this disease. Over the past decade, with claims of reduced side effects and advances in technology—including the use of special X-ray and ultrasound techniques to guide placement—brachytherapy has become a very valuable treatment option in the management of prostate cancer.

Brachytherapy involves the placement of small pieces (called *seeds*) of radioactive materials directly into the prostate—sometimes referred to as the *seed implants*. Most often, radioactive iodine (Iodine-125) seeds are used, though radioactive palladium (Pd-103) is used more often in the treatment of high-grade tumors or cancers that have more than one foci within the prostate. The brachytherapy technique is an option available to men who have early-stage prostate cancer (T1 or T2 tumors) who have a life expectancy of more than five years. Men who are not candidates for brachytherapy treatment would be those who have already undergone a TURP or who have very large prostate glands.

Much effort goes into the treatment planning process. A transrectal ultrasound study is done to accurately outline the shape of the prostate and the cancerous tissue, then with computer assistance a plan is devised that tells the doctor exactly where the radioactive seeds are to be placed.

The Seed Implant Procedure Brachytherapy can be done while the man is under general anesthesia, but is increasingly done as an outpatient procedure under spinal anesthesia. The man is placed in what is called the *lithotomy* position on the operating table, lying on his back with this knees bent

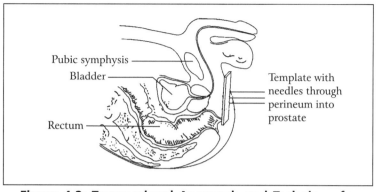

Figure 4.2: Transperineal Approach and Technique for Radioactive Seed Implants in the Prostate

Reprinted with permission Cash & Dattoli, *Oncology Nursing Forum*, 1997

up towards his chest (women will recognize this as the "feet in the stirrups" position they are placed in for a pelvic examination or the delivery of a baby). A plastic template is placed on the perineal area, the area that extends from the rectum to the scrotum (see Figure 4.2). Under fluoroscopy (X-ray) and ultrasound guidance, steel or plastic needles are placed through the perineum and rectum into the targeted area of the prostate. Radioactive seeds arc threaded into the prostate through the needles. Typically, any-where from 100 to 150 radioactive seeds will be placed, or *implanted*.

After the seeds are in place, the needles and template are removed. The seeds are permanently implanted; they will remain in place for the rest of the man's life. An indwelling (Foley) catheter is then inserted through the penis and urethra into the bladder just before the man is taken from the operating room to the recovery room. At some point within two hours post-implant, the man will undergo a CT scan of the prostate and/or other types of X-ray exams such as the *cystourethroscopy*, to assure the accuracy of seed placement.

The man's urine output will be watched closely. The nursing staff in the recovery room will check the volume and color of the urine, and will especially watch for blood clots. While each treatment center will probably have minor variations in procedure, the catheter will be removed within one to two hours if blood clots are not a problem. Just before removing the catheter, a nurse or technician will instill a small amount—usually, about one cup—of sterile saline. This liquid will partially fill the bladder, which hopefully, will help the man urinate more quickly on his own. As soon as it is determined that the man can void on his own—usually by urinating on two or three separate voidings with a volume of over 100 cc each time—he can leave the recovery room and return home.

Obviously, the man will need a designated driver to take him home and make sure he is safe in his home surroundings. Most treatment centers also ask the man to strain all of his urine for two weeks post-implant, just in case there are radioactive seeds in the urine. Should a seed be discovered, it should *not* be handled. Remove the seed from the strainer using a forceps or tweezers, wrap it in aluminum foil or place it in a metal container, and take it to the radiation therapy doctor so that it can be disposed of safely.

The brachytherapy technique has many advantages over external beam therapy. The radiation dose is very concentrated in and around the actual site of the cancer, such that exposure and subsequent damage to surrounding tissues and organs is minimized or eliminated. The procedure is done as a one-time, outpatient treatment. Recovery time is minimized, and the odds are that continence and potency will be preserved.

Post-Implant Side Effects The man who has undergone the implant procedure will experience some side effects during the immediate post-implant period. He might have discomfort and pain in the perineal area as well as urinary symptoms including inability to urinate, decreased urine stream, and urgency. Blood in the urine can be expected during the first forty-eight hours, and blood clots can cause urinary obstruction. For this reason, it will be important to monitor urinary output through the first seventy-two hours. Sometimes, an indwelling or Foley catheter is left in place for a short time post-implant.

Other common side effects such as urinary obstruction, urinary tract irritation, a need to urinate often (*frequency*), a need to urinate during the night (*nocturia*), and pain or burning with urination (*dysuria*) could appear around seven to ten days post-implant. These side effects are temporary and seem to peak or be at their worst within two to three weeks after the implant. Most of these side effects are easily treated. Some men will have some rectal side effects such as soft stools and increased number of bowel movements. The development of sores or ulcers in the rectum is rare.

Post-Implant Care at Home Since brachytherapy is usually done as an outpatient procedure, most of the post-implant "nursing care" will be done by the man himself or a caregiver. Men who live a great distance from the treatment facility are generally asked to stay within close range for at least twenty-four hours post-implant. After that, the development of a major problem is unlikely, and it is safe for the man to be more on his own. Still, it's important to know what to expect, what to do in case problems develop, and how to manage symptoms that occur.

It should be stressed here that the likely symptoms are short-lived and fairly easy to manage. Most treatment facilities—the good ones—should have a routine follow-up plan. Within twenty-four hours of the implant, the treatment facility nurse or doctor should telephone the patient to make sure things are going as expected. One treatment center's procedure is that a nurse makes routine follow-up calls, at first weekly and then twice a month for two months.

Self-care considerations include:

Preventing infection: A most important aspect of post-implant care revolves around preventing the development of infection in the perineal skin. Men will be given a dose of antibiotics via the intravenous line just before the procedure, and then will be given a course of oral antibiotics (usually a seven-day prescription) post-implant. The man must understand the importance of using the antibiotics, and must complete the full prescribed course—every capsule or pill, and on the right schedule. Keeping the perineal area clean and dry is a priority. Cleaning the perineum with soap and water, followed by gently but thoroughly drying with a soft towel once or twice a day should provide protection from infection. Dressings are not recommended since bacteria or germs can grow in soiled dressings.

Minimizing swelling, bruising, and pain: Some bruising and swelling—edema—in the perineal area and scrotum is to be expected, and this is the post-implant side effect that is the biggest problem for most men. However, even this can be easily managed. Nurses in one oncology center where nearly three hundred men have undergone this procedure discovered that the simple application of an ice bag to the perineum for a period of twenty-four hours post-implant prevents the occurrence of severe swelling and bruising.

Most men who undergo an implant procedure deny that outright pain is a problem. Still, they do admit that they are quite uncomfortable and appreciate having a soft pillow to sit on. Most men are given a prescription for a mild opioid analgesic such as oxycodone and report that after the first forty-eight hours they no longer needed pain medication.

Minimizing rectal discomfort: A very small percentage of men (around 2 percent) who undergo implant procedures develop *proctitis*, an inflammation of the rectum and anus. When this occurs, it appears around four weeks post-implant and lasts less than two weeks. Symptoms of proctitis include frequent, "gassy" bowel movements, soft stool, rectal bleeding, and rectal irritation. Most of the time, proctitis can be managed through a low-residue diet. Irritation in the rectal or anal areas can be soothed by using a cortisone cream or suppository after every bowel movement and at bedtime. Sitting in the bathtub or use of a "sitz bath" can be helpful, too. Infrequently, proctitis can occur much later, even one to two years post-implant. The symptoms should be reported to the doctor immediately, and the doctor should look fully for the cause, which could relate to the development of a colon or rectal cancer or the development of a *fistula*, an abnormal tract between the bladder and rectum.

Preventing urinary problems: Blockage of urine can occur as a result of swelling around the bladder and urethra. The incidence is higher if the prostate is large, or if the man had this problem before the implant. When retention happens, a catheter can be reinserted and left in place for a period of time, often around forty-eight hours, after which the catheter is removed and the process of evaluating urinary function starts again. If urinary retention continues to be a problem, nurse experts recommend that patients use *intermittent self-catheterization* instead of continuing to use the indwelling catheter. A nurse, doctor, or urology technician can teach the man or his caregiver to perform this procedure safely. Usually, the urinary retention problem will resolve within a few weeks.

Some men with urinary symptoms can benefit from taking medicines to reduce these symptoms. Some of these medicines, called *Alpha 1 blockers*, are usually used to treat high blood pressure or hypertension, but they also relax the muscle in the urinary sphincter, which eases the flow of urine. One *Alpha 1 blocker*, a drug called *tamsulosin*, has very little effect on blood pressure but has been very effective in treating urinary symptoms and is especially valuable since a man could continue taking his regular blood pressure medicine. Some treatment centers routinely prescribe tamsulosin for a period of time before the implant to help avoid urinary retention problems.

Sexual activity: Sexual intercourse can usually be safely resumed two weeks after the implant procedure. Condoms must be used for at least two weeks during all forms of sexual activity to prevent a sexual partner's accidental exposure to a radioactive seed. The semen could be temporarily discolored—a dark brown color is most often noted—because of blood in the semen (called *hematospermia*), which does go away or resolves over time. A fair number—up to 25 percent—of men who have had implants say that for up to six months post-implant, they have pain with ejaculation. The vast majority of men who have implants are able to maintain the ability to have an erection.

Radiopharmaceutical Application

Another way in which radioactive materials are used is in a form called *radiopharmaceutical*—a liquid formulation of the radioactive substance *Strontium 89*. This substance is used to manage problems such as pain or the risk of bone fractures that occur when cancer has spread to several places in the bones. It is given via a one-time intravenous dose, but additional doses can be given every ninety days if necessary. As it moves through the bloodstream, Strontium 89 more or less fools bone cells into thinking it is calcium. When cancer cells spread into the bones (*bone metastases*), there is increased cellular activity that uses calcium. Strontium 89 moves through the bloodstream into metastatic sites and kills or at least slows down the cancer cells' growth and division. Strontium 89 can be prescribed by a radiation therapy or nuclear medicine doctor and can be given in an outpatient clinic.

When Strontium 89 is given, the man will need to use a few protective measures. He should flush the toilet twice each time he urinates as a way of diluting the radioactive substance in the sewer system for one week following administration of Strontium. During that one-week period, any clothing that gets stained with either blood or urine should be washed in a batch separate from that of other family members.

Like other uses of radiation, Strontium 89 is not without side effects. The man who receives Strontium 89 can be expected to have some decrease in his bone marrow activity resulting in reduced white blood cells and platelets. The effects on bone marrow will subside within five to six weeks, so the man will need to take extra precautions to decrease his chances of infection and injury that could cause bleeding. Some men also have a sudden increase in pain within the first forty-eight hours after the Strontium is given, but this is actually considered a good sign: it means that the Strontium is acting against the cancer cells in the bone.

One problem in the use of Strontium 89 is its expense: one dose costs over $2,000, plus another $1,000 for the costs associated with the actual administration. HMOs or insurance plans may be reluctant to authorize its use. In this case, the oncology doctor or nurse may need to expend extra effort to demonstrate the effectiveness of this treatment to the HMO or insurance-company decision maker to make sure these costs are covered.

Hormonal Therapy

Hormone therapy is mainly used to treat Stage III or IV prostate cancer when cure is not thought to be possible. When hormone therapy is compared to no treatment at all in these later stages of disease, the occurrence of problems such as bone fractures, spinal cord compression, and urinary obstruction is reduced for men who are on hormone treatment.

The use of hormones in the treatment of prostate cancer is based in the fact that prostate cancer cells are often affected by the presence or absence of hormones. Some prostate cancer cells are totally dependent on the hormone androgen (*testosterone*). When testosterone is not present, these *hormone dependent* cells die. Other cells, referred to as *hormone sensitive* cells, will not die when deprived of hormones but they will not divide, either. *Hormone independent* cells do not need or depend on hormones at all and will continue to grow and divide even in the absence of hormones. Hormone therapy is not curative by itself, but the use of hormones should be considered when the cancer is not contained within the prostate gland.

Prostate cancer cells vary in their need for or use of hormones. Testosterone, which is produced in the testes, is especially important to the growth and development of prostate cancer cells. *Luteinizing hormone-releasing hormone* (LHRH), which is released from the hypothalamus gland, stimulates the release of androgen. LHRH stimulates the pituitary gland to make *luteinizing hormone* (LH), which in turn stimulates the testes to make testosterone.

Reducing a man's androgen or testosterone level can be done in one of two ways—either by the use of medicines that block hormone production and release, or by surgically removing the testes.

Removing both testicles, a procedure called *bilateral orchiectomy* (sometimes referred to as *surgical castration*), is the oldest method of quickly reducing testosterone. As drastic as it seems, bilateral orchiectomy does have some benefits. First, the operation is relatively simple for the doctor to perform and ensures that the desired drop in hormone levels will occur quickly. The recovery period is not long, and complications are uncommon. When compared to what for some men is the nuisance and expense of buying and taking medications on a strict schedule for the remainder of their lives, orchiectomy could be viewed as the simpler route. The cons are probably obvious: for many men, the loss of both testicles can affect self-esteem. Men who have both testicles removed will also have a loss of desire for sexual activity (loss of libido), impotence, and hot flashes, and will increase their risk for osteoporosis. There is really only one person who can weigh the pros and cons that go into making this decision: the man whose lifestyle will be affected and who has and understands all the facts.

The manipulation of hormone levels with the use of hormones that counter the effects of testosterone is a less drastic but still effective way to reduce testosterone levels. The female hormone *estrogen*, in the form of *diethylstilbestrol* (DES), blocks LHRH and LH, resulting in reduced release of testosterone. One common and expected side effect of DES—breast enlargement (*gynecomastia*) and tenderness—is particularly distressing to some men, while others find it merely annoying. It can be prevented by low-dose radiation to the breasts. Because estrogen therapy also brings with it an increased risk of heart attack, stroke, and pulmonary embolism, it is prescribed less frequently today, and newer hormonal therapies avoid some of these problems.

LHRH agonists are in a relatively new class of drugs used to manipulate LHRH. At first, the LHRH agonist increases the testosterone level in what is called a *flare*; the testosterone level then drops quickly. During a flare, symptoms caused by the prostate cancer such as pain, impotence, and hot flashes can get worse, and prompt medical care is called for. The class of drugs called *antiandrogens* can be used to reduce the flare. Antiandrogens prevent the prostate cancer cells from using testosterone. In the treatment approach referred to as *total androgen ablation* (TAA), antiandrogen drugs such as flutaminde and bicalutamide are combined with the LHRH agonists leuprolide or goserelin. TAA is often used in an attempt to increase survival time or prolong the time before cancer progresses.

Most people are aware that hormones can produce side effects. Decrease in testosterone levels will cause at least some men to experience hot flashes similar to what women experience during menopause. Other side effects of hormones for men include breast tenderness, diarrhea, nausea, impotence, and decreased libido. The doctor or nurse should provide men with full descriptions of any side effects that are expected to occur when a man begins to use hormone therapy. Flutamide, generally prescribed to be taken three times a day, can cause diarrhea. But the diarrhea can be avoided if it is taken every eight hours, still three times a day, but just evenly spaced out over the twenty-four-hour day. Leuprolide and goserelin are given once a month, leuprolide by intramuscular injection and goserelin by subcutaneous injection. Positive responses to hormonal manipulation can last several years, offering men good control of cancer, sometimes throughout the rest of their natural life spans. If the disease does eventually progress, palliative use of radiation therapy or changes in hormonal manipulation might offer additional control.

Neoadjuvant hormone blockade refers to the use of hormones *before* other local therapies such as prostatectomy or external beam radiation therapy, in an attempt to slow the spread of cancer or reduce the size of the tumor, thus increasing the chance of cure.

Maximal androgen blockage (MAB) or *complete androgen blockade* refers to the combination of orchiectomy and antiandrogen therapy. A few promising case reports, where the end results seemed to increase survival time, led to the common use of this treatment strategy. Later clinical trials have not proven the strategy to be effective in increasing survival; in fact, the men studied reported decreases in their quality of life.

Instead, hormones are given to reduce tumor size, and thus relieve distressing symptoms caused by prostate cancer.

Chemotherapy

For the most part, chemotherapy as we currently know it has not been useful in the treatment of prostate cancer. The chemotherapy drugs cisplatin and etoposide have been used to treat men who have late-stage cancer or whose cancer has not been controlled with hormonal therapy, but the benefits of this treatment strategy have not been proven in clinical trials. There is ongoing research into the use of chemotherapy for prostate cancer.

Follow-Up

Following diagnosis and treatment of prostate cancer, regular checks of PSA values will help monitor the patient's response to treatment and rule out or identify early the possible reappearance or recurrence of the cancer. For those men who follow the watchful waiting (and no treatment) course, the PSA blood test and digital rectal exam should be done every six months, and another prostate biopsy should be done within one year of diagnosis. After that year, a biopsy can be done if the PSA level rises or if the man experiences problems. The National Comprehensive Cancer Network/ American Cancer Society's *Prostate Cancer Treatment Guidelines for Patients* recommends that men who were treated with prostatectomy, external beam radiation therapy, or brachytherapy should have a PSA blood test every six months for the first five years, and then yearly, plus a yearly DRE. Still, some treatment centers suggest getting a first post-treatment PSA level at two months. Even though some men might think an earlier PSA test would offer reassurance that the treatment is working, it is likely that the PSA will be elevated for a few months as a result of the physical manipulation of the prostate during the treatment.

Men with later-stage prostate cancer—men whose cancer has spread to the lymph nodes, bones, or other organs—should have the PSA and physical exam (including DRE) every three months. In addition, men who are getting

Table 4.5: Treatment Options for Recurrent Prostate Cancer

Prior Treatment	Results of Follow-Up Tests	Salvage Workup	Salvage Therapy
Radical prostatectomy	Abnormal DRE Increasing PSA level	Bone scan Pelvic CT scan Biopsy of the area where the prostate gland was	External Beam Radiation Hormone therapy Observe until symptoms appear
External beam radiation or brachytherapy	Abnormal DRE Increasing PSA level	Bone scan Prostate biopsy Pelvic CT scan	Hormone therapy Observe until symptoms appear Surgery (in some cases)
Late stage—spread beyond the prostate and nearby tissues		Bone scan	Hormone therapy

Adapted from NCCN Treatment Guidelines for Patients (1999) and NCI PDQ Treatment Statement for Prostate Cancer (1999)

antiandrogen treatment should have blood tests that check for liver problems, and men who have high PSA levels or bone pain should be checked with a bone scan.

Recurrence

Signs and symptoms of recurrence of prostate cancer include high blood PSA levels, rectal or urinary symptoms, and abnormal findings on digital rectal exam. If it is determined that the cancer has come back or *recurred*, the man will need to undergo a full evaluation, much as he did when he was first diagnosed, to determine the extent of the spread of disease. When cancer returns after treatment, doctors often refer to a second treatment attempt as *salvage therapy*. The *salvage workup* determines the extent of the cancer's spread. The treatment options available to the man with recurrence depend on his prior form of treatment, the areas where the cancer now appears (whether the recurrence is considered *local or distant*), any other medical conditions the man has that make one form of treatment more risky than others, and results of his follow-up tests. Table 4.5 lists the treatment options for recurrent prostate cancer according to stage of disease and prior treatment.

Future

Hardly a day goes by that there is not a newspaper story, a spot on a local or national television news program, or an article in a medical or nursing journal about prostate cancer. Even the U.S. Congress has gotten into the act! When it approved spending for 1999 for the National Institutes of Health (NIH), Congress asked that NIH take action regarding prostate cancer research. Specifically, Congress demands that NIH

- clearly describe its prostate cancer research activities

- evaluate the idea of a national model research, education, training, and treatment center

- increase funding to these programs

- provide Congress with a five-year plan that outlines prostate cancer research opportunities into the year 2003

The NIH increased prostate cancer research funding from $114 million a year in 1998 to $180 million in 1999. In addition to the National Cancer Institute, eight other institutes at NIH provide researchers with opportunities to explore prostate cancer–related questions. And there are so many questions.

The scope of NIH's prostate cancer research efforts reflects the full range of questions posed by prostate cancer, and almost certainly provides clues to what the approaches to prostate cancer will look like in the not-too-distant future. Research efforts are focusing on causes, prevention, screening and early detection, biology, and treatment of the various stages of prostate cancer. Effort is underway to discover the basis of the racial, ethnic, and socioeconomic aspects of prostate cancer, and the roles genetics play in this most common form of cancer. Ongoing clinical trials involve agents specifically developed for men with prostate cancer, including vaccines, a chemotherapy protocol that combines taxotere with thalidomide, other new chemotherapy drug classes, and biologic agents or monoclonal antibodies such as herceptin.

Aside from federally funded and government-led research efforts, a growing number of private corporations also focus on various questions posed by prostate cancer. A promising example is *ProctoScinct*, developed by the Cytogen Corporation, a monoclonal antibody scanning technique that its developers hope will be useful in the staging of men with both newly diagnosed prostate cancer and recurrent disease. In developmental testing, newly diagnosed men were given an IV injection of the monoclonal antibody *ProctoScinct* combined with a radioactive tracer cell called *Indium-111* that collects in tissues that have abnormal collections of cells resembling normal prostate cells. After the injection, CT scans are obtained at least twice, the first time within thirty minutes and a second time between three and five days later. The CT images highlight possible sites of cancer in lymph nodes and other organs. The *ProctoScinct* scan is believed to increase the accuracy of staging, adding to the staging information used to determine if local therapy such as prostatectomy, brachytherapy, or cryosurgery should be recommended.

In the end, there are still more questions than answers. Scientific processes such as clinical trials will help determine safe and effective ways to treat cancer. The growing number of local and national prostate cancer advocacy groups helps to define research priorities and also to convince policy-makers to allocate appropriate funding to allow researchers to make real progress in finding answers.

5

Lung Cancer

Cynthia J. Simonson, R.N., M.S., C.S., A.O.C.N.

The most important thing to know about lung cancer is that being diagnosed with it is not an automatic death sentence. Many forms of early-stage lung cancer can be cured, and many forms of later-stage lung cancer can be controlled. A second important piece of information is that, in almost all situations, having lung cancer is not an emergency. You have the time to get the expert opinions and information you need to make good decisions about treatment, and to find nurses and doctors who are experts in treating lung cancer and with whom you can have a trusting relationship.

Causes of Lung Cancer

To understand how lung cancer can be prevented, we must first discuss what causes it: namely, anything that damages lung cells and makes them grow out of control.

Many things can trigger damage to the lungs. Most are inhaled and cause chronic irritation of the lung tissue, and the most common irritants come from smoking tobacco. Currently, about 172,000 cases of lung cancer are diagnosed in the U.S. each year. Of the new cases, about 52 percent are smokers and about 40 percent are former smokers. Only the remaining 8 percent are nonsmokers. This means that over 90 percent of lung cancer cases could be avoided if we could stop people from ever smoking. Tobacco smoke has all the chemicals needed to damage the genes in lung cells and trigger uncontrolled growth.

Clearly, tobacco smoke is not the only cause of lung cancer. The genes in a cell are responsible for determining what kind of cell it is, how it works, how it grows, and for carrying information from old cells to new cells. Some families are at increased risk of lung cancer because they pass damaged genes from parent to child. If you have a family history of lung cancer, you could be at increased risk—particularly if you smoke.

Exposure to ionizing radiation, asbestos, radon, arsenic, coal, nickel and nickel compounds, cadmium, chromium and chromium compounds, polycyclic aromatic hydrocarbons, and vinyl chloride can also cause chronic irritation to lung tissue and damage genes. Most exposures to these chemicals occur in work settings. The Occupational Safety and Health Administration (OSHA) requires employers to notify employees of the dangerous chemicals in their workplace. If you work with dangerous chemicals, it is important to follow safety procedures to reduce the amount of these substances that are inhaled. Again, this is especially true for smokers. Smoking marijuana and crack cocaine can also increase the risk of developing lung cancer.

Lung Cancer Prevention

If you currently smoke, it is very important that you stop. Smoking cessation will improve your health in general and will help you recover from any surgery or other treatment that you may need. Your risk of developing lung cancer will decrease for every year you don't smoke. Your risk will not return to that of a person who has never smoked, but in ten years the risk will be 20 to 50 percent of a current smoker. There are many successful strategies you can use to quit smoking. Nicotine is very addictive and most people need help and support to quit. Talk to your nurse or doctor about what might work best for you.

There are other strategies to prevent lung cancer. Research continues about the role of carotene, and vitamins A and C, in reducing the development of lung cancer, especially in smokers. Some studies have shown promise, some have not. Another antioxidant, selenium, has also shown promise in reducing the risk of lung cancer in smokers. Still, the best prevention by far is smoking cessation. Although it is very important for adults to quit smoking, the greatest efforts should be made in preventing adolescents from ever starting to smoke.

Early Detection

Lung cancer is very difficult to find and diagnose at an early stage. Most early lung cancers are found by accident when someone is having an X-ray for another reason. The National Cancer Institute (NCI) has studied whether doing routine chest X-rays and looking for cancer cells in sputum help identify lung cancers earlier. Unfortunately, those tests have not proven helpful enough to be worth doing routinely on everyone. It may still be a good idea for people who smoke or have smoked to talk with their nurses and doctors about routine examinations.

Studies are being done to find more effective ways to find lung cancer early. A new way to use a low-dose CT scan as a screening tool, especially in high-risk groups such as smokers, is being studied and may prove to be very helpful. New ways to examine sputum from the lungs to look for damage to genes, and to look for antibodies to lung cancer, may also prove useful. Until then, it is important to keep up with your routine health examinations, to know the warning signs of lung cancer, and to see your nurse or doctor if you have any of the following symptoms:

- chronic cough or a change in a chronic cough

- chest pains around or under the ribs

- unexplained shoulder pain

- pneumonia or bronchitis that keeps coming back even with antibiotics

- shortness of breath or wheezing

- swelling of the neck or face

- coughing up blood

- trouble with or painful swallowing

- fatigue

- weight loss

If you or a member of your family have any of these symptoms, please get examined by your health care professional.

Types of Lung Cancer

Lung cancers are grouped into two main types, depending on the kind of lung tissue that has begun to grow abnormally. The two types are termed *small-cell lung cancer* (SCLC), sometimes called "oat-cell lung cancer" because the cells seen under the microscope resemble kernels of oats, and *non-small-cell lung cancer* (NSCLC). It is a common misconception that other types of cancers growing in the lungs—such as colon or prostate—are also lung cancer. They are not. If you have colon cancer and it begins to grow in the lungs, it is still colon cancer. It would be treated as colon cancer and you would want to read about colon cancer to get information about good treatments.

SCLC, which makes up only about 20 percent of diagnosed lung cancers, is more aggressive than NSCLC. It grows rapidly and has almost always spread—or metastasized—by the time it is diagnosed. It often grows in the surrounding lung tissue and lymph nodes and metastasizes to bones, bone marrow, adrenal glands, and brain. If SCLC is discovered at a very early stage, it is possible to cure it with aggressive treatment. If it is diagnosed at a later stage, most people die within two years of diagnosis and treatment. If SCLC goes untreated, the typical survival time is eight to sixteen weeks.

NSCLC is more common than SCLC, making up about 80 percent of all diagnosed lung cancers. It is actually four different kinds of lung cancers that grow and respond to treatment in about the same way. These four types of NSCLC are termed *squamous cell, adenocarcinoma, large cell*, and *mixed cell*. Two other related cancers that are also included in the NSCLC group are *carcinoid* and *mesothelioma*. In general, NSCLC grows more slowly than SCLC, tending to grow first in the area where it started (the primary site), then invading the surrounding lung tissue and ribs. It eventually spreads to other areas of the body, mainly bones, brain, and liver.

Diagnosis and Workup

Most lung cancers grow slowly, and have been developing for ten or twenty years before they can be detected by current diagnostic tests. The damage that causes lung cells to grow abnormally also prevents them from performing their normal functions. That is why it is so harmful to have lung cancer cells crowding out useful cells. Lung cancer cells only know how to grow and spread to other parts of the body. This area of spread is called a *metastasis* or *metastatic disease*. Cancer cells spread to other parts of the body through the blood stream and the lymph glands, the glands that swell when you have an infection. Lymph glands are scattered throughout the body and are an important part of the immune system, your body's infection-fighting system. Because of the rich supply of blood vessels and lymph glands in the lungs, lung cancer cells spread earlier and more easily than some other cancers.

It is not uncommon for the symptoms from metastatic disease to be what leads a person to seek health care in the first place, and to the diagnosis of lung cancer. The earlier lung cancer is found, particularly before metastatic disease develops, the more likely it is to be cured. That is why it is so important for us to find new and better tests to detect very early lung cancers, and why symptoms of lung cancer should not be ignored.

Diagnosis

Generally, a symptom such as shortness of breath, a persistent cough, or blood in the sputum gets the person to go to a doctor who, after a health history and physical examination, requests a chest X-ray, CT, MRI, or PET scan. Sputum cytology—examination of cells that are shed from the bronchi and lung and carried up the throat in the sputum—is a way to search for signs of cancer cells. Sputum can be collected by coughing up fluid from the lungs. Sputum can also be collected through a *bronchoscope*, a tube that is inserted through the throat into the lungs to obtain a sputum sample. If cancer cells are identified, additional tests are needed to determine the size and location of the cancer. Sputum cytology may not always detect cancer cells, making more testing necessary in order to determine the cause of suspicious symptoms. In this situation, a tissue sample of the mass noted in imaging tests will be needed. One way to obtain this sample is the *biopsy*.

A *biopsy*, the removal and examination of a tissue sample from the tumor, must be done to determine the cell type of the lung cancer. Depending on the size and location of the tumor, this biopsy can be done by a fine needle aspirate (FNA) under CT guidance. The doctor pinpoints the tumor precisely with a CT scan, then inserts a very thin needle into the tumor to remove cells. If a swollen lymph node in the neck or underarm can be felt, a FNA or other type of biopsy of that node may be done. Depending on what type of lung cancer you have, you may also need a bone marrow biopsy. Marrow is the tissue inside bones where blood cells are formed and stored.

Invasive procedures such as *bronchoscopy* or *mediastinoscopy* may be needed to help look directly at the tissue in the lungs or in the *mediastinum*, the part of your chest where your heart and lungs are located. Bronchoscopy involves putting a lighted tube through your throat into your lungs. It allows a doctor to look for lung cancers and to take a biopsy of any abnormal area that is found. Mediastinoscopy involves making a small incision in the upper part of the chest and inserting a lighted tube to look for lung cancers, swollen lymph nodes, or other abnormalities. It also allows a doctor to biopsy any abnormal area. Occasionally, if the only area of abnormality is deep within the lung, a surgery called a *thoracotomy* is done and an *open lung biopsy* may be needed to establish an accurate diagnosis.

A pathologist—a doctor who specializes in looking at cells under a microscope and determining what kind of disease you have—will look at any biopsy that is taken and determine what kind of lung cancer is present. When all of this information is collected, the stage of your lung cancer can be accurately determined. Staging, along with one's general health, plays an important role in determining survival time after diagnosis and the treatment that can be offered.

Staging

Another important part of the diagnostic workup is staging. It is important to know how large the lung cancer tumor is, its aggressiveness, and if it has spread to other parts of the body. These things help determine the extent, or *stage,* of the lung cancer. The stage helps determine what kind of treatment would offer the most benefit. Staging is determined by doing a biopsy, scanning X-rays, and sometimes surgery. The staging workup usually includes CT scans or MRIs of the chest, liver and abdomen, and brain. Some doctors may use PET scans or SPECT scans as well. If bone pain is present, additional scans or X-rays of the skeleton or particular bones will also be used.

Small-cell lung cancer is staged most often using a system with only two major designations: *limited stage* and *extensive stage* disease. *Limited stage* means that the cancer is found only in one lung, the mediastinum, and lymph nodes in the area close to the affected lung. If radiation therapy were used, all sites of disease could be included in one single treatment field. Limited stage corresponds with stages I–IIIB of the TNM staging system discussed later. *Extensive stage* includes any SCLC that has spread beyond the local area.

Generally, non-small-cell lung cancer is staged using the TNM classification system where T refers to the size of the tumor, N to the lymph nodes involved, and M to the distant metastasis. Table 5.1 describes the different categories as designed by the American Joint Committee on Cancer (AJCC). Your nurse or doctor may also use the more general staging system, described in Table 5.2, to describe NSCLC. Table 5.3 compares the two staging systems.

The *prognosis*—the length of time that a person is likely to survive after diagnosis—is better when the diagnosis occurs during an early stage of lung cancer. For NSCLC found at an early stage, there is a 50 to 60 percent

Table 5.1: AJCC TNM Staging System for NSCLC

T =	**Primary Tumor Characteristics**
TX	Cancer cells found in sputum or fluid, no tumor on X-ray or bronchoscopy
T0	No sign of primary tumor can be found
Tis	Carcinoma in situ (tumor growing in cells, but has not left or grown outside of the cells)
T1	Tumor smaller than 3 cm in diameter, no spreading
T2	Tumor larger than 3 cm, or tumor that is smaller but is spreading to other lung tissue
T3	Tumor of any size that is spreading into nearby tissues such as chest wall, blood vessels
T4	Tumor of any size that has spread into nearby organs
N =	**Involvement of Regional Lymph Nodes**
N0	There is no evidence of regional lymph node involvement
N1	Spread to lymph nodes around bronchi (small branches of the tubes that bring air into lungs)
N2	Spread to lymph nodes around bronchi and into mediastinum
N3	Spread to lymph nodes on opposite side of chest from tumor and just below the collar bone
M =	**Distant Metastasis**
M0	No spread to distant organs or site
M1	Spread to distant organs or site

Table 5.2: Stage 0–4 Staging System for NSCLC

Stage	Description
Occult	Cancer cells found in sputum or other lung fluid but no primary tumor can be found
Stage 0	Cancer in a local area only, has not grown through top layer of lung, incapable of spreading
Stage I	Cancer has not spread beyond its primary location. Divided into IA and IB, both of which are surgically resectable
Stage II	Cancer has spread to nearby lymph nodes in the lung. Also divided into IIA and IIB, both of which are surgically resectable
Stage III	Cancer has spread to surrounding structures and lymph nodes. Divided into IIIA and IIIB, not usually surgically resectable
Stage IV	Cancer has spread to other sites of the body, not surgically resectable

chance of being alive five years after diagnosis and treatment. If NSCLC is not treated, or if it is diagnosed at a later stage, most people do not live much longer than two years after diagnosis.

Treatment

Because both NSCLC and SCLC are often treated with a combination of surgery, chemotherapy, and radiation therapy, it is important to be seen by

Table 5.3: Comparison of Staging for Non-Small-Cell Lung Cancer

Stage	T = tumor	N = node	M = metastasis
Occult Cancer	Tx	N0	M0
Stage 0	Tis	N0	M0
Stage IA	T1	N0	M0
Stage IB	T2	N0	M0
Stage IIA	T1	N1	M0
Stage IIB	T2	N1	M0
	T3	N0	M0
Stage IIIA	T1	N2	M0
	T2	N2	M0
	T3	N1	M0
	T3	N2	M0
Stage IIIB	Any T	N3	M0
	T4	Any N	M0
Stage IV	Any T	Any N	M1

a doctor from each of these specialties before deciding on a treatment plan. A good way to accomplish this is to go through a consultative process in a multispecialty clinic. Multispecialty clinics, usually located within teaching hospital systems, are staffed by physicians and nurses with expertise in cancer and, in some clinics, in a specific type of cancer. In the clinic setting, each patient's case is reviewed by this team of specialists who will work *with* you to plan your treatment. Under ideal conditions, all needed opinions can be provided in one clinic visit. Because the doctors and nurses discuss your case together in a coordinated approach, you often end up with a better, more comprehensive, treatment plan; you may also have the best chance of being offered treatment on a clinical trial at a multispecialty clinic (see Chapter 15 for more information about clinical trials). Be sure to ask the doctors if a clinical trial is available and right for you. Even if you do not want to be treated at a multispecialty clinic, you may want to consider going to such a clinic for an opinion about what your treatment should be.

If a multispecialty cancer center or clinic is not available in your geographic area, your primary care nurse or doctor can arrange for consultations with a surgical oncologist, thoracic surgeon, medical oncologist, and radiation oncologist. It can sometimes be hard to put these medical opinions together and decide what to do; your primary doctor can help evaluate the treatment options offered by the specialists.

It is important to be evaluated by doctors who are experts in treating lung cancer. It is also important to find out if a nurse with special education and experience in oncology will be involved in providing and managing the treatment protocol. Nursing support is a critical part of cancer care. An oncology nurse understands cancer treatments and their side effects, and can offer the patient information and emotional support. Ask what oncology education and ongoing educational support the nurses at each clinic have received. A good sign of a knowledgeable oncology nurse is the designation of Oncology Certified Nurse or Advanced Oncology Certified Nurse —credentials granted by the Oncology Nursing Certification Corporation. A nurse who has this credential has at least two to three years of experience, has passed the certification examination, and has kept up on current knowledge in order to be recertified every four years.

Another important consideration about treatment is smoking. Every person with cancer is advised to do his best to quit smoking before treatment starts. Those who do not smoke will recover more easily from surgery, cough less, hurt less, and will generally feel better. Nicotine can speed up metabolism—the rate that the body burns calories—and smoking leads to the loss of the energy and nutrients that are crucial for optimal healing.

Treatment for SCLC

SCLC and NSCLC are treated differently. The treatment for SCLC is usually a combination of chemotherapy (drugs used to treat cancer) and radiation therapy (strong X-ray beams used to treat cancer); these treatments are discussed in detail in Chapters 13 and 14. Because most people with SCLC are diagnosed with extensive-stage disease, surgery is usually not an option. Only rarely is a person diagnosed with a very small area of SCLC that can be surgically removed; if performed, surgery would be followed by chemotherapy for four to six months.

Radiation therapy to the brain—*prophylactic cranial radiation*—may also be offered to try to prevent metastasis to the brain. This kind of radiation is controversial; it can cause long-term side effects, but current research shows that it can lengthen life for some lung cancer patients. Discuss the idea of prophylactic cranial irradiation fully with your nurse and doctor before it is begun.

Most people with *limited-stage* SCLC start their treatment with four to six months of chemotherapy. Several drugs can be used in the treatment of

SCLC, and different protocols use different combinations of drugs, different doses, and different schedules. Even in this one form of lung cancer, there is still no agreement among the experts about which protocol is the best or most effective. Some of these drugs can be given by mouth (oral chemotherapy), but most often they are given directly into the vein (intravenous or IV chemotherapy). Different drugs work in different ways to damage cancer cells; usually, the best results are obtained by combining drugs, thus increasing the number of cancer cells killed with each treatment. Since the combined drugs often have different side effects, you get increased effectiveness without increasing the severity of side effects. Chemotherapy goes everywhere your blood goes and affects cancer cells wherever they are growing.

Radiation therapy to the chest is combined with chemotherapy in the treatment of limited-stage SCLC. It can be given along with, alternating with, or after the chemotherapy. It works to prevent cancer cells from growing again in the lungs and the lymph nodes in the chest. It works only on the tissues in the radiation field. Prophylactic cranial radiation may also be offered.

Most people with *extensive-stage* SCLC also begin treatment with combination chemotherapy. Radiation therapy may be given to help reduce the size of lung cancer tumors, or to treat painful areas of metastases in the bones. If brain metastases are already present, radiation might be used to treat the brain before chemotherapy is given. If combination chemotherapy is successful at shrinking extensive-stage SCLC, prophylactic radiation to the chest and brain may be offered, as it would be in limited-stage disease.

Occasionally, people with very advanced disease may decide not to receive aggressive treatment with chemotherapy and radiation therapy. Instead, these therapies might be offered in lower doses to manage uncomfortable symptoms such as pain, cough, or an area of bony metastasis that is at risk for fracture. Both chemotherapy and radiation can be given in a way that provides relief without causing serious side effects.

Treatment for NSCLC

Treatment for NSCLC includes combinations of chemotherapy and radiation therapy, but surgery is also important here. It is best to be seen by a surgeon who specializes in treating lung cancer, and knows the best ways to remove the tumor with the least chance of it coming back. If surgery is right for the kind of lung cancer that has been diagnosed, it is usually performed before the chemotherapy or radiation therapy, although chemotherapy or radiation are occasionally used to help shrink a lung cancer tumor down to a size that could be successfully removed. Most often, combination chemotherapy and radiation therapy is used after surgery for about six to eight months. If surgery is not possible because of the size and location of the tumor, combined chemotherapy and radiation therapy is used. Again, the treatment generally lasts about six to eight months.

Treatment-Related Side Effects

There are both short- and long-term side effects to lung cancer treatments. The long-term side effects are discussed later in this chapter under "Survivorship Issues." Short-term side effects are reviewed here.

Postoperative pain and fatigue are the most common short-term side effects of surgery. The short-term side effects of chemotherapy depend on which drugs are used; they include hair loss, fatigue, risk of infection from lowered blood counts, some numbness and tingling in hands and feet, changes in the way food tastes, and changes in appetite. Nausea and occasionally vomiting are also common with chemotherapy, but drugs that prevent or minimize these symptoms are readily available.

Short-term side effects of radiation therapy include fatigue, change in appetite, skin irritation, and risk of infection from lowered blood counts, especially if chemotherapy is used during the same time frame. Hair loss from cranial radiation therapy will be permanent.

Treatment for lung cancer is evolving all the time. We are learning more and more about how to treat it successfully, and developing new and better treatments. The most important part of treatment is finding nurses and doctors who are experts in treating lung cancer and who you like and feel you can trust.

Symptom Management

Cough, shortness of breath, pain, and swelling of the face are a few symptoms that, while they occur in other forms of cancer, are most common among people with lung cancer. Some symptoms indicate a serious problem and warrant the immediate attention of the physician or nurse. Knowing what causes the symptom can de-mystify the problem and provide comfort and control.

Cough can be caused by a tumor that irritates the bronchi or lungs and/or increased secretion of mucus. The collection of mucus provides a place for bacteria to grow, eventually resulting in the development of pneumonia. Persistent cough can be painful, prevents adequate rest, and if there is metastatic spread into the ribs, can actually cause rib fractures. There are various interventions that should be used to promote comfort and prevent pneumonia. Smoking cigarettes and cigars is, of course, discouraged since the smoke contains irritants. Deep breathing and coughing exercises can be used to clear out secretions. Breathing humidified and warmed air can sooth irritated tissues in the airway. Inhaled medications such as bronchodilators may be helpful for people who have chronic lung disease, such as emphysema, that narrows lung passages. Narcotic medications such as codeine suppress cough and might be useful if the person has a dry, non-productive cough. Suctioning is recommended *only* if the person's cough is ineffective in removing secretions.

Hemoptysis, blood in the sputum or coughing up blood, occurs when a tumor invades blood vessels in the air passages and lungs. Hemoptysis can occur even when cough is not present, but can also be aggravated by a persistent cough. The doctor must be made aware of the presence of hemoptysis and, if hemoptysis has been present before, any increase in the amount of blood seen in the sputum. Normally, slight hemoptysis might be managed with cough suppressants, but serious bleeding can be an emergency situation that requires special positioning to avoid blood spillage into the good lung, and, in some cases, emergency surgery may be necessary to stop the bleeding.

Shortness of breath, or *dyspnea,* is a common problem for people with lung cancer for obvious reasons—a portion of lung tissue is unable to perform normal breathing function. Dyspnea can also be the result of radiation- or chemotherapy-induced damage to lung tissue or fluid collection around the lungs. Many people describe this as a sensation of being smothered and find it truly terrifying. Again, the physician and nurse must be made aware of any increase in dyspnea and initiate appropriate assessments so the most effective intervention can be recommended. There are many self-care measures that can be used to cope with this distressing symptom. The oncology nurse or physical or respiratory therapist can help patients and caregivers learn to use relaxation and controlled breathing techniques, positioning for optimal lung expansion, and ways to conserve energy. Oxygen therapy also offers another therapeutic option.

Pain is very common, and expected, among most people with lung cancer. It is more likely to occur as the cancer becomes more advanced. Chest pain occurs in about half of all people with lung cancer, and pain occurs as lung cancer metastasizes to bones. Regardless of how common it is, every attempt must be made to get pain under control. Chapter 17 offers more in-depth information about the management of cancer pain.

Swelling of the neck or face is a sign that blood flow through the major blood vessel going into the heart, the *superior vena cava*, is obstructed. The obstruction results in congestion above the obstruction and increased pressure in the blood vessels in the head, neck, arms, and chest. This problem occurs often enough that it is recognized as a "syndrome"—the superior vena cava syndrome (SVCS). Though SVCS does occur in noncancerous conditions, most of the time the cause is cancer, and the most common kind of cancer that causes SVCS is lung cancer. It occurs in up to 10 percent of all people with lung cancer but in up to 20 percent of persons with SCLC. SVCS can be present at the time of the lung cancer diagnosis, but might also occur later in the course of the disease. Another cause of SVCS can be the formation of an obstructing blood clot around the special vascular access catheters that are used by many people with cancer. Symptoms of SVCS include shortness of breath, facial and upper body swelling, and distention of blood vessels in the neck and chest. Other, generally later, symptoms include cough, hoarseness, changes in vision, and headache. Any of these symptoms must be reported to the doctor immediately. The treatment of SVCS is determined by the cause of the obstruction, how severe the symptoms are, the patient's prognosis, goals of treatment, and, of course, the patient's preferences. The medical management of SVCS can involve chemotherapy, radiation therapy, the placement of a stent to relieve obstruction, and/or surgery. Self-care strategies that help to promote safety and comfort include frequent assessment for existing and developing symptoms. Dyspnea can be relieved by positioning, such as raising the head of the bed or placement of pillows, and oxygen therapy. Steroids, diuretics, and a low-salt diet are sometimes prescribed to manage swelling. If arms are swollen, they should not be used to obtain blood samples or to take blood pressure. Rings should be removed. The increase in venous pressure that occurs when a person holds his breath to "push" during bowel movements can be minimized by avoiding constipation, and the use of stool softeners can be helpful. SVCS can be successfully treated, but it can also develop again. The patient and his family need to continue watching for its signs and symptoms.

Follow-Up

Treatment follow-up visits with the doctor or other members of the cancer care team will be scheduled, initially, about every three months. The oncology nurse practitioner or doctor will perform a physical exam to assess recovery from treatment and to check for signs of recurrence, with particular attention paid to the lungs, lymph nodes, liver, and brain. It is important to discuss general status: how you feel, including any new symptoms of pain, fatigue, or loss of appetite. Chest scans and labwork may be done about every six months. Generally, at two years after treatment, follow-up visits are scheduled about every six months. After five years, expect annual follow-up exams.

Survivorship Issues

People can and do survive lung cancer and its treatment. At times, it takes a lot of patience, courage, support, faith, and persistence to get through the treatment and cope with the side effects. When treatment is first finished, the focus is often on regaining strength and energy, recovering from side effects, and getting on with life. At first, each follow-up visit with the nurse practitioner or physician is an anxious time, because fear of recurrence is high. As more time passes and the fear subsides, life really can resume a more normal pattern.

Late-Term Side Effects

There are some permanent side effects caused by the treatments used for lung cancer, and some side effects may not show up for years. These are called *late-term side effects*. These side effects come from permanent damage done to normal cells and tissue by the treatment.

Decreased Lung Function If surgery has been required and a significant amount of lung has been removed, shortness of breath, especially upon exertion, can be a problem. Anything that compromises the remaining lung tissue such as infection, asthma, or emphysema can be dangerous and make breathing more difficult, since there is less healthy lung tissue in reserve. Radiation treatment can also reduce the reserve of healthy lung tissue, make breathing difficult, and make other lung problems more serious. Treated lung tissue becomes stiff or less elastic, a condition called *radiation fibrosis*. These problems are all made worse by smoking.

Pain A possible problem related to surgery, especially if ribs have been cut in a thoracotomy, is chronic nerve pain along the incision line. This kind of pain, called *neuropathic pain* or nerve damage pain, can require special pain medicines for effective management.

Hair Loss If hair loss occurs during or just after chemotherapy treatments, it will grow back when the treatment is finished. If radiation has been used to treat or prevent brain metastases, the hair loss is more likely to be permanent.

Changes in Mental Status Radiation to the brain can cause short-term memory loss and slower thinking. This gradually worsens as time goes on. There are many strategies to help cope with changes in mental status. Talk with your nurse or doctor about how to learn about these problems and coping strategies. Personality changes, confusion, and dementia are also possible late-term side effects from radiation to the brain.

Secondary Cancers One of the late-term side effects that can occur after radiation or chemotherapy is the development of a secondary cancer. The risk is greater if chemotherapy and radiation were used together. Leukemia is the most common secondary cancer, usually occurring about six or seven years after treatment. It would be treated just like a primary leukemia, but often does not respond well to treatment. People who have been treated for lung cancer and continue to smoke are at risk for developing a second lung cancer. Again, it is important to stop smoking and to avoid being around other smokers.

The nurse or doctor should be prepared to discuss potential late-term side effects a person might expect, how he will be monitored for these problems, and available and appropriate management strategies.

Recurrence

The news that lung cancer has come back or *recurred* is frightening. It is generally impossible to cure lung cancer when it recurs; however, treatment can slow down the growth of the cancer and control any uncomfortable symptoms. Some of the same chemotherapy drugs used to treat the initial lung cancer might be used again, or a different or new lung cancer drug may be used. Radiation therapy can be used alone or with the chemotherapy. Surgery is almost never used for a recurrence unless the area is very small and no lymph nodes or other tissues are involved, in which case it would be appropriate to remove the tumor. A clinical trial for people with recurrent lung cancer might be available.

Although lung cancer that has recurred cannot usually be cured, slowing it down provides the opportunity to make plans for the time that is left. Chapter 19 provides a useful overview of palliative care and other end-of-life issues.

Future Directions

We are in a time when new and hopeful developments are occurring quickly, and new treatments are being developed to improve the treatment of lung cancer. The development of technologies that have helped us look more closely at the genetics of lung cancer cells and understand more about how they grow and spread are being used to create drugs that more precisely attack cancer cells, killing them without doing as much damage to normal cells.

Some of the new groups of drugs under development include *antiangiogenesis drugs, tyrosine kinase inhibitors*, and *antibody-mediated drugs*. The promising antiangiogenesis drugs block a cancer cell's ability to grow its own blood vessels. If a small lung cancer tumor cannot grow its own blood vessels, it cannot continue to grow or spread. The tyrosine kinase inhibitors block one of the ways that cells grow. Most normal cells do not respond to this kind of blocking, so the treatment mainly targets cancer cells to keep them from growing out of control. These drugs are just beginning to be tested on people. Because scientists are beginning to understand more and more about genetic engineering, they are able to create antibody-mediated drugs that are taken directly inside cancer cells and then released to damage them. Normal cells are not affected by these antibody-mediated drugs, and are therefore spared any damaging effects. Many of these new technologies that help stop the growth of cancer cells without damaging normal cells will make treatments for lung cancer more effective and easier to tolerate.

6

◆ ◆ ◆

Colorectal Cancer

Jody Pelusi, R.N., F.N.P., A.O.C.N., Ph.D.

You hear a lot about breast and prostate cancer from the media, but only recently have there been concerted efforts to get the word out about colorectal cancers, possibly because they arise in an area of the body that is rarely discussed. The screening tests for these cancers are not heavily covered in the media, either. This is a grave mistake, as colorectal cancers are a major health problem in developed countries. They are the third most commonly diagnosed cancers and, in the United States, the third leading cause of cancer-related deaths for both men and women.

Screening for colorectal cancer is highly effective, in fact vital. Routine screening tests can actually reduce the number of cancers that develop, as precancerous lesions can be removed before they turn into cancer. If a cancer has already developed, early detection can reduce the treatment required and improve the overall outcome of this disease. Colorectal cancers are very curable if found and treated in early stages.

The good news is that after 1985 there was a decrease in the overall incidence of colorectal cancers, as more people began to undergo routine colorectal cancer screenings. In addition, more people are becoming long-term survivors of colorectal cancers, thanks to new technology and treatment options.

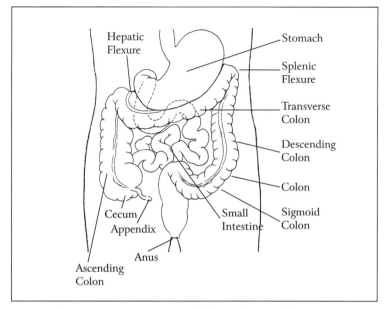

Figure 6.1: Anatomy of the Colon and Rectum

Adapted from NIH Publication No. 99-1552: What You Need To Know about Cancer
of the Colon and Rectum

Anatomy and Physiology

The colon and rectum are part of the digestive tract system. Although cancers that arise in either of these areas are reported together as *colorectal* cancers, colon cancer and rectal cancer are distinct diseases. Each has different presenting signs and symptoms and requires different types of treatment. Colon cancer is the more common of the two, accounting for about three-quarters of the cancers in the colorectal category.

The entire digestive tract consists of the mouth, esophagus, stomach, liver, gall bladder, pancreas, small intestine, and large intestine. The large intestine—also referred to as the large bowel—is a long, muscular tube comprising the colon, rectum, and anus. The function of the large bowel is to absorb water and vitamins from digested food and fluids; the remaining material is compacted into waste we call feces or stool, which is eliminated from the body.

The colon—the upper five to six feet of the large bowel—is divided into the four sections shown in Figure 6.1:

- The *ascending* colon is on the right side and goes up.

- The *transverse* colon goes across the abdomen.

- The *descending* colon is on the left side and goes down.

- The *sigmoid* colon is shaped like an "S."

The sigmoid colon connects to the rectum. The rectum is only six to eight inches in length and is connected to the anus. Over half of colorectal cancers arise in the rectal and sigmoid areas—sometimes called the *rectosigmoid*—of the large bowel.

The large bowel itself is made up of several layers of tissue, the innermost layer being the *mucosa* or lining of the bowel, then the *submucosa*, followed by the *muscularis* (see Figure 6.2).

Abdominal and pelvic lymph nodes lie outside the bowel itself. Understanding the anatomy of the large bowel will help a man understand treatment options. Colorectal cancer treatments are selected on the basis of how deep the cancer penetrates the different layers of the bowel wall and if it has spread to any other areas outside the bowel itself.

Risk Factors and Protective Factors

All people are at risk for colorectal cancer. Three-fourths of all individuals diagnosed with colorectal cancer have no known risk factors, which makes routine screening of everyone over the age of fifty all the more vital.

The following risk factors may increase a person's chances of developing colorectal cancer:

Advancing Age

Age is the most common risk factor for colorectal cancer. As one's age increasers, so does the risk for developing cancer. Most colorectal cancers develop in people over the age of sixty-five.

A History of Adenomatous Polyps

Ninety to ninety-five percent of colorectal cancers arise from the mucosa (the innermost layer of the bowel wall) and are classified as *adenocarcinoma*. This type of colorectal cancer can arise from a type of growth called a polyp. A polyp is a benign tumor that grows inward from the wall of the colon or rectum (see Figure 6.3).

Over time, certain types of polyps—*adenomatous polyps*—can develop into

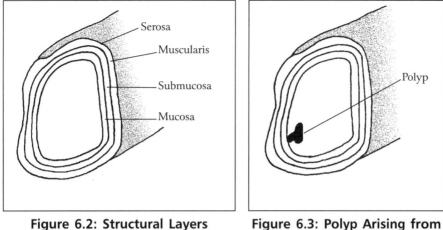

Figure 6.2: Structural Layers of the Colon

Figure 6.3: Polyp Arising from the Bowel Mucosa

cancer. The larger these polyps grow, the more likely they are to turn into cancer. Removing them while they are small will greatly reduce the chances of developing colorectal cancer. Thus, having the colon and rectum examined regularly can help determine what, if any, types of polyps exist and which ones should be removed.

Adenomatous polyps, which are premalignant, account for about half to two-thirds of all colorectal polyps. They are found in about 25 percent of the population by the age of fifty. Men have a 60 percent chance of having an adenomatous polyp by the time they reach eighty years of age. The likelihood that an adenomatous polyp will progress to cancer or that the person will develop other adenomatous polyps or cancer somewhere else in the colon and rectum can be estimated from the characteristics of the first-discovered, or *index,* polyp. During one's first colorectal examination, the size of the index adenomatous polyp seems to be directly related to the individual's future potential of developing malignant colorectal growths. Thus, the larger the size of the index adenomatous polyp, the more likely it will be that a cancer will develop. There are other nonmalignant growths— *hyperplastic polyps* and *mucosal tags*—that can develop in the colorectal area, but they are not believed to affect one's overall health (see Table 6.1).

A History of Adenomatous Polyposis Coli

A few young people inherit the potential to develop hundreds of adenomatous polyps throughout their entire colon very early in their lives. This condition is called *adenomatous polyposis coli* (APC). Treatment for APC must

Table 6.1: Nonmalignant Growths That Occur in the Colon

Non-malignant Growth	Incidence	Significance
Hyperplastic Polyps	10 to 30 percent of all polyps	• Generally small (-0.5 cm in diameter) • Tend to be predominantly in the distal bowel • Are of no clinical importance
Mucosal Tags	10 to 30 percent of colorectal polyps	• Small • A variety of other histologic types, such as lipomas and hamartomas, are uncommon • None are believed to be of clinical importance

be done at an early age (teenage or young adult), as colorectal cancer is very likely to occur. Only about 10 to 15 percent of people who eventually develop colorectal cancer have APC. Currently, new medications are being designed and used to reduce the number of polyps and ultimately delay or prevent the occurrence of cancer in people with APC.

A History of Inflammatory Bowel Disease

Individuals who have a history of inflammatory bowel disease (a disease that causes inflammation and irritation to the lining of the colon), such as *ulcerative colitis* and *Crohn's disease,* are at a higher risk for developing cancer. The risk for these individuals increases if they have had the disease for longer than thirty years. The irritation and chronic inflammation of the bowel lining leads to the development of dysplasia, where normal cells develop abnormal characteristics over time. These dysplastic or abnormal areas arise on the surface of the bowel lining; they can be seen on screening examinations and treated before they cause physical symptoms.

Family History of Colorectal Cancer

A family history of colorectal cancer in a first-degree relative (mother, father, sister, brother, or child) is also a risk factor, if that individual was diagnosed at an early age (younger than fifty). Some families may have only one member with a history of colorectal cancer diagnosed after the age of fifty; this is called *sporadic occurrence* and does not increase cancer risk for other family members. Other families may have several family members with colorectal cancers, a condition called *hereditary nonpolyposis colorectal cancer*, or HNPCC. In HNPCC, colon tumors usually occur in the right side, in the ascending colon; some health care professionals classify this as *HNPCC-A*. If other types of cancers in addition to colorectal cancer are seen in multiple family members—such as breast, ovarian, uterus, and kidney cancer—the condition is then referred to as *HNPCC-B*.

A Personal History of Colorectal Cancer

If an individual has had the diagnosis of colorectal cancer, he or she may be at risk for developing another colon cancer. Thus, routine screening remains necessary even after successful treatment for colorectal cancer. Just because a person has had one type of cancer doesn't mean another, totally unrelated type of cancer won't occur.

Diet and Other Considerations

A possible but unproven risk factor includes diets that are high in fat and cholesterol. Although the direct mechanism is not understood, a connection seems to exist between diet, environmental exposure, and the development of colorectal cancer: When people from countries with a low incidence of colorectal cancer move to the United States, their risk for colorectal cancer eventually (within ten years) becomes identical to that of people who have lived in the U.S. all their lives.

It is important to remember that most colorectal cancers are sporadic in nature and occur in people over the age of fifty. About 75 percent of all colorectal cancers occur in people who have *no* known risk factors. For this reason, general screening and detection activities are vital in fighting these diseases.

Potential Protective Factors

Although scientific studies have yet to determine specific ways to prevent or decrease the risk of colorectal cancer, several recent studies show that there may be some benefit to taking an aspirin or nonsteroidal anti-inflammatory (NSAID) drug daily. More studies are underway to determine if this will be truly effective. Before taking any medication, discuss this issue with a health care professional.

Diet also seems to be associated with colorectal cancer; however, no specific diet has been found to alter the course of the disease. Health experts encourage a low-fat, well-balanced diet with at least five servings of fruit and vegetables per day for overall good health.

Screening and Early Detection

The primary strategy for preventing colorectal cancer is to detect and remove any precursors of the disease *before* they have the chance to develop into cancer. If cancer starts to grow, it can become quite large before physical signs or symptoms occur.

Remember, routine colorectal screenings can prevent, as well as detect, cancers at their earliest and most curable stages. Although this sounds simple, most Americans are not screened routinely for colorectal cancer. In 1992, just over 17 percent of people fifty years and older had undergone routine screening. Even fewer (9.4 percent) had undergone screening three years prior to that. In order to change the dismal statistics of this cancer, each of us must get screening tests when they are appropriate and encourage our family, friends, and coworkers to do the same.

Colorectal Screening Guidelines

Both men and women with no risk factors for developing colorectal cancers and no suspicious symptoms should begin routine screening at the age of fifty. Different combinations of tests are available based on personal and family risk factors as well as preference; the tests include fecal occult blood test (FOBT), digital rectal examination (DRE), sigmoidoscopy, colonoscopy, and double-contrast barium enema (see Table 6.2). A growing number of experts recommend colonoscopy be used instead of sigmoidoscopy, believing that having only sigmoidoscopy is like having a mammogram only on one breast (only half of the colon is examined). It would not be surprising to see sigmoidoscopy eliminated from the screening guidelines in the near future.

The American Cancer Society's current guidelines encourage individuals to undergo an FOBT and a flexible sigmoidoscopy starting at age fifty. If both tests show no signs for adenomatous polyps or colorectal cancer, the recommendation is to follow one of these three regimens:

- yearly FOBT and DRE with a flexible sigmoidoscopy every five years

- yearly FOBT and DRE with a colonoscopy every ten years

- yearly FOBT and DRE with double-contrast barium enema every five to ten years

A DRE should be performed prior to a flexible sigmoidoscopy or colonoscopy for correlation with findings.

If a patient is at high risk for developing colorectal cancer, these exami-

Table 6.2: Routine Screening Tests for Colorectal Cancer

Fecal occult blood test

FOBT examines the stool for any signs of blood. Cancerous tumors, certain types of polyps, and chronic irritations of the bowel lining can lead to occasional blood in or on the stool itself. You may take home a test kit to obtain the specimens, or the health care provider may obtain the specimen when performing a rectal examination. The test consists of taking a small portion of stool and placing it on a specimen card. Then the health care provider or laboratory applies a liquid to the card to test for the presence of blood. To ensure the most accurate results, the patient must follow certain dietary and medication guidelines prior to undergoing the FOBT. Dietary and medication information will be given to you by your health care provider.

Digital rectal examination

DRE is an examination to detect a mass in the rectal area. The health care provider inserts a lubricated, gloved finger into the rectum to feel for irregular or abnormal areas. Although DRE is useful in detecting some polyps and cancers, the DRE only examines the rectal area.

60 cm flexible sigmoidoscopy

Sigmoidoscopy is an examination to visually explore the distal portion (descending colon, sigmoid colon, and rectum) of the colon. During the examination, the health care provider uses a slender, flexible, hollow, lighted tube (called a sigmoidoscope) to check for cancer and/or suspicious polyps in the rectum and lower portion of the colon. A sigmoidoscopy can identify nearly all cancers and polyps larger than 1 cm in diameter. Seventy-five to 80 percent of polyps are located in this distal portion of the colon. If a cancer or a suspicious polyp is found, the person needs to have a colonoscopy examination so that a biopsy or polypectomy (removal of a polyp) can be done. They will also examine the remainder of the colon that the sigmoidoscopy cannot reach.

Colonoscopy

A colonoscopy is a procedure that uses a colonoscope, an instrument that is similar to the sigmoidoscope but slightly larger and longer. It, too, is inserted through the rectum. The colonoscope is connected to a video camera. The video display allows the health care provider to look closely at the inside of the colon and rectum. If a suspicious polyp is found, it can be removed by passing a wire loop through the colonoscope to cut the polyp away from the wall of the colon using an electrical current. Colonoscopy usually does not cause pain, although it may be uncomfortable; people are sedated before and during the examination.

Double-contrast barium enema

Also known as a barium enema with air contrast, an enema of barium sulfate is given to partially fill and open up the colon. Once the barium sulfate coats the colon, air is introduced to partially inflate the area, expanding the colon and increasing the contrast and quality of the X-rays being taken. A barium enema with air contrast helps find those lesions that alter the structure of the colon itself.

nations must be started at a younger age, and the frequency of testing will be determined by personal and family risk factors.

Colorectal Screening Guidelines for High-Risk Individuals

The American Cancer Society (ACS), American College of Gastroenterology (ACG), and the American Gastroenterological Association (AGA) endorse the following recommendations for those people who are at high risk for developing colorectal cancer—individuals who have a personal history of colorectal cancer or a parent, sibling, or child with an adenomatous polyp or invasive colorectal cancer.

- A colonoscopy is recommended within one year of surgery for colorectal cancer if the individual did not have one prior to surgery.

- For family members with a history of HNPCC, genetic counseling is suggested, along with a colonoscopy every one to two years between the ages of twenty and thirty, and annually after age forty.

- For family members with a history of familial adenomatous polyposis, genetic counseling is suggested.

- A colonoscopy three years after the initial colonoscopy is recommended if large (>1cm) or multiple adenomatous polyps were found on the original test.

- A colonoscopy is recommended every one to two years for those individuals with inflammatory bowel disease.

Diagnosis and Workup

Signs and Symptoms of Colorectal Cancers

The location of the cancer determines the types of symptoms an individual will have. Most people with precancerous lesions and early-stage cancers will have no symptoms. However, if symptoms do occur from a colorectal cancer, they can include:

- a change in bowel habits (unexplained diarrhea, constipation, frequency, or consistency of stool)

- a change in the shape of the stool (narrower than usual)

- blood in or on the stool (bright red, very dark, or black)

- unexplained general stomach discomfort (bloating, fullness, and/or cramps)

- frequent gas pains

- a feeling that the bowel does not empty completely during bowel movements

- pressure, spasm, or pain in the rectal area

- unexplained weight loss

- unexplained and persistent fatigue

Although these symptoms can be associated with other health problems—such as ulcers, inflammation of the colon, or hemorrhoids—be sure to follow up on these symptoms instead of waiting to see if they go away on their own. "Don't treat thyself—get it checked out!"

Later symptoms could include:

- nausea (with or without vomiting)

- cough and/or shortness of breath

- bone pain

- jaundice—"yellowing" of the eyes and/or skin

Any of these symptoms should prompt a man to see his primary care provider, whether he or she is a doctor, nurse practitioner, or physician's assistant. At this first visit, the man can expect to undergo a complete medical history and thorough physical examination. The medical history should include questions about the man's individual and family risk factors, diet, occupational history, and any previous cancers. If there is a history of cancer, any previous cancer treatment will be significant to discuss. The symptoms will need to be assessed, including weight changes, changes in appetite and diet, changes in the size and shape of stools, abdominal discomfort, skin color changes, nausea and vomiting, unusual itching, and fatigue.

Initial laboratory tests will most likely include a baseline carcinoembryonic antigen (CEA) level and possibly a CA 19-9 (both tumor markers), tests that assess liver and kidney functions, and a complete blood count. Imaging studies will include a chest X-ray, CT scan, sigmoidoscopy or colonoscopy (depending on the location and type of any polyps), and an air contrast barium enema. If any polyp is seen during the colonoscopy, it can be removed and used for pathologic examination. A small piece of any tumor that is seen during a colonoscopy can be removed, or *biopsied,* and will be used for pathologic examination. Endoscopic ultrasound (EUS) is used to stage tumors located in the rectum.

Getting the Diagnosis

The pathologist looks at the polyp or biopsy specimen under a microscope to determine whether cancer is present. If it is, it will be classified as to its type. There are five general types or categories of colorectal cancer:

- adenocarcinoma (the most common type)

- mucinous (colloid) adenocarcinoma

- signet ring adenocarcinoma

- scirrhous tumor

- neuroendocrine tumor

The type or category of tumor tells us from which type of cells the cancer originated. Despite differences in cell type, the medical management of these cancers is essentially the same.

The Stage of Cancer

Once the cancer has been classified, it is necessary to identify the *stage*—extent and location—of the cancer, as this will help determine the most appropriate treatment options. Each stage of cancer is treated differently and has different outcomes. The stages of colorectal cancers are determined by the size of the cancer, depth of penetration of the tumor into the bowel wall, and any spread of disease outside the bowel itself.

Staging tests for colorectal cancer can include a lower GI barium enema to look at the outline of the colon and rectum, a colonoscopy to evaluate the entire colon (if a colonoscopy was not done as part of the initial workup), chest X-ray, and CAT scans of the chest, abdomen, and pelvis. Laboratory testing will include a complete blood count (CBC), platelet count, blood chemistry, and a carcinoembryonic antigen (CEA) test. These tests assess the effect of the cancer on different organs of the body. They may also be used on an ongoing basis to determine the response to treatment.

Although different types of staging systems are used for colorectal cancer—including Dukes' and Modified Astler-Coller (MAC)—treatment decisions should be made with reference to the TNM Classification System (see Table 6.3). The TNM system describes the tumor in terms of T (tumor size and depth of penetration of the bowel wall), N (whether regional lymph nodes contain any cancer), and M (whether the cancer has spread or metastasized to other organs).

Each individual diagnosed with colorectal cancer will be classified as having either stage 0, 1, 2, 3, or 4 disease, which in layman's terms relates to early and local disease, regional disease, or distant and advanced disease (see Table 6.4 for a comparison of the TNM and staging systems; Table 6.5 gives the treatment options available at the different stages).

About 65 percent of patients present with advanced disease, probably due to their lack of routine screening. Five-year survival for early and local

Table 6.3: TNM Classification System

Primary Tumor (T)

TX	Primary tumor cannot be assessed
T0	No evidence of primary tumor
Tis	Carcinoma in situ; intraepithelial or invasion of lamina propria*
T1	Tumor invades submucosa
T2	Tumor invades muscularis propria
T3	Tumor invades through muscularis propria into subserosa or into nonperitonealized pericolic or perirectal tissues
T4	Tumor directly invades other organs or structures and/or perforates visceral peritoneum**

*	Tis includes cancer cells confined within the glandular basement membrane (intraepithelial) or lamina propria (intramucosal) with no extension through the muscularis mucosae into the submucosa
**	Direct invasion in T4 includes invasion of other segments of the colorectum by way of the serosa; for example, invasion of the sigmoid colon by a carcinoma of the cecum

Table 6.4: Comparison of Staging Systems

Staging Grouping

Stage 0	Tis	N0	M0	Dukes'
Stage 1	T1	N0	M0	A
	T2	N0	M0	
Stage 2	T3	N0	M0	B
	T4	N0	M0	
Stage 3	Any T	N1	M0	C
	Any T	N2	M0	
Stage 4	Any T	Any N	M1	D

stage disease (Stages 0 and 1) is close to 95 percent after treatment. The five-year survival rate drops to 35 to 60 percent when lymph nodes are involved (regional disease, Stages 2 and 3), and to 10 percent when metastatic disease is apparent (advanced disease, Stage 4). It is not known why, but prognosis is worse for men of color.

Treatment

If the cancer extensively invades the wall of the colon, a surgical resection, also called a *colectomy*, may be performed. This procedure involves removal of the cancer, some surrounding colon tissue, and the nearby lymph nodes. In rare cases, where the surgeon is unable to reconnect the remaining part

Table 6.5: Treatment Options

Stage 0 (extremely high cure rate)
- Local excision or simple polypectomy with clear margins.
- Colon resection for larger lesions not amenable to local excision.

Stage 1
- Wide surgical resection and anastomosis
- Survival at five years 91.4 percent
- Thirty-seven percent of colorectal cancers are diagnosed at this stage
- Colon cancers diagnosed at very early stages are often removed with a polypectomy (removal of polyps containing the cancer) or local excision (removal of the cancer and a small margin of nearby tissue from the inner surface of the intestine)

Stage 2
- Wide surgical resection and anastomosis
- Positive clinical trials
- Chemotherapy for Stage 2 colon cancer is a controversial issue; clinical trials are underway to determine if surgery alone or surgery plus chemotherapy should be standard therapy; some people at high risk for recurrence may be offered chemotherapy by their oncologist

Stage 3
- Wide surgical resection, anastomosis, and chemotherapy
- Clinical trials

Stage 4
- Surgical resection, anastomosis or bypass of obstructing primary lesions in selected cases
- Surgical resection of isolated metastases (liver, lung, ovaries)
- Local ablative techniques (cryosurgical ablation, embolization and radiation therapy, chemotherapy
- Chemotherapy (locally by perfusions or systemic)
- Clinical trials
- Radiation therapy in selected cases
- Hospice care

of the colon, a *colostomy*, a surgical opening that brings a part of the colon through the abdominal wall, re-routing colon contents though the opening instead of through the rectum, is necessary. The colostomy may be temporary, required only until the colon has healed, at which time it can be reconnected, or *reanastomosed*. In cases where the entire rectum is removed, a colostomy will be permanent. If the cancer has reached a very advanced stage, surgery may be performed to relieve symptoms such as blockages and bleeding, but in these cases surgery is not performed as a curative measure.

Adjuvant chemotherapy is often recommended for colon cancer, especially if the cancer has spread to nearby lymph nodes. Fluorouracil (5-FU) is the drug most commonly used in the treatment of colon and rectal cancers. 5-FU is often used in combination with other drugs such as Levamisole or Leucovorin, which enhance its effectiveness; Levamisole stimulates the patient's own immune system, and Leucovorin blocks enzymes that help cancer cells grow. Chemotherapy treatments will be given over a six- to twelve-month period, depending on the treatment plan selected. There are several combinations and schedules for the use of these drugs. Currently in development is an oral tablet that may be an alternative to intravenous medication. New chemotherapy drugs such as Irinotecan (CPT-11) have been approved by the FDA for the treatment of tumors unresponsive to 5-FU and the treatment of regional disease (Stages 2 and 3). As these drugs are being developed and introduced rapidly, getting the most up-to-date information is critical. The NCI's Cancer Information Service [(800) 4-CANCER] or the NCI website are sources for current information.

All of these medications have side effects that can be well managed. Before you receive your first doses of chemotherapy—either IV or orally— your oncology nurse will review the potential side effects and what can be done to prevent or minimize them. In addition to discussing the management of side effects, the oncology nurse can provide you with information on nutrition, exercise, stress management, local support groups, and resources so that all aspects of your illness and your overall wellness are addressed. It is important to remember that your family also needs information and support during this time.

In advanced stages, chemotherapy or radiation given to specific areas may shrink metastases and relieve some symptoms, but they have not been shown to greatly improve survival rates. There is no standard chemotherapy for patients with widespread metastatic disease. Clinical trails are underway to determine ways to improve survival and the quality of life for these patients.

Rectal Cancer Treatment

Rectal cancer diagnosed at very early stages (Stages 0 to 1) can be treated with procedures that do not require cutting into the abdomen or major surgery. A *polypectomy* may be used to remove a superficial cancer plus a small amount of nearby rectal tissue during colonoscopy.

Rectal cancers diagnosed as invasive in nature may be treated in one of the following ways:

A *low anterior resection* is used when the cancer is near the upper portion of the rectum, close to where it connects with the colon. The colon can then be attached to the anus and waste is eliminated in the usual way.

An *abdominoperineal resection* (APR) is done when the cancer is in the lower part of the rectum, close to the anus. A colostomy is needed after this procedure.

Adjuvant therapy consists of radiation therapy combined with chemotherapy and is recommended if the cancer has spread through the main muscle layer of the rectum or has spread to lymph nodes. The main chemotherapy drug used is 5-FU. This is usually administered as a continuous infusion over several weeks.

Pelvic exenteration is performed when the cancer has advanced and involves nearby organs such as the bladder or prostate. In this procedure, the rectum is removed as well as the surrounding organs that show evidence of the cancer's spread. A colostomy is needed after pelvic exenteration. Chemotherapy and radiation can shrink metastases in patients with advanced disease, but they have not improved survival rates. As in colon cancer, surgical removal of isolated liver metastases is sometimes recommended.

Colostomy   Prior to the use of modern surgical techniques, people with colon cancers, especially cancers located in the lower part of the sigmoid colon, quite often needed the surgical procedure that necessitates creation of a temporary or permanent colostomy. Even though the need for a permanent colostomy is less common today than a decade ago, some people will need a colostomy to divert feces to the outside of the body. A temporary colostomy is indicated when the surgeon wants to allow the bowel to heal properly before re-attaching (or *reanastomosis*) the two ends after removing tumor and the portion of the colon that was involved with the cancer. Or, the surgeon may think it is necessary to allow the suture line that connects the bowel to heal without the irritation caused by the flow of fecal material. A permanent colostomy will be necessary if the location or size of the tumor made removal of the rectum necessary or if remaining tumor is expected to eventually obstruct the bowel.

If creation of a temporary or permanent colostomy is expected, the expertise of the enterostomal therapy or wound ostomy continence nurse (ET nurse) can make a huge difference in the man's ability to physically and emotionally deal with the colostomy. Usually, the surgeon does have a choice about the placement of the stoma, the opening of the colostomy. The ET nurse is consulted *prior* to surgery and works with the surgeon to identify the optimal location for the stoma. Ideally, the stoma should be placed so that body folds, the umbilicus (belly button), waistline, and any surgical scars are outside of the area needed for the adhesive portion of the colostomy pouch, the disposable bag used to collect feces. After surgery, the ET nurse's role is to help the patient and, if necessary, his caregiver, learn to take care of the colostomy so that activities of daily living are disrupted as little as possible. If such a nurse expert is not "on staff" at the hospital where the surgery will be performed, there are ET nurse consultants available in most medium and large cities and through many home care agencies.

There are a growing number of helpful resources for people with ostomies. For assistance locating an ET nurse consultant in your area, contact the Wound Ostomy and Continence Nurses Society (WOCN) via its website (www.wocn.org) or telephone (888) 224-WOCN [224-9626] or the World Council of Enterostomal Therapists in the U.K by telephone at +44-127-377-5432. In addition, the United Ostomy Association (UOA) (www.uoa.org) offers information and assistance directly to consumers. WOCN, in collaboration with the UOA, produced the video "Ask the E.T. Nurse: Basic Ostomy Care Guidelines," an educational video for people with ostomies and their caregivers. The video offers easy-to-follow instructions and care tips that can be viewed at your own pace and comfort level. The video, which costs twelve dollars, can be ordered from the Information Utilization Institute (IUI) Video Library at PO Box 470392, Ft. Worth, TX 76147-0392. *The Ostomy Book*, by Mullen and McGinn, is a complete reference book on ostomies, offering a fact-filled, funny, and heartwarming account of the experience of having an ostomy.

Recurrent Colon Cancer

Recurrent cancer means that, after the initial treatment phase has ended, the cancer comes back. It has been found that 80 to 90 percent of colorectal cancer recurrences (if they do occur) will develop within the first two or three years after treatment. Treatment is dependent on the site of the recurrent disease, previous treatment, and the overall health of the patient. Options for the retreatment of recurrent disease include:

- surgical resection of locally recurrent cancer
- clinical trials
- palliative chemotherapy
- palliative radiation therapy

Questions to Ask When the Diagnosis Is Colorectal Cancer

Regardless of whether you have colon or rectal cancer, you should ask the oncology team questions in order to be informed about your treatment options. Such questions can include:

- What type of cancer do I have?

- What stage is it?

- What are my treatment options based on my personal factors?

- Are any treatments not available to me based on my personal factors? Why?

- Am I a candidate for a clinical trial? Why or why not?

- What is the expected outcome of my treatment (cure, control, palliation)?

- What are the benefits of going through the proposed treatment?

- What are the risks of going through the proposed treatment?

- What are the potential side effects of the treatment and what can you and I do to prevent or minimize them?

- Will I have a colostomy (temporary or permanent)?

- How often will I have treatment and for how long?

- Will I be in the hospital or can my treatment be done as an outpatient or in my home?

- How much time will the treatment take?

- How will I feel after the treatment?

- What types of things should I report to you?

- What is the cost, and what will my insurance cover?

- How do we know if the treatment is working? How will I be evaluated and how often?

- What can I do to stay healthy during the treatment?

- At the end of the treatment, how will I be seen for follow-up, and how often?

- How will the treatment impact my daily life and my family and friends?

- Will I have any restrictions related to work, sexual activity, diet, etc.?

- What type of support (emotional and educational) is available to me and my family and friends?

- If I or a family member need to talk to you, how can we reach you?

- If I decide to get a second opinion, are you willing to discuss my case with another provider?

- If the cancer is going to come back, when would I expect it to do so and how would I know that it may have returned?

Follow-Up

To date, there is no large-scale research study or consensus in the medical community about how best to follow a person after treatment for colorectal cancer. However, many patients are followed by yearly evaluations that include a head-to-toe physical examination, CBC, platelet count, other blood chemistry tests, CEA blood test, and chest X-ray. A detailed history will be done with special attention given to nutrition, appetite, and weight. Unexplained weight loss or gain, increasing unexplained fatigue, alteration in bowel function or type of stools, persistent abdominal or pelvic pain, and unexplained cough are symptoms that require special attention and, most likely, further testing.

Your doctor may recommend periodic colonoscopy as well as CT scans of the abdomen and pelvis. The timing and extent of the follow-up examinations are based solely on your case; others who also have been treated for colorectal cancer may be on a different follow-up schedule. Although you may have undergone treatment for colorectal cancer, you should not forget to be screened for other health problems, such as heart disease and other cancers. These tests, based on your personal and family history and your age, should be incorporated into your wellness plan.

Resources for You and Your Family

Regardless of the type and extent of your cancer, many resources are available to you. The Resources section at the back of this book is an excellent place to start. Each person responds differently to different forms of material and support. Describe to your health care team members how you like information given to you and what type of information you are interested in, and they can help you find the resources that will be the most useful to you.

7

♦ ♦ ♦

Testicular Cancer

Fred Fanchaly, R.N.

"Testicular cancer? What's that? I didn't know you could get cancer there!"

This is not an uncommon response to a diagnosis of testicular cancer. Just ask Scott Hamilton, Olympic ice skater; Lance Armstrong, world champion cyclist; or actor Mathew Ward. All three men are survivors of testicular cancer.

Testicular cancer occurs in the reproductive organs called the testicles, and affects young men on into adulthood. According to National Cancer Institute data, approximately 7,400 Americans are diagnosed with cancer of the testicle each year.

Young men and adult males are generally reluctant to focus on possible medical problems. Some men mistakenly discount the possibility that a problem exists because their testicles don't hurt. Unexplained bumps and bruises are usually attributed to sports injuries or other random events. Real men don't spend a lot of time examining their privates; yet in 40 percent of the men with testicular cancer, the cancer has already spread at the time of diagnosis.

The cure rate for testicular cancer has improved dramatically over the past five years. Twenty years ago, the cure rate was a dismal 25 percent; now it is close to 90 percent. One drug—Cis-Platin, also known as Platinol—is the single cancer-killing medication responsible for the dramatic increase in the successful treatment of cancer of the testicles. We'll talk more about this medication in the section on treatment.

The goal of this chapter is to talk frankly about testicular cancer, from the normal structure and function of the testicles to life after a diagnosis of testicular cancer and everything in between. Emphasis will be placed on prevention and detection, particularly testicular self-exam, the two-minute key to early detection of testicular cancer.

Normal Structure and Function of the Testicles

The testicles are two egg-shaped sex glands located in the scrotum, the loose sack of skin just under the base of the penis (see Figure 7.1). They may vary in size from one individual to another, but all perform the same functions. The front of the testicle is smooth. There is a rubbery-feeling cordlike structure on the top and back of each testicle called the epididymis; it stores and transports the sperm. It is important during testicular self-exam (TSE) that young men can distinguish the normal features of their genitals from something that is not normal. TSE is described in detail later in this chapter.

The testicles are the primary sex glands of reproduction in men, just as the ovaries are the primary glands of reproduction in women. The testicles are the incubators for the production and storage of sperm. During sexual intercourse, the sperm are mixed with fluid produced by the prostate gland and forcefully ejected from the penis into the vagina of the female, where the sperm seek out the egg (also called the ovum) to begin the process of fertilization.

Production of the androgen hormone called testosterone is the second major function of the testicles, also called gonads or testes. Testosterone, one of many hormones produced in

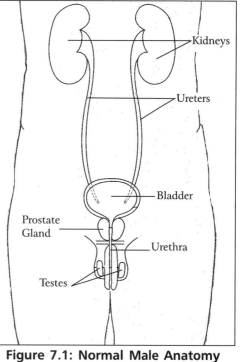

Figure 7.1: Normal Male Anatomy

Reprinted courtesy of the National Cancer Institute

the human body, is responsible for the development of secondary sex characteristics during puberty and adolescence. Increased levels of testosterone in the blood trigger the appearance of body and pubic hair, the change in voice, and the increase in body mass and musculature.

The testicles are not just physical organs of reproduction and hormone synthesis. They represent a man's masculinity on a psychological and social level. Euphemisms for the testicles are numerous—"nuts," "family jewels," "balls"—and often associate a man's masculinity with power and achievement, not to mention sexual prowess. How often have you heard an expression like "Boy, that took balls!"? Frankly speaking, we're talking about a pretty sensitive issue here, literally and figuratively.

Statistics and Risk Factors

Each year, over seven thousand Americans develop testicular cancer. Cancer of the testicle strikes men between the ages of fifteen and thirty-five, but is most often diagnosed when a man is in his mid-thirties. It is the most common cancer for men in this age range, and accounts for one percent of all cancers in men, and one in seven deaths in this age group. While this is the age group at highest risk, cancer of the testicle can occur in men at any age. It is most common in Caucasians, followed by Hispanics, Japanese, Chinese, and Filipinos. The incidence rate is lowest in African Americans.

A number of factors place young men at risk for developing cancer of the testicle. Men who have experienced a condition called cryptorchidism —an undescended testicle—are at the highest risk for development of the disease. With cryptorchidism, one of the testicles remains in the lower abdomen rather than moving down into the scrotum. Eighty to 85 percent of testicular tumors occur in the undescended testicle, while 15 to 20 percent occur in the opposite testicle. The risk exists even if surgery has been performed to mechanically place the undescended testicle in the scrotum.

Other risk factors include:

- A previous history of testicular cancer.

- A history of *mumps orchitis* (an inflammation of the testicle) or other viral infection during childhood or early adolescence.

- A history of an *inguinal hernia* (a condition in which a small part of the intestine slips through a hole in the abdomen down into the scrotum) or *hydrocele* (a condition in which fluid accumulates in the scrotum) during childhood. Both the hernia and hydrocele are easily repaired surgically; doctors are unsure why they place a man at higher risk for development of testicular cancer.

- A father or brother with a history of cancer of the testicle.

- High socioeconomic status.

One additional possible factor is worth mentioning. During the 1940s, 1950s, and 1960s, a drug called diethylstilbestrol (DES) was given to women to prevent complications of pregnancy. Daughters of women who were given this medication during pregnancy are at a higher risk of developing vaginal cancer than women whose mothers did not receive the drug. For this reason, the Food and Drug Administration banned the use of DES in 1971. An article in the May 25, 1999, edition of *The New England Journal of Medicine* reports that DES sons have a higher rate of minor genital-tract abnormalities such as an undescended testicle. Whether DES exposure increases the risk of testicular cancer is still controversial; even if exposure does increase the risk, it is unlikely that the risk is great.

Early Detection

"And the survey says . . . "

A recent survey, published in the September/October 1998 issue of *Cancer Practice*, revealed that less than half of the physicians interviewed said they routinely performed testicular exams on their male patients, and less than 30 percent said they taught their patients how to check their testicles for suspicious lumps.

Most men are unaware of testicular cancer or prefer to ignore it, and only 3 percent regularly check their testicles. "Men should check their testicles every month," says Donald E. Engen, M.D., a urologist at the Mayo Clinic in Rochester, Minnesota. "I think adolescent boys should be taught how to examine themselves in junior high school gym class; it is important to get to know the testicles so that you will know when there is a change."

If found early, testicular cancer is highly curable. The American Cancer Society and American Academy of Family Physicians recommend teaching monthly TSE to all young men between the ages of thirteen and eighteen. The best way to learn how to examine your testicles is by asking your doctor or other health care provider to show you and tell you what you are looking for. If you are too embarrassed, you can call the American Cancer Society and ask for a free, waterproof testicular self-examination card you can hang in your shower.

Performing Testicular Self-Exam (TSE)

TSE is best performed after a warm bath or shower, when the skin of the scrotum is relaxed and both testicles can be felt. When possible, perform the exam standing in front of a mirror so you can see visible changes in your body.

Examine each testicle, one at a time. The index and middle fingers should be placed underneath, with the thumbs on top. Roll each testicle gently back and forth and feel for the normal structures. Remember, the epididymis is the C-shaped, cordlike structure on the top and back of the testicle that stores and transports the sperm. Do not confuse the epididymis with an abnormal lump (see Figure 7.2).

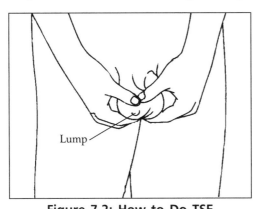

Figure 7.2: How to Do TSE

Reprinted Courtesy of the National Cancer Institute

Feel each testicle for any abnormal lump on the front or side of the testicle, the size of a pea or larger. These lumps are usually painless—a painless lump is a major warning sign.

If you discover a lump, *call your doctor*. The lump might be caused by an infection or other abnormality; then again, it might be a cancer. Only your doctor can decide.

"So How Do I Know If Something Is Wrong?"

There is no single 100 percent definitive sign of testicular cancer. Even the most common signs, taken individually, can still be linked to problems that are *not* cancer. Cancerlike symptoms are often caused by infections or inflammation of the testes, torsion of the testes, accumulation of fluid in the scrotum (*hydrocele*), or engorged veins of the scrotum (*varicocele*). As is the case with all forms of cancer, finding and treating testicular cancer as soon as possible is key to successful treatment. The most common signs and symptoms of testicular cancer listed here should not be ignored and *are* reasons to consult a doctor right away:

- a small painless lump on the testicle

- an enlarged testicle (feels bigger than it used to)

- a feeling of heaviness in the testicle or groin—as one young man explained, "It felt like there was a hand holding and slightly tugging on one of my balls, all the time."

- pain in the testicle, or no pain at all with the presence of a lump (big warning sign here!)

- a sudden feeling of puffiness in the scrotum

- a change in the nipples or increase in the size of the male breast not associated with obesity

- the sudden appearance of blood in the urine

Other more subtle signs and symptoms include urinary problems, an abdominal mass or pain in the abdomen or lower back, a decrease in weight or loss of appetite, and increased fatigue not associated with an increase in physical activity. Although other diseases may be the cause, the NCI recommends that a physician be consulted if these symptoms persist for more than two weeks.

Most men discover testicular cancer themselves, either unintentionally or while doing testicular self-exam. More than one cancer has been discovered by the man's partner while engaging in sexual activity.

Diagnosis and Workup

Initial Tests

When the symptoms suggest that there might be cancer in a testicle, a personal and family history is taken and a complete physical examination is conducted. The scrotum and testicles are carefully examined. A testicular mass should be *transilluminated* to help distinguish between a solid mass and a cyst. Transillumination—an assessment technique that basically involves shining a bright light on the scrotum and determining the light's ability to shine through the tissue—is simple and painless.

Your doctor may order blood and urine tests, a chest X-ray, and a *sonogram*, also called *ultrasound*. This painless exam bounces high-frequency sound waves off the testicles; the returning echoes are converted into pictures. Tissues of different density reflect these sound waves differently. Most testicular tumors are verified using ultrasound and appear as solid masses (as opposed to cysts, which appear as fluid-filled masses). These tests provide good clues as to the likelihood that a cancer is present or if the symptoms can be attributed to some other cause. If there is high suspicion of cancer, confirmation can only be made by looking at a specimen under a microscope.

Surgical Steps

Unlike other tumors, those found in a testicle are never biopsied, because of the very high risk of local spread of the disease if the tumor is cancerous. The *only* way to confirm or rule out cancer is to remove the affected testicle so that a pathologist can look at the tumor cells under a microscope.

The surgical procedure to remove the testicle is called an *inguinal orchiectomy*. It is performed not only to diagnose cancer but also because chemotherapy is not readily taken in or absorbed by the testicles, and it is absolutely necessary to remove the primary tumor. The patient receives a general anesthetic and will have no recollection of the surgery. The surgeon makes a small incision in the groin and removes the whole testicle from the scrotum. The specimen is sent to the pathologist for a thorough microscopic examination. The postoperative pain associated with the procedure is similar to what one feels after an appendectomy.

Staging Workup

As soon as the diagnosis of testicular cancer is confirmed, the patient is usually referred to an oncologist, a physician with special training and expertise in the treatment of cancer. Initially, a series of tests will be performed to determine the *stage* of the disease.

Staging determines if the cancer is localized or if it has spread to the lymph nodes in the lower abdomen and other parts of the body. Lymph nodes are small, bean-shaped structures linked together by tubes called lymph vessels. They exist throughout the body, and their function is to trap bacteria or cancer cells and produce and store cells that fight infection.

The information obtained during staging will assist the doctor in planning treatment. Many patients will have a CT (or CAT) scan performed, a series of painless X-rays of various sections of the body. The doctor might also order an intravenous pyelogram (IVP). During an IVP, special dye is injected into a vein, the kidneys collect this dye and excrete it from the body in the urine, and X-rays are taken to outline the structure of the urinary system and identify any abnormalities. Additional tests may reveal the presence of tumor markers—substances detectable in the blood or urine that suggest the presence of cancer. Seventy to 80 percent of patients with testicular cancer have elevated marker levels. Treatment of the cancer results in a decline in the blood level of the marker. Some examples of tumor markers related to testicular cancer are alpha-fetoprotein (AFP), human chorionic gonadotropin (HCG), placental alkaline phosphatase (PAP), and lactate dehydrogenase (LDH).

The oncologist will review the pathologist's detailed microscopic examination of the testicle removed during surgery. It is important to know the cell type of the tumor, as this will guide the oncologist in planning treatment. Ninety-five percent of all testicular tumors are germ-cell tumors, which arise from the testicular cells that divide to produce immature sperm cells.

Non-germ-cell tumors of the testes are quite rare, particularly in young men. As men get older, a variety of non-germ-cell tumors can occur—the most common is lymphoma—but these are rare as well. A man with a non-germ-cell tumor would benefit from consultation with a urologic group with experience in all aspects of testicular tumors.

There are two main types of germ-cell testicular cancers:

- *Seminomas* are tumors that arise from the germ cells. These tumors make up 30 to 40 percent of all testicular cancers and are very sensitive to radiation therapy.

- *Non-seminoma tumors* are a class of cancers that arise in the same germ cells but may contain several different cell types within one tumor. They are also called mixed-cell tumors, and the degree of variation in the cells is an important factor the oncologist uses to plan treatment. These tumors may contain a combination of cells called embryonal carcinoma, teratoma, yolk sac carcinoma, and choriocarcinoma.

Once all the exam results are complete, the oncologist will determine the stage of the disease. The three stages are:

Stage I: The cancer is confined to one testicle.

Stage II: The cancer has spread to lymph nodes in the lower abdomen.

Stage III: The cancer has spread beyond the lymph nodes in the abdomen to other parts of the body, including the lungs and the liver.

When staging is complete, the oncologist will discuss treatment options with the patient and family members.

Treatment

In general, men with early and limited disease—accounting for about 70 percent of all men who are diagnosed with testicular cancer—are highly curable. Men who have Stage I seminoma undergo surgery and generally have radiation therapy after surgery; nearly all—over 95 percent—will survive their cancer. Those with Stage II seminoma have just slightly lower survival rates; up to 90 percent survive. Statistics are similar for men with Stage I and II non-seminoma germ-cell tumors.

Testicular cancer may be treated with surgery, radiation therapy, and chemotherapy. These treatments may be used alone or in combination with each other. An additional promising new direction in the treatment of testicular cancer is bone marrow transplant. No one treatment protocol is effective for all kinds of testicular cancer; different cell types require different treatment strategies. For example, seminomas and non-seminomas differ in their patterns of spread and response to therapy.

Decisions about treatment for testicular cancer are complex. Sometimes it is helpful to have more than one doctor's opinion about the diagnosis and treatment plan; it is every patient's right to be fully informed of his options for treatment, and getting a second or third opinion gives him greater confidence in the decision he eventually makes. It may take a week or two to get an appointment for a second opinion, but in most cases this will not delay treatment, nor make treatment any less effective. In the United States and abroad, there are recognized centers of excellence for the treatment of testicular cancer. Centers of excellence for the management of testicular cancer are listed in the Resources section at the end of this book.

Surgery

Surgery to remove the affected testicle and the primary (original) tumor is the first phase of treatment for testicular cancer, in addition to being essential for accurate diagnosis. Nearly 90 percent of men with Stage I testicular cancer—determined by *pathologic staging* at the time of surgery—can be cured with surgery alone.

Depending on the stage and type of the disease, additional surgery may be necessary. *Radical peritoneal lymph node dissection* (RPLND) is indicated when the diagnostic tests reveal that the cancer is Stage II and has spread to the lymph nodes in the abdomen. The patient is given a general anesthetic, and the surgeon surgically removes the chains of lymph nodes that stretch from the groin up into the abdomen along the spine. The main objective of the surgery is to remove as much tumor as possible, increasing the effectiveness of the adjuvant therapy (chemotherapy) and preventing further spread of the cancer. Improved surgical techniques have made it possible to spare the nerves responsible for sexual arousal and orgasm; however, the operation may cause sterility, as it interferes with ejaculation. Medication may treat this problem, although some cases do not respond.

Young men who anticipate getting married—or those who are already married and want to start a family—should consider preserving their sperm in a sperm bank before undergoing this procedure.

Radiation Therapy

Radiation therapy uses high-energy rays to damage cancer cells and stop their growth. It affects the ability of all cells to regenerate themselves and reproduce, but normal healthy cells are better able to recover from the radiation damage than cancer cells. Radiation treatments are very carefully planned for each individual. Special shields are made to protect the remaining testicle and other important organs from the radiation. Seminomas are highly sensitive to radiation; non-seminomas are less responsive and require other treatment strategies. The major side effects of treatment are nausea and fatigue (see Chapter 13 for more information about radiation therapy and the management of side effects).

Chemotherapy

Chemotherapy treatment for testicular cancer has advanced rapidly in the last five years. A combination of cancer-killing drugs may be given orally by pill, injected into the muscle, or injected into the vein so that it circulates throughout the body to reach the cancer cells. The five main drugs used to treat testicular cancer are:

- Ifex (ifosfamide)

- Vepesid (etoposide)

- Velban (vinblastine sulfate)

- Blenoxane (bleomycin sulfate)

- Platinol (cisplatin)

Many oncologists regard Platinol as the "magic bullet" for the treatment of various forms of testicular cancer. Much of the pioneering research using Platinol was conducted by Lawrence Einhorn, M.D., in collaboration with with John Donohue, M.D., at the Indiana University Cancer Center in the 1970s. These two physicians created the framework for treating advanced germ cell tumors with the modern combined approach of effective chemotherapy and aggressive integration of surgery.

Platinol used in combination with other drugs has dramatically cut the death rate from testicular cancer and boosted the cure rate; as a result, according to the NCI, about 70 percent of men with advanced disease can be cured. The most common and well-studied regimen is the three-drug combination of bleomycin, etoposide, and cisplatin (Platinol)—BEP—given in three twenty-one-day cycles with a ten-day rest period between each cycle, meaning the man can expect to be in treatment for three months.

Other Treatments

Bone marrow transplant is the newest treatment for testicular cancer and continues to be studied as a way to manage patients whose cancer does not respond well to cisplatin-based chemotherapy protocol or whose cancer recurs after chemotherapy. In this procedure, bone marrow is taken from the patient and treated with drugs to kill any cancer cells that might be present. The marrow is frozen and stored while the patient receives high-dose chemotherapy with or without radiation therapy. The goal is to destroy any remaining marrow. The healthy frozen marrow is then thawed and given back to the patient intravenously; it circulates through the body and finds its way to the empty marrow spaces in the bones and begins to grow and produce healthy red and white blood cells.

Peripheral stem cell therapy is being studied at several cancer centers. Memorial Sloan Kettering Cancer Center in New York City has developed a regimen for use as the initial therapy for patients with advanced disease, and also in the treatment of testicular cancer that has not responded well to the standard chemotherapy treatment. The early studies look promising; clinical trials will need to be completed to determine the overall value of this form of treatment.

"What Does the Future Hold?"

The recovery and personal triumphs of testicular cancer survivors Scott Hamilton and Lance Armstrong attest to the fact that there is definitely "life after testicular cancer." New or additional self-care responsibilities will enhance the quality of survival and also ensure that a problem or even recurrence is discovered early, when treatment will be most effective.

Regular follow-up exams are very important for anyone who has been treated for testicular cancer. The plan varies for the different types and stages of the cancer; for most patients, blood tests to measure the presence and levels of tumor markers may be done every month or two for two to three years after treatment has finished. Chest X-rays and CT scans may be done at intervals. Once a patient is three years post-treatment, checkups may be reduced to once or twice a year. Men should continue to perform TSE every month on the remaining testicle.

Body image changes are certain to affect some men with the removal of one testicle. Those men concerned with sexual function and body image will benefit from the coping mechanisms discussed in Chapter 18, "Cancer, Sexuality, and Sex." Joining a support group for men with testicular cancer allows for open exchange of concerns about living with the disease. One resource for groups is the Testicular Cancer Resource Center (www.acor.org/diseases/TC). There are chat rooms on the Internet created specifically for men with testicular cancer; for more Internet listings, see the Resources section at the end of this book.

The removal of one testicle does not make a man sterile, and advances in treatment attempt to preserve the potency of the remaining testicle. It should be mentioned here that, as a result of the problems encountered with silicon breast implants in women, artificial testicle implants are not generally offered in the United States. However, several companies manufacture saline-filled testicular implants available from international suppliers, and one California company, Mentor Corporation, is waiting for FDA approval for a saline-filled implant that would be available in the U.S. The Testicular Cancer Resource Center, however, does not recommend testicular implants for cosmetic reasons. The surgical fee for a testicular implant can run from $2,400 to $3,600; public or private insurance plans are unlikely to pay for this kind of surgical procedure.

The outlook for men with testicular cancer is excellent. Due in part to early detection and improved staging methods, a large majority of testicular cancer patients are cured with initial treatment. Researchers continue to investigate the cause, prevention, diagnosis, and treatment of the disease. Specific research is directed at as yet undiscovered tumor markers that may be present in abnormal amounts in the blood or urine of a person with the very early stages of testicular cancer. Research continues to study new drugs and combinations of existing drugs in varying doses and schedules to increase the effectiveness and decrease the side effects of treatment. The remarkable improvements in dealing with this disease may lead to new advances in treatment of other cancers.

Young men with testicular cancer have more resources available to them today than ever before. The World Wide Web has created an instantaneous resource for all kinds of patient information, from finding a local support group to choosing a center of excellence to discussing treatment options and getting answers to insurance and financial questions. Testicular cancer is no longer the death sentence that it was many years ago. Today, men with testicular cancer have a bright future ahead of them.

8

◆ ◆ ◆

Penile Cancer

Pamela J. Haylock, R.N., M.A.

Most of the time, cancer of the penis is in fact a form of skin cancer that just happens to occur on the skin covering the penis. Penile cancer occurs very infrequently: fewer than one thousand U.S. men are diagnosed with cancer affecting the penis each year, accounting for less than 1 percent of all men's cancers in this country. However, in cultures and populations where circumcision is not a common practice and personal cleanliness is not ideal, cancer of the penis can account for up to 12 percent of all cancers in men. Countries with higher rates of penile cancer include Uganda, Mexico, China, India, and Puerto Rico, and men who come from these countries could be at higher risk as well.

Since a man's penis is symbolic of his masculinity, the mere thought of cancer affecting the penis—and the resulting threat to sexual and physical function—is very frightening to most men. In fact, when diagnosed early, penile cancer is very curable, although most doctors have little experience with this disease. Men who are concerned about a possible cancer of the penis or who have been diagnosed with it are advised to get medical care from a doctor who is knowledgeable about penile cancer and skilled in its management.

Risk Factors

The causes of cancer of the penis are not clear, though there is a connection between the human papillomavirus (HPV)—the virus that causes genital warts and is also linked to cancer of the uterine cervix in women—and cancer of the penis. There is some thought that penile cancer might be linked to the cervical cancer of female sexual partners, but this is so far unproven. Other than its association with HPV, there is no proven link between cancer of the penis and the other sexually transmitted diseases, syphilis, gonorrhea, granuloma inguinale, and chancroid.

There is a connection between the development of penile cancer and men who were not circumcised as infants. This link is especially important when boys and men are not accustomed to regularly cleaning *smegma* (the substance created by the collection of skin cells shed from the penis and foreskin and bacteria) from the fold of skin over the tip of the penis, the *preputial sac*. Smegma is carcinogenic—it causes cancer—in some animals, but the actual factor responsible for its causing cancer in human males has not been found.

Prevention and Early Detection

It seems clear that the simple act of routinely cleaning the penis and under the foreskin is an important preventive measure. When parents make the decision to forego circumcision for a son, it then becomes their responsibility to teach the young boy how to do the simple cleaning procedure. In communities where circumcision is not commonly used, health care providers and lay people can share the responsibility of teaching basic hygiene to boys, thereby reducing the number of men who might otherwise develop penile cancer later in their lives.

To clean the penis and under the foreskin:

- Pull back, or "retract," the foreskin from the tip of the penis.

- If the foreskin is too "tight" and doesn't fully retract, consult a urologist for instructions on dilating or stretching the foreskin.

- Using soap and water, wash the penis thoroughly, rinse, and dry.

- Allow the foreskin to return to its normal position.

Penile cancer usually affects men between forty and sixty years old. It most commonly starts in the *glans*—the tip—but cancer can develop anywhere along the shaft of the penis. The most common signs of this cancer include:

- a painless nodule—small lump or growth—on the penis

- a sore or ulcer, sometimes with bleeding, under the foreskin or anywhere on the penis

- a discharge from the sore or the penis

- swelling

- swollen lymph nodes in the groin area

Perhaps because it is so uncommon or because of the fear of what these symptoms could mean, cancer of the penis is quite often diagnosed late, when it has already spread to the lymph nodes.

Diagnosis and Workup

Any time changes or sores are noted on the penis, a biopsy must be done either to confirm the exact diagnosis or to rule out other possible problems. Some important precancerous skin changes can affect the penis. Failure to treat these conditions in the precancerous stage can result in the development of cancer. These conditions include:

- *Buschke-Lowenstein*: A large warty-looking change. It can be treated by local excision—cutting it away.

- *Erythroplasia of Queyrat*: A raised, red area that looks almost like velvet. It is treated with fluouracil cream applications twice a day, or by local excision.

- *Paget's disease*: A red, inflamed area. It is treated with local excision.

- *Leukoplakia*: A white, crusty area. Treated with local excision.

Once a diagnosis of cancer is confirmed, the doctor will examine the area closely to determine the exact location and size of the lesion, whether it is attached to underlying penile structures, and whether it has spread to the base of the penis or the scrotal area.

Types of Penile Cancer

Almost all cancers involving the penis are the *squamous cell carcinoma* type. Squamous cell cancers start in and involve the top level of the skin, the epidermis. Though extremely rare, melanoma and sarcoma can also affect the penis. In some cases, cancer from other organs such as the bladder, prostate, rectum, or kidney can spread to the penis, and in some very rare cases leukemia can involve the penis. Cancers involving the penile urethra—

the part of the urinary tract that lies within the penis—are also rare: fewer than five hundred cases have ever been reported in the world's medical literature.

Stage and Grade

Even though there is no staging system specific to cancer of the penis, the TNM system is used by many experts. Table 8.1 outlines the TNM system with respect to squamous cell carcinoma of the penis.

Table 8.1: TNM Staging System for Squamous Cell Carcinoma of the Penis

T	N	M
T0—No evidence of primary tumor	N0—No evidence of lymph node involvement	M0—No evidence of distant metastases
TIS—Carcinoma *in situ* (Bowen's disease, Erythroplasia of Queyrat)	N1—Involvement of a single regional lymph node	M1—Distant metastases present
T1—Tumor not more than 1 cm and affecting only the outer layer of skin	N2—Involvement of single nodes on both the right and left groin or several nodes on either side	M1a—Evidence of hidden metastases based on blood tests or other findings
T2—Tumor 1 cm and affecting only the outer layer of skin	N3—Nodes are fixed to underlying tissues or there are skin ulcers over the involved nodes	M1b—Single metastasis in a single organ site
T3—Tumor of any size invading underlying tissues	N4—Involvement of lymph nodes in the regional area	M1c—Several areas of metastasis in a single site
T4—Tumor invading nearby structures such as the corpus, urethra, symphysis, perineum		M1d—Metastases in several organ sites

A common and more simple staging system for penile cancer uses Stages I through IV:

Stage I: Cancer is limited to the tip (glans) and the foreskin, but does not involve the shaft of the penis or the corpora cavernosa.

Stage II: Cancer has invaded the corpora cavernosa but has not spread to the lymph nodes.

Stage III: Cancer has spread to the lymph nodes in the groin.

Stage IV: Cancer has spread to local and regional lymph nodes and to other more distant organs.

Treatment

The forms of treatment available to treat cancer of the penis will depend on the size of the cancer, its exact location on the penis, how deeply it has invaded the skin of the penis, and the extent of the cancer's spread. Treatment for cancers of the penis can include removing all or part of the penis (called *total* or *partial penectomy*), radiation therapy, and topical chemotherapy.

Stage I penile cancer is cured by removing the cancer. When cancer involves only the foreskin, removing the cancer itself along with the foreskin is commonly recommended. Carcinoma *in situ*—also called Erythroplasia of Queyrat or Bowen's disease of the penis—is managed with a chemotherapy cream that is applied directly onto the site or use of microscopic surgical techniques. Even in Stage I cancers, total or partial penectomy may be needed to provide cure. Other possible treatment options include the use of external beam radiation or brachytherapy techniques (see chapter 13, "Radiation Therapy"). The value of laser techniques for the treatment of early stage penile cancer is not yet proven, but it seems to offer hope for cure or at least control of the cancer while maintaining near-normal appearance and function of the penis.

In Stage II penile cancer, penectomy offers the best chance of cure. Whether the penectomy is partial or total depends on the extent and location of the cancer. In some cases, external beam radiation therapy followed by surgery might be offered as a treatment option. Here again, the value of laser therapy is under study.

Stage III penile cancer is removed with surgery. Lymph nodes might be swollen as a result of infection, rather than as a result of spread of the cancer. When nodes are swollen, a course of antibiotics is prescribed. If the nodes are still swollen after three weeks, additional surgery will be needed to explore and, if cancer is found, to remove lymph nodes in the groin area. For men who cannot undergo surgery, radiation therapy to the lymph nodes might be used. Radiation therapy following surgery may decrease the chance of cancer reappearing in the nodes of the groin area.

There really is no curative therapy for late stage—Stage IV—or recurrent penile cancer. Any treatment offered will target the management of distressing symptoms and help the man achieve comfort during the last stages of his life. Surgery might be used to control infection and bleeding, and radiation therapy can offer hope for control of pain caused by lymph node involvement and the spread of cancer to bones.

Effects of Treatment

The change in appearance and function of the penis following therapy for penile cancer depends on the amount of tissue removed in the course of treatment. Men who are treated with radiation therapy have fewer problems with sexual activity than men treated with surgery. Men who undergo partial penectomy will not lose the ability to achieve erection, ejaculate, or reach orgasm. Men who have had total penectomy obviously lose the ability to have erections, but can retain the desire for sexual activity, enjoy stimulation in the genital and perineal region, and still have orgasms.

After a total penectomy, urine is expelled through a newly created opening in the perineum, the *perineal urethrostomy*. Ejaculation can occur through this opening as well. Some specialty centers with extremely skilled reconstructive and urologic surgeons, such as the Mayo Clinic in Minnesota, use techniques to create a new penis after a total penectomy. A semirigid or inflatable penile prosthesis allows the man to achieve erection and have sexual intercourse.

Follow-Up

Men who have been diagnosed and treated for penile cancer will need to learn how to watch for signs and symptoms that the cancer has reappeared or spread. In addition, these men need to be followed by their doctor on a regular basis—at least every six months for the first two years, then yearly for the remainder of their lives.

Future

Because penile cancer is quite rare, at least in the U.S., it has been difficult to determine the advantage of one treatment form over another. For this reason, men who develop this disease should consider taking part in a clinical trial process, if one is available. It seems reasonable to assume that this form of cancer is largely preventable. Public health efforts such as teaching simple personal hygiene in high-risk communities must be a priority.

9

♦ ♦ ♦

Male Breast Cancer

Jean Lynn, R.N., B.S.N., O.C.N.

When we hear the words "breast cancer," we usually think of a disease that affects women. Breast cancer very rarely occurs in men, but the incidence of male breast cancer is on the rise, and men should be aware that they might be at risk of developing this disease.

About Breast Cancer in Men

The recognition of breast cancer in men dates back to ancient Egyptian times. However, the first documented report of male breast cancer in medical literature is from the fourteenth century by a British physician, John of Ardene, who noted an enlarging breast mass on a priest. A local barber surgeon promised cure, but John "would let no cutting come there nigh."

The cause of breast cancer is unknown for men as well as for women. The incidence of male breast cancer in the United States remained stable for approximately fifty years, began to increase in the late 1980s, and has risen sharply since 1991. The reason for this is unclear. We do know that male breast cancer is a predominately hormonally sensitive tumor, as it is in females; the role of estrogen as an etiologic factor is being explored. At the start of the twenty-first century, according to the American Cancer Society, approximately fourteen hundred men will develop breast cancer and four hundred men will most likely die from the disease every year.

Globally, the incidence of male breast cancer varies. This cancer occurs more often in northern Europe and North America than it does among men in Japan and Finland. The incidence is much higher in Egypt because of a disease called schistosomiasis, transmitted through a parasite that causes inflammation around the liver and subsequently leads to hyperestrogenism (elevated estrogen levels).

In the United States, Jewish men seem to have a higher risk, though the increased risk is not thought to be statistically significant. African-American men in the United States have a higher incidence and have a higher death rate than Caucasian males in this country.

Risk Factors

There is limited information about breast cancer in males because it is a relatively uncommon problem. When it does occur, it seems to go unnoticed until it has advanced to a stage that is difficult if not impossible to cure. For this reason, men should be aware of factors that might place them at risk for developing the disease.

Family History Family history is especially significant if breast cancer is diagnosed in any first-degree relative (mother, brother, sister, or daughter). Sixty percent of men with breast cancer have at least one female family member with the disease. Multiple cases of male breast cancer in a family are unusual, but have been reported among siblings, uncles, and nephews. The mutation of the BRCA-2 gene (a gene linked to breast cancer) may be a causative factor in about one-third of familial breast cancer in females, and it has been noted that these families also have a high incidence of male breast cancer.

Age The incidence of breast cancer increases steadily after men reach the age of thirty-five; the average age of diagnosis is sixty-three.

Kleinfelter's Syndrome One of the strongest risk factors is Kleinfelter's Syndrome, a condition that results in an extra sex chromosome. Men with this condition do not produce enough testosterone and often experience testicular insufficiency and atrophy, gynecomastia (breast enlargement), an increase in the secretion of follicle-stimulating hormone (FSH), and obesity. They are also likely to have low levels of androsterone (a male sex hormone that contributes to the deepening of the voice and the growth and development of the genitals, armpit and pubic hair, and sweat glands), resulting in high estrogen-to-androgen ratios. Kleinfelter's Syndrome occurs in about one or two of every one thousand men. Approximately 4 to 6 percent of men with breast cancer also have Kleinfelter's Syndrome.

Gynecomastia (Breast Enlargement) There is a causal though unproven relationship between the gynecomastia—abnormal breast enlargement in men—and the development of breast cancer. Gynecomastia is noted in anywhere from 1 to 40 percent of males with breast cancer.

Testicular Abnormalities Undescended testes (cryptorchidism) have been implicated as a possible cause of breast cancer. This condition frequently causes testicular insufficiency, which can result in higher estrogen levels.

Other Associated Risk Factors Even though data is not conclusive, a few other factors also seem to increase a man's chances of developing breast cancer. Among these are:

- infertility
- radiation exposure, especially if exposure occurred at a young age in relationship to treatment of another malignancy such as Hodgkin's lymphoma, thymus enlargement, or puberty gynecomastia (breast enlargement that occurs during puberty); breast cancer seems to occur in these men twelve to thirty-six years after exposure to radiation
- history of head injury associated with direct or indirect injury to the hypothalamus resulting in hyperprolactinemia (stimulation of milk production)
- occupational risks such as chronic work exposure to heat (suggesting that increased environmental temperatures may be associated with testicular dysfunction); telephone workers and men working in the electromagnetic fields may be at higher risk
- late puberty
- hypercholesteremia (elevated cholesterol levels)
- synthetic estrogen use
- male to female transsexual (three cases reported in the literature)

Clinical Presentation

The average age of men diagnosed with breast cancer is sixty-three years—ten years older than the average age of women at the time of breast cancer diagnosis. Male breast cancer most often occurs in the left breast, commonly appearing as a mass or lump just beneath the nipple. This mass is usually in a fixed position, attached to the skin or the chest wall because of the small size of the male breast. Male breast cancer may also occur in the upper, outer quadrant of the breast or as a mass in the axilla (armpit). The mass is usually painless, unilateral (occurring on just one side), irregularly shaped, firm, and approximately 4 to 5 cm (about 2 inches) in diameter at presentation.

Half of men with breast cancer have disease that has spread to the axilla at the time the diagnosis is made. Seventy to 80 percent of all men have a discharge—often bloody—at the time of diagnosis. About one in five men with breast cancer have nipple and areolar abnormalities such as scaling, irritation, redness, or inverted nipples. These men are likely to have had symptoms for three to eighteen months, which is why male breast cancer is most often diagnosed at an advanced stage of disease. Gynecomastia is present in about a fourth of all cases, which can complicate the diagnostic process.

Diagnosis

Mammography can be useful in diagnosing male breast cancer—revealing the difference between a diagnosis of cancer and gynecomastia, although the procedure is difficult because of the limited size of the breast. Most often, the mass appears calcified or as a *spiculated,* or starlike, lesion. Fine needle aspiration of the breast is done to collect cells, or tissue is removed to confirm a diagnosis.

Ninety-six percent of male breast cancer is infiltrating ductal carcinoma; the remaining 4 percent are sarcomas. Preinvasive breast cancer is only rarely detected in men. Since men do not have lobules (milk-producing ducts) in their breasts, they do not develop lobular cancer, although there have been some rare reported instances cited in the literature. Eighty percent of these cancers are dependent on estrogen and progesterone to stimulate their growth, suggesting that a man's lower estrogen environment leaves receptor sites more often available for binding with tumor cells.

Treatment and Prognosis

The current trend in treatment of male breast cancer is to do a modified radical mastectomy, removing all of the breast tissue and the lymph nodes closest to the breast under the arm. Breast-conserving surgery, increasingly used in female breast cancer, is not used because of the small size of the male breast. Radiation therapy may be used if there is a good deal of lymph node involvement either in the axilla or the internal mammary nodes (closest to the breastbone).

Chemotherapy is usually offered to men with locally advanced disease (involving the lymph nodes). The usual chemotherapy regimen is given over four to eight cycles, one cycle at approximately one-month intervals. Since most male breast cancer is hormonally sensitive, tamoxifen (Nolvadex) is given after chemotherapy for a period of five years. Side effects from the chemotherapy are similar to those that women experience. Weight gain, decreased libido, fatigue, and nausea are the most common. Hair loss occurs with the most common chemotherapy regimens.

Survival rates for male breast cancer are affected by three critical factors: (1) age at diagnosis; (2) size of the tumor; and (3) involvement of the lymph nodes, the most important factor.

For men with hormonally sensitive tumors, the treatment response rates can be as high as 80 percent. In those men who have node-positive disease, the addition of chemotherapy improves their disease-free survival rate. If the breast cancer returns, the most common sites of recurrence are bones, lung, brain, liver, and skin.

Male breast cancer is on the rise. Survival rates are similar, stage for stage, to those of women. However, male breast cancer is most often diagnosed at a later stage, which substantially reduces long-term survival for men with this disease. Men with a strong family history of breast cancer should have an annual clinical breast exam. Genetic screening of high-risk individuals for the BRCA-2 gene should also be considered for men in this category. Early detection is the key to prolonging survival rates.

Support

Men with breast cancer can feel quite isolated and embarrassed in addition to experiencing the fear and anxiety associated with any cancer diagnosis. The Y-Me National Breast Cancer Organization has a twenty-four-hour hotline that can be reached at (800) 221-2141. The Y-Me website (www.yme.org) has several links to male breast cancer resources. The Komen Foundation's website (www.komen.org) also lists resources for men with breast cancer.

10

♦ ♦ ♦

The Boy with Cancer

Marcia Rostad, R.N., M.S.

Approximately eight thousand children who are fifteen years old or younger will be diagnosed with cancer in the United States each year. The incidence of cancer increases in adolescence with nearly thirty-five hundred teenagers between the ages of fifteen and nineteen years diagnosed annually. These numbers account for less than 1 percent of all cancers reported in the United States, making childhood cancer a rare disease. Accidents continue to lead the childhood mortality rate at over 40 percent; in contrast, approximately 10 percent of all childhood deaths are caused by cancer.

Childhood cancer is diagnosed more often in boys than girls, although only by a small ratio (1.2:1). The predominance of cancer in boys varies by the type of cancer, the age of the boy, and race. For example, leukemia occurs more often in boys than girls between birth to four years and ten to fourteen years. Boys also have a higher rate of lymphoma and medulloblastoma (a tumor of the central nervous system) throughout childhood than do girls. African-American boys have a lower rate of leukemias, brain tumors, and bone tumors than African-American girls.

Types of Cancers That Affect Children

Cancer that occurs in children—and its treatment as well—differs in many ways from similar cancers occurring in adults. An adult with leukemia has a much different disease than a boy with leukemia.

In children, the vast majority of cancer comes from the *mesodermal germ layer* of tissue. The mesodermal germ layer is the substance from which a child develops his bones, cartilage, muscle, blood, blood vessels, sex organs, kidneys and other body structures. Childhood cancers also come from *neuroectodermal tissue*, which forms the child's nervous system. In adults, all the body structures and systems are completely formed and matured. Adult cancers, called *carcinomas*, occur when the mature structures of the body develop cancers from tissues of superficial, or epithelial, origins.

Children are subject to cancers that do not occur in adulthood. Wilms' tumor, neuroblastoma, and retinoblastoma occur solely in the very young. Cancers occurring in childhood have almost no known prevention, whereas 80 percent of adult cancers are preventable.

The most important difference between adult and childhood cancers is that childhood cancer is more responsive to current treatment. Proportionately, more children are cured of their cancer than adults. The survival rate for children with all types of cancer exceeds 60 percent; the adult survival rate just approaches 50 percent. It is important for parents and family to remember these encouraging statistics as their loved ones go through treatment. It will help them to remain hopeful and optimistic.

Cancers That Occur More Frequently in Boys

Several types of cancer can occur in boys more often than in girls. This section will focus briefly on the childhood cancers that are of special concern for boys and their parents.

Acute Lymphocytic Leukemia

Leukemia is the most common cancer in children. More boys than girls are diagnosed with common childhood leukemia, or *acute lymphocytic leukemia* (ALL). The highest number of cases occur at four years of age. While it seems tragic for a young boy, only four years old, to be diagnosed with this life-threatening illness, his chances for cure are much better than if he were diagnosed at a younger age or as a teenager. Boys diagnosed with ALL three decades ago had only a 5 percent chance of survival. Today, those chances are as high as 75 to 90 percent, with the right kind of therapy. When a boy is diagnosed with ALL, or any other type of cancer, being in the care of childhood cancer specialists will give him his best chance for survival.

Acute lymphocytic leukemia, also known as *acute lymphoblastic leukemia*, is a cancer of the white blood cells. These cells are formed inside the bones in tissue called *bone marrow*. Normally, white blood cells go through different steps of maturation in the bone marrow. When the white blood cells have "grown up" and can be useful to the body, they leave the marrow and enter the bloodstream. The white blood cell's job, once in the blood, is to fight infection. In ALL, something goes wrong and white blood cells in the bone marrow don't completely mature. The bone marrow tries to make mature white blood cells but never succeeds; instead, it makes immature white blood cells by the thousands, to the point that they spill out into the blood. As a result, the body becomes full of useless white blood cells. Because the blood goes everywhere in the body, the useless white blood cells go into every organ and tissue and interfere with their normal functions. Kidney function, circulation, and immunity are examples of body functions that can be impaired by the abnormal influx of immature white blood cells.

The purpose of leukemia treatment is to return the bone marrow to normal function by stopping the overproduction of immature white blood cells. Boys with ALL are treated with an aggressive course of chemotherapy that attacks and destroys the fast growing leukemia cells in the blood and bone marrow, eventually stopping the process altogether. It is not possible for a few doses of chemotherapy to achieve permanent results; therefore, the boy must go through two to three years of therapy. This therapy includes a variety of chemotherapy medications that are given by intravenous injections, or sometimes in pill form. Because leukemia may spread into the spinal fluid that surrounds the brain, the boy must also have frequent spinal taps to inject chemotherapy directly into the spinal fluid. This is the only way that appropriate doses of chemotherapy can enter the central nervous system.

For boys, the spread of leukemia to the testes is a major concern. The testes are regularly examined and monitored throughout treatment for any enlargement or mass. Should spread of leukemia be suspected, the boy must have a testicular biopsy. It is very important to help the boy understand how this procedure is done and why it is necessary. Any genital examination on a boy of any age can be embarrassing and frightening. Young boys are especially prone to imagining harmful things may be done to their genitals during these exams or from surgery. The testicular biopsy is generally done as an outpatient procedure by a pediatric surgeon. A tiny incision is made into the testes where the mass has been found, and a very small sample of the mass is removed. Afterwards, the boy may experience mild discomfort and swelling; these symptoms will go away in a few days.

The treatment for testicular leukemia is radiation. Because the leukemia will, in a short time, spread to both testicles, radiation treatments are given to both testes even if only one is enlarged. The radiation treatment will leave the boy permanently sterile, although he will still be able to engage in sex and have ejaculations when he matures. Sexually mature adolescents and their parents who are concerned about the permanent effects of sterility should consult reproductive specialists about the possibility of sperm banking. It is likely the adolescent will prefer to speak to the reproduction specialist in private, and parents should honor this request. The donation discussion can be quite difficult and awkward to initiate. Specially trained counselors can help prepare the family and teen with making this decision. For more on sperm banking, see Chapter 18.

Boys and girls with leukemia are at equal risk for the spread of the disease to the central nervous system. When this happens, the leukemia cells have mysteriously eluded the chemotherapy and stayed alive by seeking refuge in the spinal fluid, sometimes even when the child has received chemotherapy given by spinal tap. If leukemia spreads to the central nervous system, the boy must receive radiation therapy to the brain and the entire length of the spinal column.

Radiation to the brain has many side effects, including nausea and vomiting, extreme tiredness after the treatment ends, and the risk of learning disabilities later in life. Parents need to advocate for special testing if they suspect their son has learning disabilities as a consequence of cancer therapy. Children with documented learning disabilities have certain government-protected educational rights, including the development of an Individualized Education Program. Parents are encouraged to check with their local school district for further information about their son's educational rights.

Lymphoma

Lymphoma is a cancer of the lymphoid system, a system that helps with immunity and the circulation of certain fluids. There are two different types of lymphoma: *Hodgkin's disease* (HD) and *non-Hodgkin's lymphoma* (NHL). Lymphomas can be confused with leukemia, since both diseases are a cancer of a blood cell. In leukemia, the blood cell that becomes cancerous is located in the bone marrow. In lymphoma, the blood cell is located in the lymph tissue and is called a lymphoid cell. Both types of cells play a role in fighting infection, although their roles are unique.

Lymphoma occurs more frequently in boys than in girls. It mostly strikes between the ages of seven and fourteen years. Certain genetic, immunological, viral, and environmental factors are suspected of having a part in its occurrence.

Boys who develop a lymphoma usually have a variety of symptoms, depending upon the location of the tumor or tumors. These may include enlarged lymph nodes in the neck and upper chest region, an enlarged spleen and liver, loss of appetite, weight loss, tiredness, night sweats, abdominal pain, and trouble with the respiratory system. The disease can develop very rapidly and the enlarged lymph nodes can become quite obvious. In a few cases, masses in the abdomen and lungs become so enlarged and grow so rapidly that the child becomes critically ill. These situations are treated as an emergency, and treatment must be started very quickly.

Therapy for lymphomas includes chemotherapy and radiation therapy. Some boys, because of the location and small size of the lymphoma, receive only radiation or chemotherapy. Other boys will need both forms of treatment. Chemotherapy consists of several different types of drugs, all given according to a specific plan or protocol. The duration of therapy depends on the type of lymphoma and whether the lymphoma has spread to other areas of the body. Treatment may last for only a few months or as long as two years. The prognosis for survival varies greatly. When a lymphoma is treated in its earliest stage, the chance for cure is quite high. Advanced disease is very hard to treat and the outcome is much less predictable.

Boys who develop a lymphoma are at a very active age. Many are involved in sports and other group activities, and the effects of the illness and treatment can complicate their continued participation. It is important to help the boy remain a part of his circle of friends and be as involved in their activities as possible while going through therapy. The boy may have just become interested in expanding his social circle to include activities with girls. The diagnosis of cancer at this youthful age can assault his courage to develop these relationships. It is very important, during these formative years, for the boy with cancer to remain in school, participate in peer activities, and expand his social circle.

Medulloblastoma

Brain tumors occur more often in childhood than in later life, striking nearly 1,500 children each year. There are several types of brain tumors that occur at different ages in childhood and in different areas of the brain. Twenty-five percent of all childhood brain tumors are *medulloblastomas*, which are diagnosed more often in boys than in girls. This brain tumor is located in the lower part of the posterior brain known as the cerebellum. In pediatrics, most brain tumors occur in the posterior regions—or back part—of the brain while adult brain tumors rarely occur in this area. The cause of childhood brain tumors is unknown, but the role of heredity and prenatal/perinatal exposure to harmful environmental agents are being investigated.

Medulloblastoma is a rapidly growing tumor that can cause *hydro-cephalus* or swelling of the brain. The boy may complain of headaches and vomiting (which are usually worse in the morning), tiredness, double vision, and an unsteady walk. In infants, the head circumference may become enlarged.

The treatment for medulloblastoma includes radiation and chemotherapy. For a boy who is under the age of two or three years, chemotherapy alone is the preferred treatment until he grows older. Radiation is delayed in infants and toddlers to help prevent unnecessary brain injury and damage to the bones that make up the spine. Unfortunately, progression of the brain tumor despite chemotherapy may make radiation therapy necessary despite its risks to the small child.

Radiation therapy must include the brain and the entire length of the spine because the cancerous cells have likely spread into the cerebral spinal fluid. The radiation dose to the brain and spine must be high enough to destroy the tumor. Unfortunately, this results in harmful effects, which become apparent as the boy goes through childhood. He will have some learning deficiencies, endocrine or hormonal dysfunctions, and growth abnormalities. The boy must be carefully followed by medical specialists and placed on appropriate hormonal replacement therapies. Because the spine was irradiated, normal growth of the spinal bones will not occur. As a result, the boy's torso will be disproportionately short in comparison to the rest of his body. The physical disfigurement may be quite plain to see.

Boys who become long-term survivors of brain tumors face difficult futures. They will need assistance in dealing with their abnormal physical stature and their learning deficiencies, and should be tested for possible placement in special school programs for children with unique educational needs. They may also be eligible for disability assistance programs. These boys may not develop adequate self-esteem and may become self-conscience and reclusive, or they may act out and be rejected by their peers. The family will need to work hard to provide this boy with the acceptance and socialization he may not receive from his peer group.

Rhabdomyosarcoma

A cancer that develops from certain types of muscle tissue is called *rhab-domyosarcoma* (RMS) or *undifferentiated sarcoma*. It occurs slightly more often in males during peak years of two to six and at fifteen to nineteen years of age. Frequent sites for occurrence are the head and neck region and the bladder and prostate area. Although its cause is unknown, RMS has been associated with familial cancer syndromes.

The signs and symptoms of RMS vary depending upon the location of the tumor. In general, the tumor mass presses upon local blood vessels and organs, causing pain and swelling. Rhabdomyosarcoma of the eye region will cause the eye to droop or bulge, RMS of the *paranasal sinuses* can cause nasal obstruction, and RMS of the bladder can cause urinary difficulties. A biopsy of the tumor is necessary to make the proper diagnosis and determine appropriate therapy.

Treatment of RMS includes surgery, chemotherapy, and radiation therapy. The purpose of surgery is to remove the tumor totally or, if that is impossible, partially. Surgery is followed by a specific plan of chemotherapy plus radiation therapy to the primary site of the tumor. This treatment regimen is very intense but its rewards can be great. Over 70 percent of cases have long-term survival rates if there was no spread of the cancer at the time of diagnosis. Because RMS is a cancer of many subtypes, a prediction of outcomes must be made on an individual basis.

The long-term effects of cancer therapy in boys treated for RMS can be distressing. Radiation to facial bones of a young boy can result in an uneven growth that requires corrective plastic surgery. Radiation and surgery to the lower pelvis and genitourinary tract can result in ejaculatory dysfunction, scarring of the ureters, and bowel or bladder obstruction. Radiation therapy for orbital RMS can eventually lead to cataracts. The boy will require regular medical follow-up once treatment is over so that problems that arise are quickly managed and corrected.

Osteosarcoma

Adolescent boys are at risk for a type of bone tumor called *osteosarcoma* (OS). These tumors usually occur during the teen years when boys are growing rapidly. The bones most at risk include the end of the femur nearest the knee, the upper end of the tibia, and the humerus nearest the shoulder. Certain genetic illnesses including *osteogenesis imperfecta* and *Paget's disease* put the boy at risk for the development of OS. Trauma does not cause this cancer, but trauma to the site usually draws attention to the problem.

Boys with OS will eventually have pain, with or without swelling, and a mass at the site of pain. The pain can be so severe it makes activities, including walking, too painful to do. At the time the tumor is diagnosed, 20 percent of these cancers will have spread into the lungs or nearby organs. There are different subtypes of OS, so a biopsy of the tumor is necessary for an accurate diagnosis.

Surgery is very important in the management of OS. Chemotherapy is administered before and after surgery. Before surgery, chemotherapy is given either by vein or through a catheter inserted directly into the tumor. Surgery may involve either amputation or limb salvage. Decisions around amputation depend greatly upon the size of the tumor, the extent of tumor spread, the age of the child, and whether the boy is likely to have acceptable function either from limb salvage or from an artificial limb. In certain limb salvage procedures, the boy will not be able to bend the knee of the affected leg, and the growth plate of the opposite leg will be stapled to stop it from growing. Newer limb salvage techniques and extraordinary artificial limbs are being developed. The family and teen need to work closely with the orthopedic surgeon in making the best decision.

The teenage years are years of expanding social circles, developing relationships, and participation in physical activities and mark the beginning of freedom from one's parents. The challenges of OS threaten a young man's ability to participate thoroughly in these milestone achievements. Strong psychosocial support, a faithful community of friends, and a supportive school system are very helpful.

Cancers Specific to Childhood

Several cancers occur only in childhood. Their rate of occurrence may be equal between boys and girls, but since they do not occur in adulthood they are worth discussing.

Neuroblastoma

Neuroblastoma is a cancer that occurs in about five hundred infants and very young children each year. The malignant cells come from neural crest cells, cells found in an embryo, which normally give rise to the adrenal glands and central nervous system. For unknown reasons, these beginning cells either are delayed or do not complete their maturation process. There may be a genetic component contributing to the cancer's development.

Tumors can occur in the abdomen, spine, chest, pelvis, and wherever the central nervous system is located. Newborns may be quite ill from this tumor at birth and need to be cared for in a Neonatal Intensive Care Unit. An older baby may develop an enlarged abdomen related to the tumor. An affected toddler may refuse to walk because of pain from a tumor near the spinal cord. Some children have no symptoms at all and the neuroblastoma is discovered during normal baby checkups.

Neuroblastoma is a mysterious disease. The tumor can, in the first several months of the baby's life, disappear by itself without the need for medical attention. It is believed that some babies have neuroblastoma that spontaneously goes away without ever being discovered. In these cases, the baby experiences a delay in its development and the maturation is completed after birth rather than before.

The treatment for neuroblastoma varies. Some babies require no treatment; the tumor shrinks and disappears on its own. Some children will require only surgery to remove the tumor, while others will need aggressive treatment with surgery, chemotherapy, and radiation therapy. Children who are older than twelve months of age, have a tumor that has spread to other parts of the body, and whose tumor cells contain specific cellular disorders are at high risk for responding poorly to therapy. Unfortunately, most children with neuroblastoma fall into this category.

Even if the child has a poor prognosis, in most cases it is very worthwhile to begin therapy. Therapy can help to reduce the size of the tumor and decrease the severity of the child's symptoms. Treatment can help the child feel better, have less pain, and enjoy a reasonable quality of life. Children with a good prognosis can expect a cure from therapy.

Wilms' Tumor

Wilms' tumor is a tumor of the kidney. Four hundred cases occur every year, mostly in children two to three years of age. The cause is unknown, but some cases are familial or associated with genetic abnormalities. Most children have few symptoms except for a painless enlargement of the abdomen, which is most commonly discovered by family members. The tumor can spread to other parts of the body including the liver and lungs.

Surgery is the mainstay of treatment. The entire kidney, with the tumor attached, is carefully removed by the pediatric surgeon. The surrounding area, including the opposite kidney, is checked for cancer spread. Afterward, the child is treated with chemotherapy to destroy cancer cells that may have spread to other areas of the body. The child may also receive radiation therapy. The size of the tumor, the specific subtype of Wilms' tumor, and whether the cancer has spread determines if radiation therapy is added to the child's treatment plan.

Most children do well after treatment for Wilms' tumor. A survival rate of 80 to 90 percent is common, even in children whose cancer has spread to other parts of the body.

Retinoblastoma

Retinoblastoma is a cancerous embryonic tumor of the retina of the eye. This very rare tumor occurs in two forms: *hereditary*, which accounts for 40 percent of all cases, and *sporadic*. In the hereditary form of retinoblastoma, the disease is inherited from either parent. It makes its appearance in the first few months of life. Tumors may occur in both eyes. In children with sporadic retinoblastoma, the tumor appears between the ages of two to three years and is usually confined to one eye.

Both men and women can carrying the gene for retinoblastoma. The parent who carries the gene has a 40 percent chance of passing on the disease to offspring. People who know they carry this gene are advised to have genetic counseling before starting a family.

Retinoblastoma can be a localized tumor affecting only the retina, or it can spread to the optic nerve, the lining of the brain, and the central nervous system. The diagnosis is made during a complete fundoscopic examination the doctor performs while the child is sedated or under general anesthesia. Children with retinoblastoma may develop a white light in the pupil called *leukocoria*, have strabismus (cross-eye) of the involved eye, or red, painful eyes. Treatment is begun immediately after diagnoses.

Treatment is individualized but commonly includes *enucleation*, or surgical removal of the eye. However, a clear understanding of this disease and starting treatment during early stages can, in some cases, save the child's eye. Three to six weeks after enucleation, the socket is fitted for an artificial eye. A new artificial eye will be required about every five years. If the child has the disease in both eyes, the best eye will not be removed but will be treated using other methods. If the remaining eye does not respond to therapy, an enucleation of the remaining eye must be considered.

Radiation therapy is very effective in the treatment of retinoblastoma. It can help control the tumor, thus saving the child's useful vision. Because the child is so young at the time retinoblastoma occurs, it frequently becomes necessary to sedate the child or use general anesthesia to keep the child still during radiation treatments. Other therapies include the use of *photocoagulation* to destroy the blood vessels that supply the tumor. *Cryotherapy*, or the application of extreme cold, has the same effect. These treatments will have a scaring effect on parts of the eye structure, which will have an impact upon vision. The remaining vision may be satisfactorily correctable but some children will be challenged by some degree of blindness for their entire lives.

Chemotherapy is useful if the cancer has spread to the lining of the brain or the central nervous system. However, the prognosis for the child is poor when this occurs.

The five-year survival rate for children with retinoblastoma is 90 percent if diagnosed and treated early. Useful vision can be retained if enucleation can be avoided and the tumor does not spread to the macula. Unfortunately, retinoblastoma increases the child's risk of developing other forms of cancer early in adult life. These include cancers of the bone, breast, prostate, and bladder. These cancers are often resistant to therapy.

The Challenges of Childhood Cancer

Issues of Physical and Emotional Development

Children in their early years are going through major stages of rapid physical and emotional development. Playing and learning social skills through organized activities can be threatened by the isolation the boy with cancer frequently experiences. Young boys in cancer therapy are often kept away from other children as a means to minimize exposure to infections. It is important for parents to include their son in playgroups and activities during the days blood counts are not low and the boy is feeling well.

School

School-age boys can have frequent absences from school because of cancer treatments and illness. It is important that the boy continues his studies at home or is enrolled in a home-bound education program. In this way, he will keep up with his peers and maintain normal milestones of development.

Peer Relationships

The adolescent is particularly burdened with the consequences of cancer and cancer therapy. The boy must deal with physical changes such as hair loss, limb amputation, acne, and weight gain from steroid therapy that make him different from other boys. It is not uncommon for high schools to prohibit the wearing of hats, a common strategy to cover hair loss, making it difficult for the adolescent to hide his illness. Classmates can be very exclusive when they learn a boy has cancer. It is difficult for the boy to deal with these rejections during the time in his life when being a member of a group and participating in group activities are so important. Efforts to date and establish personal relationships with others builds self-esteem and self-worth. But it is hard for the boy with cancer to be successful in this during the time of cancer treatment.

Family Issues

Family life is changed by the cancer diagnosis, and the boy may feel responsible and guilty for these changes. The family will need to define a new "normal" and discourage any suggestions that the boy is at fault. Family dynamics can be strained during stressful moments of cancer therapy, and siblings very often feel ignored and forgotten. Parents need to devote special time to the siblings and to each other throughout the experience.

Long-Term Survivorship

Becoming a long-term survivor of cancer does not mean the disease is forever in the past. The boy needs to be prepared for a life with a history of cancer. This includes regular examinations by a doctor for the rest of his life. The boy must be forthcoming with future health care providers about his cancer history so that proper follow-up examinations and screenings can be conducted. Cancers that arise from cancer treatments are a possibility for some, and diligent monitoring for these possible problems is essential.

Today, more and more young boys and adolescents are surviving cancer and becoming productive members of society. However, society is not necessarily ready to receive them. Discrimination may occur; the survivor may have difficulty getting and keeping health insurance or life insurance, being admitted to college, or finding employment. These discriminatory acts must be brought to the attention of lawmakers; legal counsel can assist in challenging these acts.

Cancer is a life-threatening disease, but today's advancements in therapy have made it possible for many young boys and adolescents to survive. Future research will help increase survival and improve quality of life.

Resources for Children with Cancer and Their Families

There are many wish, philanthropic, or charitable organizations throughout the country that exist to grant wishes to children with certain illnesses. These organizations either serve all qualified children or limit their assistance to children who live within their locale. Children eligible for wishes do *not* need to be terminally ill; this is a common misconception. Generally, all children who have life-threatening illnesses or chronic diseases are eligible.

In most cases, it is better to wait until the child is stable and feeling well before a wish is granted. This way, the child can fully enjoy the experience. In some situations, the wish organization may need to act quickly if the child is critically ill. Most wish organizations limit the age of children who are eligible, usually age two years to seventeen years. There are too many wish organizations to list and some are better funded than others. Please contact social services at the major treatment center for a more complete list.

Wish Organizations

B.A.S.E. Camp Children's Cancer Foundation
4651 North Pine Hills Rd.
Orlando FL 32808   (407) 297-9648   (407) 298-3928 fax

Does not grant wishes but does help obtain free or reduced price tickets to central Florida attractions including Walt Disney World and Universal Studios.

The Lisa Madonia Memorial Fund
409 Veloit
Forest Park IL 60130   (708) 366-2057   (708) 366-2065 fax

Grants wishes to those eighteen to twenty-five years old with cancer.

Make-A-Wish Foundation of America
100 W. Clarendon, Suite 2200   (602) 279-WISH
Phoenix AZ 85013   (800) 722-WISH (602) 279-0855 fax

U.S. and international chapters and affiliates. A well-funded organization.

Starlight Foundation
10920 Wilshire Blvd., Suite 1640
Los Angeles CA 90024   (213) 208-5885   (213) 824-9624 fax

Grants approximately one hundred wishes each month to children throughout the U.S., U.K., Australia, and Canada

Sunshine Foundation
PO Box 255
5400 County Rd. 547 N
Loughman FL 33858   (813) 424-4188 (800) 457-1976

Grants wishes to children ages three to twenty-one years.

There are also a great many camps for children with cancer and their siblings, and some camps that are open to entire families. Many of these camps are local, but some are open to children from all over. Some camps—

those that are especially well funded—are able to cover the expense of the child to travel to and from camp. Please check with social services at a major treatment center for a list of camps your child may be eligible to attend.

Part III

◆◆◆

Treatment and Management of Cancer

11

◆◆◆

An Overview of Cancer Treatment

Pamela J. Haylock, R.N., M.A., and Kerry A. McGinn, R.N., M.A., N.P.

Cancer treatment plans are developed specific to each person, his type of cancer, what is known about the natural history of that kind of cancer, the tumor cells' known sensitivity to different forms of treatment, and the man's general health status.

Cancer treatments are either *local* or *systemic*. Local therapies are directed to only a very defined or local part of the body. The two most commonly used local cancer therapies are surgery and radiation therapy. *Systemic* therapies, such as chemotherapy and the use of biologic modifiers, are given through the blood's circulatory system and will eventually be distributed through the entire body.

Goals of Cancer Treatment

The goals of treating cancer, no matter what kind of cancer or what form of treatment, fit into one of three major categories:

1. **Cure**: The goal of treatment is the destruction of all cancer cells, including areas of microscopic metastatic tumors. There are four categories of curative therapy:

   • **Primary therapy**: The first and major therapeutic attempt to cure the cancer

- **Neoadjuvant therapy**: Chemotherapy or radiation therapy used to reduce the size of the tumor before the primary therapy
- **Adjuvant therapy**: Therapy given to supplement the primary therapy to increase the chances of cure
- **Salvage therapy**: Therapy used to treat patients who have persistent or progressive disease remaining after primary therapy

2. **Control**: When cure is not a realistic goal, cancer can often be controlled for an extended period of time, offering increased survival and quality of life.

3. **Palliation**: When cure or control are no longer possible, palliative-care protocols can reduce tumor size, extend life, or improve the quality of life through minimizing distressing symptoms.

It is important for the man and his health care team to be in complete agreement about what, exactly, is the goal of his cancer treatment.

Sequence of Cancer Therapy

After the cancer diagnosis, the man, the family members or friends he wishes to include, and his doctor or doctors will discuss the options for treatment that best fit his particular situation. Whether the goal is cure, control, or palliation, the man must be fully informed about the desired outcome of the treatment, what the treatment regimen will entail, how long it will take, his or his family's responsibilities for self-care, and the risks and benefits of following the proposed course of treatment. It is at this time, before any course of treatment is finalized, that a man may want to consider taking part in a clinical trial. Information about cancer clinical trials is provided in Chapter 15.

When cure or control is the goal, treatment generally follows a course that starts with the *primary* treatment and is followed by an *adjuvant therapy*. In the most typical situation, surgery is the primary therapy, followed by either chemotherapy, radiation therapy alone, or a sequence that uses both. Most oncology experts agree that the success or failure of primary therapy provides a fairly reliable indicator of how successful the entire course of treatment will be. In other words, if cure is a goal, the primary therapy offers the best shot. For this reason, it is critically important that the doctor who manages the primary treatment be at the top of his or her game. This is not to say that a man should travel great distances to see a doctor who is world renowned, but it will be in his best interest to be assured of the doctor's skill in the procedure or treatment modality being suggested. Chapter 3, "Your Cancer Care Team," offers suggestions on how to assemble a health care team that offers the man his best chance of achieving the best outcome possible.

When cure or control is no longer possible, the man can still hope to control the distressing symptoms of cancer and maintain the quality of the time remaining to him through various forms of *palliation*. Palliative care is reviewed more fully in Chapter 19.

Making Treatment Decisions

Making a decision about which form of treatment to have requires a good deal of thought. An important thing to keep in mind is that, for most men, *cancer is not an emergency*. There is time to get all of the information needed so that the decision is well thought out. After all, this decision will no doubt affect the rest of this man's life and perhaps affect his family and other loved ones as well.

"How do I choose?" "What treatment is best?" For most people, these are complicated questions. Some people wish for "the good old days," when the doctor made all the decisions. One thing that many people forget is that in those "good old days," there were no real treatment options. Instead, there was one accepted standard therapy that all or at least most cancer experts agreed was the way to treat a particular kind of cancer. With the exception of a man's choice to forego treatment at all, there was no real choice, no decision to be made. If he wanted to be treated for his cancer, then he agreed to undergo the standard therapy. Certainly, the decision-making process was much more clear when there were no real choices.

Here at the beginning of the twenty-first century most men who are diagnosed with cancer will be confronted with two, three, four, or even more treatment options depending on the type of cancer and his unique situation. Customs of medical practice have changed as well: doctors are no longer expected to make decisions for their patients. Doctors are, however, expected to provide all of the information necessary to allow patients to make *fully-informed* decisions.

As people travel through life, they learn to make decisions in their own ways. A man's style of decision making is unique to him, but will be formed by his family experience, his culture, his educational level, and his role in life. The emotional impact of being diagnosed with cancer quite often interferes with a man's ability to make decisions, even simple day-to-day decisions. Still, studies of cancer survivors tell us that the man's involvement in the decision-making process is important and will make a difference in how he copes with the side effects of treatment.

There are basically three kinds of decision-makers: (1) those who want the doctor to make all the decisions; (2) those who make decisions after talking with others; and (3) those who make decisions totally on their own. If the man, his family, and the health care team have a good understanding of the man's decision-making style, he will be better able to make decisions he can comfortably live with literally for the rest of his life. A man who customarily has relied on others to make decisions for him will most likely need some coaching, and perhaps a little extra time, to feel right about the decisions he needs to make. A man who feels the need to talk to others must balance time with the available options; the more options that are presented, the more time will probably be needed for the man to reach a final decision. The man who is used to going it alone may face a good deal of confusion as he tries to sort out the "what ifs" inherent in each option.

Expert second opinions are sometimes very helpful in the decision-making process. Support groups or individual cancer survivors can also be helpful. Many men at first find it difficult to talk to other men about such an intimate topic as cancer, but what survivors have to say about their treatment choices, their experiences, and their outcomes can offer much different perspectives than doctors'.

The Cancer Survival Toolbox offers this simple exercise as a way to help get started with making decisions:

- At the top of a sheet of paper, list things in life that are important in your life.

- Draw a line down the middle of the paper. On one side, write the positive things (the "pros") about the treatment option being considered. On the other side, write the negative things (the "cons").

- Look at the list of the pros and cons and think about how they relate to those things that are important in your life.

- Put this paper away for a day or two. Then take it out and think over your lists again. At this time, you might want to make changes in the pros and cons in the lists.

- If there are other people in your life, it might be helpful to share this list with them, and to use the list as a guide to talking about the decisions that are ahead.

To summarize, the basic elements of decision making are:

- Learn the facts. The health care team needs to provide most of the factual information: What kind of cancer? What stage? What are the treatment options? What expertise is available?

- How much time is available in which to make a decision?

- Consider what is important in life. How might each treatment option affect what's important?

- What are the pros and cons of each treatment option and how do these fit with what is important to the man and his family, his lifestyle, his plans for the future?

- If a course of treatment is chosen, what is expected of the man who has the cancer, his family or other caregivers, his doctor, and the other members of the health care team?

Making decisions will always be an important part of life. Most men— and women, too—feel that the element of control is one of the most important aspects of living with cancer. Having a say in the way one's cancer is managed is critical. When a person follows the basic elements of good decision making, he helps ensure that his wishes are followed.

Where Treatment Occurs

Increasingly, cancer treatment occurs in an outpatient clinic or a doctor's office. Some estimates indicate that over 80 percent of all cancer treatment now occurs outside of the hospital setting. Still, the safety net that is, at least theoretically, offered within the confines of a hospital is preferred for some complex cancer treatment situations. Many times, the first cycle of a new chemotherapy protocol is given in a hospital, particularly if the doctor's office is not equipped to handle potentially complex and/or severe treatment-related side effects. Many surgical procedures, including biopsies, can be done in an ambulatory surgical center or a well-equipped doctor's office. On the other hand, major operations still require the technical support and expert care that a hospital provides.

The Hospital Experience

Many men have never been patients in a hospital. Although some men with cancer never need hospitalization, if hospitalization will be part of your cancer experience, you need to know what to expect.

For insurance reasons, most patients now stay in the hospital for the shortest possible time. This means that anything that can be done before admission (such as blood work, X-rays, and physical examination) may be done on an outpatient basis. It also means that hospitalized patients may be discharged from the hospital before they feel they are fully recovered. Because patients are not hospitalized unless they truly need acute care, and because the number of hospital staff may not reflect the intense level of care needed, hospital personnel are often stretched—and stressed.

Read and carefully follow any preadmission instructions from the hospital. Valuables are best left at home, except for a few dollars perhaps and a wedding ring or watch, which the hospital staff will lock up for safekeeping. Bring a list of any medications you are taking at home, including the name of the drug, the dosage, and the frequency, but not the pills themselves. Hospitals must follow strict fire safety regulations and may have special rules for small electrical appliances such as shavers or hair dryers.

Hospitals provide gowns and sometimes slippers and robes. A second hospital gown can be worn opening in front in place of a robe. Some men prefer to bring their own pajamas. Some men also like to bring a photograph of family members or someone else special to place on the bedside table. This marks their spot, reminds them of life outside the hospital, and sometimes serves as a communication-starter with hospital personnel.

If you have your surgery or treatment in a teaching hospital, you may tell your story to, be examined by, and receive much of your everyday treatment from *house staff*, residents and interns who have finished medical school and are licensed physicians, but are honing their clinical skills under the supervision of more experienced doctors. (Interns are not the same as internists, doctors who have taken specialty training in internal medicine.) A man may have "his" intern or resident, with primary house-staff responsibility for his case.

The surgeon, urologist, or other cancer doctor acts as an *attending* doctor, supervising the house staff. The attending doctor may see each patient once or twice a day or have a covering doctor see his patients (on weekends, perhaps). If a problem requiring medical attention arises at another time, the nurse usually notifies the intern or resident in a teaching hospital; if this doctor cannot resolve the problem, the attending doctor is notified.

A fairly new development in some hospitals is the *hospitalist*, an experienced doctor, usually an internist, who specializes in the care of people in the hospital. If your hospital uses a hospitalist, he may be the attending doctor with primary responsibility for any nonsurgical, non-cancer-related care you need in the hospital. The hospitalist communicates with your other "outside" doctors so that they can plan care together; the arrangement saves the outside doctors from hospital trips.

Hospitals have their own vocabulary, and it is always okay to ask what something means. Some common terms include *PRN*, an abbreviation for a Latin phrase meaning "as needed," referring to medicines or treatments given only at the patient's request or if the nurse or doctor thinks there is a need. PRN dosing has been used often for pain medications, but its application as a valid pain management strategy is now being questioned by pain experts. *NPO* is an abbreviation for "nothing by mouth," meaning the patient is not supposed to eat or drink anything. The word *void* refers to emptying the bladder, or urinating.

The man in the hospital deserves considerate and respectful care, information about his diagnosis and treatment in words he can understand, and concern for his privacy. His rights are further spelled out in the Patient's Bill of Rights, formulated by the American Hospital Association and often given to a patient at admission or on request.

Consideration works both ways. For example, you should use the nurse call bell when you need help, but first ask yourself, "Is this a necessary request, something I need a nurse for?" "Could I combine two or more requests into one?" Of course, if there is any question about safety, use the call bell. Too many men, reluctant to "bother" anyone when they have to get up for the first time after surgery to use the toilet, climb over the side rails and fall. Any nurse would rather be "bothered."

A few hospitals encourage interested patients to read and contribute information to their own medical charts. This is a small but growing movement and reinforces the concept of patient and health care workers as members of a team sharing responsibility for a man's health.

The confinement of the hospital setting offers the advantage of concentrating the health care experts in one place. A good cancer treatment facility will have readily available—or at least readily accessible through a responsive referral system—the help that is most often needed by people facing cancer. Nutritional experts, physical and occupational therapists, financial counselors (to help sort through a man's insurance plans and find financial assistance when necessary), experts in comfort management, and social workers should also be available to the man and his family and friends.

The Physician's Office

Increasingly, elements of the diagnostic workup, and sometimes the entire treatment plan, are provided in the doctor's office. A growing number of office settings offer very sophisticated, systematic approaches to cancer care.

The office setting has several advantages over a hospital or clinic. First, it is usually simpler to access. For many people with cancer, access to cancer treatment in one's home community is a very real need. When facing potentially difficult treatment and side effects, the convenience of being treated close to home becomes an important consideration. Personally knowing the doctor, nurses, and other staff who are members of the community can be encouraging. The waiting rooms are usually not nearly as busy or chaotic as waiting areas in the hospital or clinic, and check-in is usually a simple affair.

The downside of an office-based treatment setting can include lack of skilled staff—sometimes there is not even a registered nurse, let alone a knowledgeable, certified oncology nurse—and minimal or no access to other health care experts such as social workers, nutritionists, and psychologists. If this is the case, the man and his family need to take more active, assertive, and creative roles in identifying their needs and finding ways to have those needs be met.

Finding Resources

Most communities, even in rural settings, have community resources that can provide needed assistance to patients and families. The growing electronic linkages offered by telecommunications and the Internet are opening channels of communication and assistance to persons in previously underserved and isolated areas. A social worker, a hospital discharge planner, the financial counselor, or your nurse or doctor should be able to provide at least a beginning list of resources available in your local area. The Resources section of this book is another good place to look for assistance.

A growing number of hospitals and public libraries offer health resource centers and the assistance of a health educator or health science librarian. People who have felt left to drift with all their questions quite often express great surprise when they discover the wealth of resources and information available to them once they really start to search. For some, finding and accessing resources might take some effort, but the effort is most often rewarding, and the result can be the feeling of at last having some control of one's life.

12

◆◆◆

Surgery

Patricia J. Kroft, R.N., B.S.N.

This chapter describes what needs to happen before, during, and after surgery. It is very general, so be sure to read the section of this book that addresses the type of cancer that concerns you, as well.

Surgery can be used in all phases of cancer. Until the advent of radiation therapy and chemotherapy, surgery was the only form of cancer treatment. Today, it is still the primary method for curing about a third of all people with localized cancers.

Surgery is used in the management of cancer in the following ways:

Prevention Surgical procedures are often used to remove precancerous lesions such as colon polyps or skin moles.

Diagnosis Any procedure that is done for the purpose of getting a sample of suspicious cells—such as a biopsy—is technically a form of surgery. *Local excision* is the removal of all local tumor and can be curative for some forms of cancer. Sometimes, major surgery that is being done for other medical problems results in an accidental, or at least unexpected, finding of cancer.

Cure Surgery is the most common approach to cure for many forms of cancer. Curative surgery is possible when the cancer is known to be contained in a specific organ or part of the body and can be totally removed without greatly endangering the patient. Adjacent affected organs or tissues, or nearby lymph nodes, may also be removed. In curative surgery, the surgeon (or surgeons) also attempts to make sure that the margins or edges of the tissue removed are free of cancerous tissue. Surgery alone cannot cure cancers that have spread beyond the primary site of cancer.

De-bulking   A surgical procedure to remove the biggest part of a tumor or to reduce the amount of cancer (the *tumor burden*) present in the body, when it is known that the cancer cannot be entirely removed, is called *de-bulking* surgery. De-bulking surgery is done before other forms of therapy are used and is a way to increase the effectiveness of adjuvant therapies.

Staging   On occasion, the actual extent, or *stage*, of cancer cannot be determined until the primary site—or *tumor bed*—is examined by the surgeon during surgery. The pathologist also examines the tumor and other tissues removed during surgery and may discover that the tumor has spread beyond what was initially believed to be the case. Staging that is determined as a result of surgical findings is referred to as *surgical staging*, whereas staging that is done on the basis of clinical examinations is *clinical staging*.

Palliation   Quite often, surgery can help reduce distressing symptoms caused by cancer that cannot be cured or controlled. In palliative surgery, an attempt is made to remove as much of the cancer as possible. This is done to allow other vital organs room to function normally and allow the patient to be more comfortable. For example, a tumor that is pressing on a nerve and causing pain, obstruction, or other symptoms might be reduced in size during a surgical procedure.

Before Surgery

Maybe the most important preparation any man can make for surgery is to be absolutely sure he is comfortable with the decision to *have* surgery. Confidence with the decision and faith in the surgical team's abilities are essential for a comfortable and speedy recovery. The man considering surgery needs to understand exactly what surgery is planned and how the operation will help him begin to recover.

Surgery

Once a decision is made, several meetings with the surgeon and at least some of his or her surgical care team will occur in the weeks or days before the actual operation is scheduled. Each of these meetings provides opportunities to ask questions about anything that is not clear or fully understood. In preparation for the operation, additional tests are performed so that the surgical team is completely aware of the patient's overall health status, including whether vital organs such as kidneys, heart, lungs, and liver are functioning normally. Blood samples are likely to be taken, and a urine sample will probably be needed as well. Other preoperative testing may include breathing tests and an electrocardiogram (EKG). In addition, the surgeon may want additional scans and X-rays.

If there is a possibility of blood loss associated with the planned surgery, the surgeon may suggest that the patient donate some of his own blood. This blood is stored in the blood bank and can be transfused back during or after the surgery, when blood counts might be low. Another option is to ask a friend or relative with the same blood type to donate a unit of blood. This blood is also stored in the blood bank, designated for *only* this one patient.

Informed Consent

At some point during the preoperative period, the surgeon will ask the patient to sign an *informed consent* or *surgical permit* for surgery. The only time someone other than the patient can sign the consent form is when the patient is physically unable, or his mental status makes his full understanding of the implications of surgery questionable. Except in cases of emergency (usually not the situation with regard to cancer-related surgeries), the patient must have an advanced directive or health care proxy that allows another person to provide permission to operate.

Before the consent is signed, risks and possible complications will again be explained in detail. By this time, the patient and his family should be well aware of any complications or unusual occurrences that may occur during and after surgery. If the patient or his family members do not feel totally informed, or for some reason feel uncomfortable with the decision to have surgery, this is an opportunity to get answers to questions or have other concerns allayed to the extent possible. Actually, a patient can ask questions, get clarification, and even cancel surgery up to the point of the first surgical incision, even though the permit has been signed.

Possible Surgical Complications

Modern surgical techniques have become almost routine and reasonably safe. Still, as a part of the informed consent process, the surgeon is ethically and legally obligated to explain the risks, even the risks that would be *very unlikely* to occur, that go along with the planned surgical procedure, including unexpected complications during or as a result of the surgery. Also, it is very important for men and their family members to know about and understand expected changes. For men having cancer surgery, surgical outcomes such as impotence, urinary incontinence, and changes in self-image are not unusual. Bodily function and body image changes are expected when the surgery requires creation of a stoma—an opening into the body that allows waste to drain to the outside. The man and his family or caregivers need to have a full understanding about the self-care requirements this kind of operation will entail.

Complications and expected changes can be permanent or temporary. Feeding tubes, drainage tubes, or long intravenous lines placed during surgery may stay in place for several days, weeks, or even months. These devices entail new skills that the patient—or his caregiver—must learn and perfect. Any of these changes may affect a man's lifestyle and the way he socializes with friends or family. Sometimes, the counseling of a social worker or nurse, or other emotional support, can help a man and his family work through this period. The man's signature on the informed consent form implies that he understands potential changes and complications and agrees to have the surgery performed.

Men who have any special requests for treatment during surgery should make sure these wishes are clearly stated in the consent. Some patients, Jehovah's Witnesses for example, may have strong feelings about receiving blood transfusions. Any wish regarding blood transfusions should be made clear to the surgical team and appear on the consent.

The Surgery Experience

Preparing for Surgery

In the few days just before the surgery and depending on the type of surgery, a man might be on a special diet. Bowel surgery, for example, requires that the bowel be "clean" and essentially empty. Laxatives or enemas are often used to clear the bowel of any stool.

People who have been taking aspirin, ibuprofen, or certain other anti-inflammatory drugs can expect to be asked to stop taking them for a week or so before surgery, to guard against prolonged blood-clotting times resulting in excess bleeding during the operation. The surgeon and anesthesiologist should be reminded about any other medicines that are used on a daily basis. Some drugs should *not* be stopped and need to be taken on the day of surgery. The doctor or nurse will tell you what drugs, if any, should be taken and at what time; they should be swallowed with just a sip of water. In general, men preparing for surgery can be expected to be asked not to drink or eat anything after midnight on the night before surgery. These precautions are important to prevent food or water from accidentally going into the lungs during the time the patient is under anesthesia.

The Day of Surgery

The current trend is for the patient to be admitted to the hospital early in the morning on the day of surgery. Most people appreciate the company of a family member or friend during the admission process and in the waiting period before surgery. Usually, a patient goes to a preoperative holding area to be admitted. If the recovery period is expected to be more than twenty-four hours, he will probably be admitted to the nursing care unit where he will stay after surgery.

For men who will go home immediately after surgery or within twenty-four hours, the admission procedure often takes place in a room near the operating room. Either way, a surgical nurse will conduct an admission interview and assess weight and vital signs, including temperature, pulse, and respiration or breathing rate. It is likely that an intravenous line will be placed in the patient's arm.

It's wise to leave valuables including money, wallet, and jewelry at home. Bring hearing aids, glasses, prosthetics, and dentures to the hospital. The admitting nurse needs to know what personal items have been brought along. These items will probably not go into the operating room, but the patient may need them in the early recovery period, in which case the nurse will place them in a safe place until they are needed postoperatively.

Personal clothing will be stored somewhere safe and hospital pajamas will be provided. The look would not be complete without paper shoes and a paper bonnet to cover the hair; the nurse may also ask that special elastic stockings, designed to prevent blood from pooling in leg veins during long periods of immobility, be used. The man will be allowed to rest in bed or on a gurney until he is escorted to surgery. Family members are usually allowed to wait in the pre-op holding area.

A man who takes a regular dose of pain medication at home should discuss pain management with his surgeon before coming to the hospital. Arrangements should be made that allow the pain control program to continue before and after surgery, perhaps by using a different dose and route of administration.

If the man is already hospitalized when surgery becomes necessary, hospital personnel will handle most of the preoperative tasks; the man does not have to worry about what he should eat and when, what medicines to take, when to wake up the morning of surgery in order to arrive at the hospital in time, or transportation to and from the hospital. Still, it is always best to be well informed about the surgery agenda and to ask questions if events seem to be off schedule. The hospitalized person is escorted from his hospital room directly to the operating room or preoperative holding area when it is time for surgery.

Preanesthetic Interview

Whether the surgery occurs during a hospitalization or as an outpatient surgical procedure, someone from the anesthesia care team will visit before surgery. The anesthesia care team is a group of anesthesiologists and possibly nurse-anesthetists that provides anesthesia to patients in surgery. Along with the patient, the anesthesia provider will make a decision about what type of anesthetic is needed for the operation. The preanesthesia assessment will include questions about the patient's general health, any allergies, and routinely used medicines. Prescription drugs, over-the-counter drugs, vitamins or herbal supplements, and illegal drugs need to be reported to the anesthesia provider. Some preparations that people might not consider to be drugs—such as St. John's Wort—can be quite dangerous when combined with certain anesthetics. Even if these substances are not taken on the day of surgery, the anesthesia provider needs to know they have been used recently. Be sure to remind your anesthesia provider of any drugs that you took with just a sip of water the morning of surgery.

The anesthesia provider will ask about any history of heart or lung problems, stroke, diabetes, smoking, or alcohol use. He or she will listen to the heart and lungs with a stethoscope and look inside the mouth. It is very important that the anesthesia provider knows about loose teeth or removable dental work. Past surgical history can provide important information, too, especially if a past surgical experience involved any problems. A personal or even family history of high fever during or immediately after surgery offers an important clue regarding a hereditary condition that can cause fever to develop. Since fever is also an indication of infection or reactions to blood products and some medications, knowing that a patient could have this condition helps the anesthesiologist understand and manage the symptom in the correct way. The preanesthetic interview also offers the patient and family the opportunity to learn how vital signs are to be monitored during the surgery.

By the time the interview takes place, an intravenous catheter (IV line) will probably have been inserted in an arm or leg. If not, the anesthesia provider may put one in place during the interview. All patients need an IV line before they get to the operating room; it is used to administer not only drugs for anesthesia but also postoperative fluids to provide hydration, antibiotics, sedatives, pain killers, and possibly blood transfusions. Some surgeries require that a catheter be placed in a large vein in the neck or in an artery to allow proper and accurate monitoring throughout surgery and during the immediate postoperative time. Some men, depending on the type of surgery, need to have a tube (often called a *Foley catheter*) inserted into the penis. The function of this catheter is to drain urine from the bladder; it is usually placed while the patient is asleep, so he will not feel discomfort. Even if the surgeon has been informed about preferences for blood transfusions, the anesthesia provider needs to know this information as well since he or she is the person who will administer any blood products during surgery.

Anesthesia

All surgeries require some form of anesthetic. A few of the surgeries done for cancer, such as relatively simple biopsies and removal of the testicle (an *orchiectomy*), can be done with a local anesthetic. The surgeon injects a very small amount of a numbing drug into the surgical area, and the services of the anesthesia team may not be required.

Major surgeries, however, require an anesthesia care provider to administer the anesthetic. The risks of anesthesia will have been explained during the anesthesia interview, but questions can still be asked until anesthesia is actually started. The choice of anesthetic can be a general anesthetic, a regional anesthetic, or a combination of both. No matter what form of anesthesia is selected, the anesthesia care provider remains with the patient throughout the entire surgery, monitoring vital signs and giving additional anesthesia and fluids as they become necessary. After surgery, during the immediate recovery period, the anesthesia provider is available to help with any additional pain relief that is needed once the anesthetic wears off.

If a general anesthetic is used, the patient is essentially asleep, breathing through a mask or a tube placed in the throat. Since the breathing tube is placed after the patient has gone to sleep, he won't be aware of the procedure. A combination of drugs and gases provides the anesthesia, and the anesthesia care provider controls the patient's breathing. When the surgery is completed, he or she reverses the anesthesia to awaken the patient.

With some types of surgeries, a regional anesthetic, sometimes referred to as a regional block, can be used. The anesthesia provider injects drugs, similar to the Novocain used by a dentist, near the nerves in the surgical area. The anesthetized area becomes numb and the patient is unable to move. After surgery, once the medicine in the regional block has worn off, feeling and mobility should return to normal. With a regional anesthetic, the patient can be awake, but most patients who have this type of anesthesia feel more comfortable not listening to the constant noise and commotion in operating room. The anesthesia provider can use an intravenous sedative that allows the patient to take a little "nap" during surgery. The sedative wears off while the patient is in the recovery area.

The Operating Room

Before going into the operating room, the patient will be interviewed by one of the nurses who will be present during the surgery. The nurse confirms the patient's name and the type of surgery, inquires about allergies, and verifies that the patient has not had food or drink during the preceding hours. She or he also needs to know about any medications that were taken by the patient prior to surgery and any current or past skin problems, including sensitivity to soaps (especially soaps that contain betadine or iodine) or skin irritation following Latex use. At some time right before surgery, a nurse or technician will shave all body hair from the incision site.

When the patient enters the operating room, he will most likely be awake. The room will probably be cold and seem very foreign. There will be several machines, many instruments, and many people in the operating room. Even the simplest of surgeries is typically staffed by at least two surgeons, two nurses, and the anesthesia care provider. In addition, members of the departments of pathology, radiology, nuclear medicine, and radiation oncology are often called in to the operating room to assist. If it is frightening to see all the members of the surgical team, just remember that they are there for just one reason—to ensure your safety and well-being. After the patient is positioned on the operating room table, the anesthesia provider attaches monitoring devices and begins the process of sedation that comes just before general or regional anesthetic.

There is a designated area of the hospital where family members can wait as the surgery is being done. When the surgeon is finished, he or she will usually look for family members to give them a report of what happened during the surgery and provide an update of the patient's condition. Family or friends are usually not allowed to visit until the patient leaves the recovery area.

The Postoperative Period

After surgery is completed, patients wake up in the operating room or recovery room. Most do not remember waking up, since some of the drugs used can cause partial amnesia. The first memory after surgery is usually the voices of nurses in the recovery area. Many patients feel they have lost all sense of time; some feel as if they have not yet been to surgery. Often, patients are very cold and shiver as they wake up. All of these reactions are common, expected, and need not be a source of concern.

The recovery nurses will provide warm blankets and do what they can to make the patient comfortable. They will check vital signs and bandages or dressings frequently. Extra oxygen from a nasal cannula or an oxygen mask might be given during this time. Nurses will monitor the blood's oxygen content (called *oxygen saturation*) with a *pulse oximeter*, which is attached to a finger, toe, or ear. The nurses frequently assess the patient's mental status by asking him the date, his name, and to describe where he is. Inability to remember these things is expected and not a cause for worry; memory will improve as the anesthetic wears off. The nurses should be informed of any discomfort, pain, or nausea so that appropriate symptom management can be put into action.

As drowsiness subsides, the patient will be asked to *cough* and *deep breathe*. During surgery and when a person is on bed rest, parts of the lungs can collapse. Taking very deep breaths and coughing restore the lungs to their normal capacity. It is a good idea to begin breathing exercises even before surgery. Take a deep, slow breath in through the mouth. Hold it for three to four seconds and then breathe out slowly. Practice this technique at home, and do it ten times every waking hour after surgery. If the exercise causes dizziness, take more time between each breath. The nurses or a respiratory therapist may offer a plastic machine that assists the patient to take big, full breaths. A schedule of hourly deep breathing exercises should continue through the first several days following surgery.

The patient must remain in the recovery area until he is fully awake or until the effects of the regional anesthetic have worn off. As soon as the recovery nurse determines that the anesthetic has dissipated and vital signs are stable, the patient will be discharged from the recovery area.

After discharge from the recovery area, the patient goes to a postrecovery area if the plan is for him to return home the day of surgery. He can dress in his own clothes and begin eating and drinking. Usually the patient is allowed to go home when he meets criteria set up by the ambulatory surgical center or come-and-go surgery unit. These criteria vary from center to center; generally, postoperative pain or nausea should be under control and the man should be able to eat, drink, and urinate before he is released.

Patients who plan to go home on the day of surgery should not expect to drive themselves. Whenever possible, they should also not be alone the first night and day after surgery. Men who live alone and have no one who can stay with them would be wise to make this information known early in the planning stages so that home care services might be arranged, or arrangements might be made for the man to stay in the hospital an extra day. When the man is released, the nurses should provide a list of signs and symptoms to watch for or monitor, as well as a telephone number to call to report symptoms of dizziness, excessive pain or nausea, fever, or increasing redness or drainage at the dressing site, or to ask questions regarding post-op recovery.

Men who are not ready to go home right after surgery will go to a nursing care unit specializing in postoperative care or to an intensive care unit (ICU). Sometimes, the ICU admission occurs directly from the operating room, bypassing the recovery area.

Some surgeries for cancer are extensive. The more difficult the surgery, the longer the surgical procedure takes. Large surgeries are more likely to have more blood loss and bigger fluid shifts, which will affect blood pressure, heart rate, and other aspects of the cardiovascular system. The man who undergoes extensive surgery typically requires more postoperative care and monitoring than regular surgical unit facilities and nurse staffing can provide. If this is the case, the surgeon may routinely reserve a bed in the ICU. The surgical staff expects patients with certain surgeries always to be admitted to the ICU even if they experienced no problems in the operating room.

The Intensive Care Unit (ICU)

Most intensive care units are very busy, noisy places. Every patient is connected to a monitoring device that, at a minimum, continually displays the cardiogram, blood pressure, and oxygen saturation. Conditions can change very quickly, and monitors help nursing personnel notice the changes as soon as they occur. The monitors have alarms that sound when something is amiss and beep when the patient moves about in the bed or becomes disconnected from the wires.

While an ICU patient, a man will usually have a Foley catheter in his penis to help collect and monitor the amount and color of urine. A tube inserted through the nose into the stomach (the *nasogastric tube*) drains stomach contents. Depending on the type of surgery, other drainage tubes may be in place; lung surgery typically requires the use of tubes in the chest cavity, called *chest tubes*, that aide in reexpanding the lungs. For more explicit information on the immediate postoperative routines or surgeries designed to fight your specific kind of cancer, be sure to read the applicable chapter of this book.

ICU patients are allowed visitors, usually restricted to the immediate family or significant other. Visitors are instructed to keep the visits short; five to ten minutes every hour is a common routine. Visitors are usually expected to check with the nurse before entering.

The ICU might be a frightening place. Most patients there spend a good deal of time sedated, napping, or sleeping. The nurse awakens the patient when it is time for bathing, receiving treatments, deep breathing and coughing, having dressings checked, changing positions, and so forth. Frequent sampling of blood for chemical analysis is expected; some patients have a catheter in an artery that allows the ICU staff to take a blood sample without having to insert another needle. Supplemental oxygen is provided via a nasal tube or a mask. Typically, patients in an ICU have frequent visits from their doctors and frequent X-rays and other studies. Because the nurses perform the same functions around the clock, and because there may be no windows in the ICU room or cubicle, patients often become disoriented and confused. For example, a patient may wake up, see that it is five o'clock, and feel convinced that it is morning and the start of a new day, when actually it is five o'clock in the evening. ICU patients at times hallucinate. If it is frightening to be a patient in an ICU, it is perhaps even more frightening for family and friends who visit. As the need for pain medication diminishes, normal sleep and activity resumes and patients should again look and act as they did before surgery.

If your surgeon recommends a stay in an ICU, it is because he or she knows you need technical monitoring and the kind of care and attention that only the highly skilled ICU staff can provide. ICUs also have a high ratio of nurses per patient, allowing each patient to get the attention he needs. Every effort is made to stabilize the cardiovascular system, to remove as many tubes as possible, and to get the patient up and moving around as quickly as possible in order to transfer him to the more comfortable step-down unit or post-op surgical unit.

Postoperative Surgical Unit

For a patient on the post-op surgical unit, the main goal is for him to regain his independence. A typical postoperative day involves being awakened early for vital signs and maybe a bed bath. Deep breathing and coughing exercises will continue every waking hour. Staff members use stethoscopes to listen to the abdomen; when they can hear rumblings indicating that the bowel is attempting to resume normal function, the patient will be allowed to eat and drink. Once a normal diet is resumed, bowels should begin working properly, and bowel movements should resume as well.

Leg exercises will consist of pointing and flexing toes and doing leg lifts.

As a result of continued immobility, blood tends to pool in the veins of the legs, causing circulation problems. Exercises can help, but the best way to prevent circulation problems and also to get lungs and digestion back to normal is to begin walking the halls of the surgical floor—and walking as much as possible.

The Foley catheter will be removed as soon as it is determined that the patient is strong enough to walk to the bathroom and can urinate on his own. Periods of urinary incontinence after your catheter is removed can be expected. It is important, however, to keep the nurse and doctor informed about any problems with urinary function. For most men, this problem will go away with time.

Many hospital personnel enter a patient's room unannounced. The surgeon can be expected to visit frequently and a nurse who specializes in cancer care may visit as well. Staff from the lab will stop by for blood samples, and a portable chest X-ray might be taken. A respiratory therapist will come by once or twice a day to provide breathing treatments. A nutritionist might visit to discuss diet. If a stoma was created, a nurse who specializes in stoma care will visit and teach the patient or his caregiver how to manage it appropriately. The oncologist can also be expected to visit. Some men, while they are still in the hospital and if they are feeling well, may begin radiation or chemotherapy if the treatment plan calls for either of these. Many other hospital personnel are there for you, if you ask to see them. The hospital chaplain can offer prayers and spiritual support. Most hospitals also employ a social worker who has special knowledge and skills that cancer survivors will find particularly helpful. The social worker can help solve problems, prepare for discharge, and arrange for access to other resources in the community. He or she can also help you arrange home care to assist with treatments and recovery.

Postoperative Pain Control

For most people, postoperative pain is one of the greatest fears. Fortunately, pain is fairly easy to control during an inpatient hospital stay. Initially, the nurses can give pain drugs via an injection or through IV tubing. Another option is *patient-controlled analgesia* (PCA), in which a metered dose of a pain-killing drug—an *analgesic*—is automatically injected into an intravenous line when the patient pushes a button. PCA is set up on a machine that will not allow more analgesic medicine than is safe.

While in surgery, particularly in extensive surgeries involving the abdomen or pelvis, the anesthesia care provider may have placed a special catheter, called an *epidural catheter*, near the spinal column. After surgery, the anesthesia provider can inject narcotics into the catheter to relieve surgical pain. As the patient's condition begins to improve, he will be ready to take pain medication by mouth. Getting pain under control after surgery contributes to recovery. For more information about the management of pain, see Chapter 17.

Going Home

Discharge from the hospital occurs when the surgeon's criteria for safe discharge are met. The surgical incision must be dry and not inflamed. There should be no sign of fever or infection, and pain should be under control with medication you can take by mouth. Usually, all of the tubes and the intravenous line are discontinued before discharge, but some patients may go home with one or more of these; home care nurses or a designated family care giver may be needed to manage these tubes or lines if the patient has not been prepared to manage these kinds of equipment himself.

By the time of discharge, bodily functions such as eating, drinking, urinating, and having a bowel movement should be close to normal. The nurse should provide a list of signs of possible postoperative problems, as well as a telephone number the patient can call if he has any questions. Any changes needed in daily activities should be known and expected, and the patient should clearly understand when it is safe for him to drive, have sex, or lift heavy objects.

After discharge from the hospital, follow-up office visits with both the surgeon and the oncologist can be expected. The follow-up schedule should be made very clear, and the man must know when and with whom to schedule follow-up appointments.

Survivor Support

If they haven't done so already, the members of the cancer care team can help get you involved with appropriate support groups, advocacy groups, and other forms of educational offerings. Quite often, a newly diagnosed cancer survivor is visited by a member of a support group while still a patient in the hospital. This will most likely be a man who has been diagnosed with the same type of cancer, someone who has experienced similar feelings and fears. Although the patient may find it difficult to talk to a stranger or may not initially be interested in support groups, many men choose to use the information later, and attend group sessions as part of their healing process. Staying in touch with other cancer survivors and the cancer nurses and social workers who moderate these support groups can increase awareness of any new treatments or ways to handle possible postoperative problems such as incontinence or fatigue. Your wife, partner, or close friend may also benefit from a support group.

Postoperative Healing

Many cancer survivors are surprised at how long it takes to feel normal again following surgery. One man might claim that he feels fit after a few short weeks, while another needs one month, two months, or sometimes more to feel back to his old self. The start of *adjuvant therapy*—postoperative chemotherapy and/or radiation therapy—adds to the stress of the recovery period. This is also the time that many men begin to come to terms with their cancer and the emotional strain that cancer survivorship entails. All of these mental and physical processes are a part of the natural healing process, the process of getting well.

13

♦♦♦

Radiation Therapy

Pamela J. Haylock, R.N., M.A.

Radiation is a form of *local* therapy that is used at some point in the therapy of at least half of all people with cancer. Radiation can be used to cure, control, and palliate cancers, and, depending on the circumstances, can be used alone or in combination with chemotherapy and/or surgery. Radiation as cancer therapy was introduced in Vienna, in 1896, when it was used to reduce a tumor on the nose of a young girl. Between then and now, the technological advances, including computer technologies, have reduced or minimized toxicities, while the accuracy and effectiveness of this treatment modality offer control and even cure for thousands of people.

How Radiation Works Against Cancer

Radiation therapy, or *radiotherapy*, refers to the therapeutic use of high-energy rays in the treatment of cancer or other forms of neoplasia. When high voltage is applied to an electronic vacuum tube, high-speed molecules call *electrons* are produced. These electrons hit a target, and, while most of the energy is transformed into heat, some form a beam of energy. *Gamma rays* are formed when the source of radiation is a radioactive material such as cobalt 60 or cesium 137. Cobalt units commonly used in radiotherapy contain a radioactive cobalt source. Linear accelerator units accelerate the electrons, thereby producing high-energy radiation. As the energy increases, so does its penetrating ability, allowing the radiation to go into deeper levels of tissue.

Radiation acts on live cells at the molecular level, affecting only those cells and tissues that lie in the path of the beam. The biologic effect of radiation is produced by the *ionization* of various parts of the cell, hence the term *ionizing radiation*. The energy of the beam frees electrons from the cell's atoms, causing ionization. The freed electrons cause more ionization until the energy is used up or depleted. The end result of the damage to the cell is the disruption of the cell cycle and cell functions, affecting cells that are the most rapidly dividing. The extent of the interaction between the radiation and the part of the cell that is in the path of the beam depends on the energy of the beam.

The action of ionizing radiation is the same on both normal and cancer cells. An early effect of radiation on cells is the delay of cell division. Permanent effects include damage to the chromosomes and disruption of cell division. Some cells will recover from a certain level of damage and continue to live, grow, and divide. But, when another injury occurs—say, from another exposure to radiation—damaged cells are unable to recover. The cumulative effect of all of this damage is the death of the affected cells.

A feedback system initiated by the death of cells "tells" the body that some repairs are needed—this is the normal healing process—but cancer cells seem to be unaffected by this reparative stimulus. Normal cells that survive an initial but sub-lethal dose usually recover within twenty-four hours. The interruption of exposure to radiation, allowing for repair of normal cells, is the rationale for *fractionation*—the division of a total dose into even, daily *fractions*—of therapeutic exposure to radiation. While the normal cells can and do repair themselves during the interruption, cancer cells cannot recover and will be exposed to the radiation energy as additional fractions are given, adding further injury and finally resulting in cell death.

The effect of radiation on the cells is in direct proportion to the *dose* or amount of radiation to which cells are exposed. Radiation dose is calculated by the measurement units called *gray* (Gy) or *centigray* (cGy) or *rad* (one gray = 100 rad; one rad = one centigray). In 1985, the term *rad* (acronym for *radiation absorbed dose*) was officially replaced by the term *gray*, and current scientific literature consistently uses *grays* or *centigrays*.

The vulnerability of cells, their *radiosensitivity*, varies throughout the body. Cells are sensitive to radiation in direct proportion to their reproductive or mitotic activity and in inverse proportion to their level of specialization. This is true of both cancer and noncancer cells. In other words, cells that are dividing rapidly are generally more sensitive to the effects of radiation. And cells that are highly specialized, such as nerve cells, are usually *not* very sensitive to the effects of radiation.

Radiation Therapy Techniques

Radiation is administered in two ways. In *external* radiation, sometimes also called *teletherapy*, radiation is delivered by a radioactive source or electro-magnetic energy from a machine that is placed at a distance from the targeted site. Therapeutic radiation is also administered when radioactive sources are placed on or in a tumor. These techniques are called *internal radiation therapy, implant therapy*, or *brachytherapy*.

External Beam Radiation

The most common method of delivering radiation is by the *external* method, also referred to as *external beam* radiation therapy. External beam radiation is further categorized according to the level of energy of the beam and by the ability of the radiation to penetrate into deeper layers of tissue. Table 13.1 lists the various kinds of external beam equipment and the most common uses of each.

Table 13.1: Types of External Beam Radiation Equipment and their Clinical Uses

Equipment	Clinical Uses
Kilovoltage	Superficial penetration: Good for skin cancers.
Orthovoltage	Deeper penetration: Most often used to treat cancers involving head and neck. Results in a high dose to the skin in order to achieve the desired penetration to the tumor.
Megavoltage/ Supervoltage (Cobalt)	Deep penetration that spares the skin, and is used to treat deep-seated tumors—those that are deep within the body.
Linear Accelerator	The most common system used to deliver radiation today. Allows for deep penetration that spares the skin.
Photons	Used to treat deep-seated tumors.
Electrons	Most Linear Accelerators have the capacity to use electrons, which give the maximum dose to the skin and the tissues just under the skin. Electrons are useful in the treatment of skin tumors and lymph nodes that are just under the skin.

Treatment Planning Treatment planning is the process of figuring out how to achieve the maximum destruction of cancer cells while protecting normal cells, tissues, and organs. Accurate treatment planning is crucial to the safe delivery of external radiation therapy. The radiation oncologist prescribes the treatment plan, which includes the treatment site, the number of fields to be treated, the daily dose and number of fractions, total dose, any blocks or beam modifications that will be needed, and the kind of radiation therapy equipment to be used.

Just as in other forms of cancer treatment, there is an approximate *dose* of radiation that is known to be effective against different types of cancer. It is also known that one dose of radiation has more effect on tissues than that same dose when it is divided into several smaller doses, or *fractions*. Fractionation of the total desired dose is coordinated to take advantage of the cellular effects of radiation, the fact that injured cells generally attempt to repair damage within twenty-four hours. Normal cells repair themselves during the interval between daily doses, while cancer cells lack this reparative ability. In this way, fractionation is a factor in protecting, or *sparing*, normal tissues.

After staging is completed but *before* treatment starts, information gathered from the clinical examination, staging workup, and imaging studies are used to precisely outline the targeted area, or *treatment field*, and in this way minimize exposure of normal tissues that surround the area being treated. Planning machines called *simulators* mimic the functions of the type of radiation equipment that will be used, without actually delivering therapeutic doses of radiation. Some modern simulators use CT-simulation—combining computerized axial tomographic scanning capability (CT or CAT scans) with simulation. This allows the patient's anatomy to be viewed from the same vantage point as the radiation beam. During simulation, X-ray or CT images simulate the treatment field that will be targeted. Sometimes, customized blocks that shield vital organs and other normal tissues are designed and constructed during the simulation process. During treatments, the radiation therapy technician attaches these blocks to the radiation therapy equipment, thereby shielding the patient from unnecessary exposure of normal structures.

Using computerized technology, a medical or radiation physicist or dosimetrist determines the best way of distributing a given radiation dose for each patient. Optimal dose distribution is managed by using devices such as blocks or wedges to filter or shift the path of the beam. Sometimes, several fields are used so that the tumor gets the desired dose and normal tissues and structures are spared.

X-ray images of the treatment field—called *port films*—generated on the radiation therapy machine are usually taken on the first day of treatment as a way to confirm the final plan. Weekly port films are used to ensure that the radiation beams and blocks are being positioned correctly throughout the course of treatment.

External Beam Radiation Treatments Most of the time, the desired total, or *cumulative,* dose is divided into even fractions. Each fraction is given during one scheduled appointment. So, depending on the goals of treatment and the desired cumulative dose, a course of radiation therapy will be completed over a period of weeks, with treatments usually given on a Monday-through-Friday schedule. Radiation therapy used to control symptoms rather than achieve a cure usually calls for a shorter, less intensive treatment plan. After the process of simulation is completed and the first day's port films confirm the final plan, the time needed for daily treatments is usually between fifteen and thirty minutes.

Recent Advances in External Beam Radiation Therapy

The therapeutic use of radiation has evolved over the last century and continues to this day. By applying new technologies, new techniques for the safe use of radioactive materials continue to evolve, resulting in breakthroughs in cancer treatment.

Conformal Radiation Therapy Made possible by CT-simulation techniques, conformal radiation therapy allows for the beam to *conform* more closely to the size and shape of a targeted tumor. This reduces exposure of normal, healthy tissues and organs that surround the tumor, resulting in the ability to deliver higher doses of radiation to the tumor without causing undue side effects.

Intensity-Modulated Radiation Therapy Intensity-modulated radiation therapy is a three-dimensional form of conformal therapy. Three-dimensional computer imaging techniques are used to plan and deliver even more tightly focused beams to tumors. Conformal and intensity-modulated radiation therapy has already been useful in the treatment of prostate cancers and head and neck cancers. Its precision helps prevent complications—such as rectal problems that occur during prostate cancer therapy or salivary gland injuries that occur with radiation of head and neck tumors that are otherwise associated with traditional delivery techniques.

Stereotactic Radiosurgery Stereotactic radiosurgery is a three-dimensional delivery technique in which the total dose is delivered all at one time, instead of being divided into the fractionated delivery system used in standard radiation therapy. Several beams deliver a high-radiation dose to small sections or a small volume of tumor. Stereotactic techniques are being used to treat vascular malformations in the brain that cannot be reached with traditional surgical approaches. Stereotactic radiosurgery is also used to treat brain tumors alone or in combination with external beam radiation therapy.

B-Mode Acquisition and Targeting B-mode acquisition and targeting is a system that combines ultrasound and a three-dimensional positioning tool to pinpoint treatment sites as radiation is being given. It is another way to greatly increase the precision targeting by the radiation beam and reduce exposure of normal tissues around the tumor.

Brachytherapy

Brachytherapy techniques are those in which a radioactive source is in direct or close contact with the targeted tumor. A major advantage of brachytherapy techniques is that the delivery of radiation does not have to go through normal tissues to get to the tumor, and high doses of radiation can be delivered to tumors while surrounding tissues are spared unnecessary exposure. The intended end result is fewer side effects and higher cure rates.

Radioactive chemical elements called "isotopes" are used in brachytherapy. As the isotope ages, it goes through a *decay* process, in which it becomes less and less powerful, losing energy over time. The decay process is measured in what is called the *half-life* of the isotope. The half-life is the amount of time it takes the isotope to lose half of its energy. For example, it takes over one thousand years for the isotope radium to decay to half of its energy level, whereas it takes just over two months for the isotope iridium to lose half its energy. Each isotope has its own, distinctive energy level and half-life, which are the determining factors in selecting a particular isotope for use in treating different forms of cancer. The most commonly used radioisotopes, their uses, and half-life are listed in table 13.2.

Brachytherapy techniques use either *temporary* or *permanent* implantation. The radioactive sources are made in several forms, including needles, seeds, and ribbons. Seeds made from isotopes that have a short half-life and low energy level are used in permanent implants. These implants are inserted into the tumor through needles. Temporary implants use sources that have long half-lives and high energy levels; leaving them in the body for a long period of time would create significant damage.

Early brachytherapy techniques required the doctor to manually apply

Table 13.2: Radioactive Materials Used in Brachytherapy

Radioactive Isotope	Cancer	Half-Life
Cesium-137	Rectum; Esophagus; Uterus; Cervix	30 years
Cobalt-60	Ocular melanoma	5.26 years
Gold-198I	Prostate	2.7 days
Iodine-125	Prostate; Ocular melanoma; Lung (bronchus)	60.2 days
Iridium-192	Breast; Head and neck; Lung (bronchus)	74.2 days
Palladium	Prostate	17 days
Radium-226 (Use has been mostly replaced by cesium, gold, and iridium)	Endometrial; Cervix	1,600 years

or load the sources into the tumor, resulting in repeated radiation exposure for medical personnel. Now, *remote afterloading devices* allow radioactive sources to be inserted or "loaded" after staff leaves the treatment area. Afterloading techniques make it possible to use isotopes with higher energy or dose rates that reduce the time needed for optimal treatment with brachytherapy.

The brachytherapy techniques call for very exact placement of radioactive sources. Even a slight displacement results in incorrect dose delivery. Staging workup, including imaging studies, provide accurate pictures of the exact location, size, and shape of the targeted tumor. The technique to be used, and the form of treatment planning required, will vary according to the tumor type being treated, and its location.

General Side Effects of Radiation and Self-Care

When the anticancer effects of radiation were first discovered in 1896, the scientific world saw this form of treatment with a great deal of hope. But, within a year, medical journals carried papers that covered distressing side effects of radiation. Skin reactions, headache, vomiting, diarrhea, high temperature, and fatigue were the most commonly mentioned problems experienced by patients getting radiation treatments.

Radiation therapy techniques used at the beginning of the twenty-first century are vastly different and improved compared with those used throughout the previous century. High-voltage equipment and more exact diagnostic testing have enhanced the planning and administration of therapeutic radiation. Precise dose and fractionation schedules allow treatment plans to be tailored to each person and to each cancer. New techniques allow for very precise targeting of the cancer while sparing vital, healthy tissues and organs that surround the cancer. Radiation-related side effects are linked to the treatment field, dose, fractionation schedule, past and present use of certain kinds of chemotherapy, preexisting conditions, and general state of health.

The most common side effects associated with modern radiation therapy are divided into acute and delayed effects. Acute side effects are those that occur during the active treatment phase. Delayed side effects can occur throughout the weeks and months after therapy is completed. As noted earlier, the expected side effects are specific to the site of disease that is being treated. Fatigue and skin reactions occur in nearly all people who undergo radiation therapy.

Skin Reactions

Skin reactions are the most common side effect of radiation therapy. Cancer survivors who went through a course of radiation therapy before skin-sparing technologies and techniques were available quite often experienced painful radiation burns. Fortunately, burns are no longer an expected side effect but instead are avoided through careful treatment planning and astute monitoring by the radiation therapy team. Meticulous skin care can minimize skin reactions.

Nevertheless, the radiation beam must go through skin to reach just about any targeted site. The outer layer of skin (the *epidermis*), hair follicles, and oil-producing glands in the deeper skin layers are injured by radiation. Acute radiation reactions affecting skin within the treatment field follow a fairly constant course. Within the first two weeks of daily treatments, the skin will react with redness called *erythema*, similar to minor sunburn. As radiation continues, *dry desquamation* will occur, in which the outer layer of skin cells—*squamous* cells—gets dry and flaky. If the skin is not treated with moisturizers and radiation treatments continue, the reaction can progress to *moist desquamation*, in which deeper layers of skin cells are disrupted and fluid escapes from the damaged cells and tissues. In moist desquamation, the outer protective layer of skin is damaged, and bacteria can enter the body through the open sores.

Late or delayed skin changes such as inflammation, severe itching, or *pruritis*, and open sores or ulcers can appear months or even years after treatment ends. These late symptoms are caused by the aftereffects of radiation, including shrinking of or damage to the oil and sweat glands, changes in pigmentation or skin color, and changes in the blood vessels that lie beneath the skin in the treated area.

Some types of chemotherapy drugs (doxorubicin, 5-fluorouracil, methotrexate, and bleomycin, for example) cause a *radiation recall* reaction. When chemotherapy is given to a person who has previously been treated with radiation, the skin over the treatment field goes through changes similar to the skin reaction the person experienced during his radiation therapy. Also, people who get chemotherapy shortly before or during a course of radiation therapy are at an increased risk for serious skin changes. For this reason, it is imperative that all members of the health care team are aware of the full treatment plan.

The following are risk factors for radiation skin reactions:

- skin folds within the treatment fields (armpit, folds under the breasts, groin, genital area)

- poor nutritional status

- chemotherapy given just before or during radiation therapy

- dose and large field size

- use of orthovoltage or megavoltage equipment

- other health conditions that increase the vulnerability of skin

Meticulous skin care can minimize the severity of skin reactions and also decrease the chances of serious delayed skin changes. Table 13.3 provides a brief overview of skin care for persons going through external beam radiation therapy.

Fatigue

Fatigue is the only side effect of radiation that is not related to a particular treatment site. Nearly all people going through radiation therapy experience fatigue; it comes on slowly, seems to progress over time, and is not usually relieved by resting. Many people begin to feel fatigue within the first few weeks of treatment, but it can occur at any time during the course of treatment and sometimes persists through weeks or even months after therapy is completed.

A fairly large radiation treatment field and dose seem to increase fatigue levels. Other factors include a treatment plan that includes both

Table 13.3: Skin Care During External Beam Radiation Therapy

Skin Reaction / Assessments	Skin Care
Skin Reaction Erythema **Skin Assessments (things to look for)** Reddening or swelling of the skin in the treatment field, especially skin in body folds such as the armpit (axilla), neck, under the breasts, in the groin, genital, and rectal areas, and areas around a surgically created stoma	Gently clean the area using mild soap, or no soap at all, and warm water; gently pat dry with soft towel Avoid mechanical friction such as rough washcloths, bath brushes, aggressive massage, constrictive clothing, scratching, rubbing, and use of tape Avoid chemical irritants such as perfumes and lotions that contain menthol or alcohol; if the treatment field includes the area under the arm, avoid using antiperspirants or deodorants with metallic ingredients; avoid use of talcum powder or talc-containing products on or over the treatment field Moisturize the skin using nonirritating lotions, creams, gels, or ointments, or a 1% hydrocortisone cream Use an electric shaver instead of a blade shaver when shaving an area included in the treatment field Avoid extremes in temperature; avoid sun exposure to the treatment field Bring changes to the attention of the radiation technologist or radiation nurse
Skin Reaction Dry desquamation **Skin Assessments** Itching and dry and flaky skin over the treatment field, especially in the high-risk areas—skin folds, groin, genitals, rectum, and around the stoma	Same as with erythema described above Noncaking cornstarch applied over the area can decrease itching A variety of skin care products specially formulated for radiated skin can be recommended by radiation therapy team members Bring changes to the attention of the radiation therapy team
Skin Reaction Moist desquamation **Skin Assessments** Skin is red, swollen, moist or weeping	Bring to the attention of the radiation therapy team Treatment goals will be to prevent infection and to improve comfort; special dressings such as hydrocolloid, hydrogel, or polyurethane films can be recommended by the treatment team; special cleansing solutions, including mixtures of hydrogen peroxide and normal saline, should also be used in attempt to minimize chances of infection Moist desquamation often signals a need to take a "rest" from treatments which can be resumed when the skin is healed
Skin Reaction Late skin changes **Skin Assessments** Redness, itching over the treated area. Open sores and black, deadened, or necrotic skin occur rarely, but can still occur several years after treatment is completed	Notify the radiation oncology nurse or physician The physician will need to determine if these skin changes are related to previous radiation exposure or recurrence of the cancer Hydrocortisone cream or oil-based moisturizers applied to the area can provide comfort Topical or systemic antibiotics might be used to prevent or treat existing infection Severe skin damage may necessitate surgical skin grafting

chemotherapy and radiation therapy, anemia, immunosuppression, diminished physical abilities before treatment starts, the use of other medications, pain that is not well controlled, emotional factors such as anxiety, depression, or family concerns, and other chronic conditions such as lung disease, diabetes, and malnutrition. The radiation therapy nurse, radiation oncology doctor, and possibly a physical or occupational therapist can help the man and his family design a plan to cope with fatigue. Such a plan will include regular exercise, a planned rest schedule, energy-conservation techniques, and changing the level of stimulation in the man's environment.

Site-Specific Side Effects

Even though new radiation therapy techniques have increased the safety of this form of treatment, side effects still occur as a result of damage to normal cells in the treatment field. As the man prepares to start radiation therapy treatments, he should learn about his specific risks for side effects and ways that he can prevent or at least minimize these problems. Table 13.4 provides an overview of the most common acute and delayed side effects associated with radiation therapy and the self-care strategies that can minimize associated problems.

The Future

Since its first therapeutic application in the treatment of cancers over a century ago, radiation has generated excitement and hope. Today, technology is exploding, and there is every reason to believe that advances in technology will result in more effective radiation therapy techniques that spare normal tissues. Combining radiation with other treatment modalities such as *hyperthermia*, medications that increase cells' vulnerability to effects of radiation (*radiosensitizers*), or other medications that protect cells against the effects of radiation (*radiation protectors*) is an exciting prospect in the scientific exploration of the uses of radiation. Radiation therapy plays a very beneficial and valuable role in the local management of many forms of cancer, and chances are the potential benefits will only increase as technologies continue to evolve.

Radiation therapy is a highly specialized and fast changing field of care. Whenever treatment is being discussed, a valuable question should always be, "Is there a role for radiation therapy in my treatment plan?"

Table 13.4: Radiation Side Effects and Self-Care Interventions

Side Effect	Occurs When:	Self-Care Intervention	Notify Doctor or Nurse If You Get:
Alopecia (hair thinning or hair loss)	Treatment Field Includes: Head Other parts of the body covered with hair	Ask the radiation nurse or doctor if hair loss is a possible side effect Select a hair piece before hair loss begins, to assure color, style Keep hair clean; use mild pH-balanced shampoo Use cream rinse and soft brush to remove tangles Cut hair short and style to cover thin spots Cover head to protect scalp from sun exposure In cool climates, cover head with a warm cap to minimize heat loss	Hair loss a source of emotional distress (or discuss with professional counselor, social worker, member of the clergy, or peer support group)
Ear inflammation (otitis media) Eye inflammation (conjunctivitis)	Treatment Field Includes: Head and neck	Ask the doctor or nurse about the potential for these side effects	Earache, dizziness Itchy eye, redness, or irritation of eyelids
Dry mouth (xerostomia) Difficulty swallowing (esophagitis)	Treatment Field Includes: Head and neck	Consult with a dietician about helpful diet changes such as drinking liquids Use artificial saliva Suck on sugar-free candies Avoid hot, spicy, acidic foods Use thorough oral hygiene program Gargle and swallow a liquid pain-relieving solution Eat small frequent meals of soft foods Take high-protein diet supplement	White patches inside the mouth Increasing difficulty swallowing Weight loss
Changes in taste or smell	Treatment Field Includes: Head and neck	Visit dentist and complete dental work prior to starting therapy Ensure dentures fit properly Use a regular and thorough oral hygiene program: *rinse mouth before and after meals and snacks *use nonalcohol mouthwash *use soft toothbrush to gently brush tongue *gently floss at least once daily Vary the smell and texture of foods with each meal Avoid cooking smells	Weight loss of more than two pounds a week A major change in appetite Reduction of food intake

Radiation Therapy

Side Effect	Occurs When:	Self-Care Intervention	Notify Doctor or Nurse If You Get:
		Ask family member or friend to prepare meals; store meal-size portions in freezer	
		Switch from hot foods to cold foods such as cottage cheese, salads	
		Arrange for assistance from community organizations such as *Meals on Wheels*	
		Consult with a dietician	
		Use plastic utensils	
		Try marinated meats	
		Experiment with seasonings for meat	
Decreased appetite (anorexia)	Treatment Field Includes: Abdomen Pelvis	Consume a high-protein, high-calorie diet; consult a dietician on how to maintain diet	Rapid weight loss Major changes in appetite
		Eat small frequent meals	
		Try acidic beverages such as lemonade, orange juice, tomato juice	
		Serve foods attractively	
		Eat with someone whenever possible	
Bloating	Treatment Field Includes: Abdomen	Eat small frequent snacks (six per day)	
		Chew food thoroughly	
		Eat slowly	
		Sit or walk after meals	
		Avoid fatty, fried, greasy foods	
		Avoid gas-inducing vegetables	
		Avoid carbonated drinks	
		Avoid chewing gum	
		Avoid milk	
Nausea or vomiting	Treatment Field Includes: Abdomen Pelvis Chest Brain	Take prescribed antinausea medication; discuss best time to take it	Nausea or vomiting that prevents eating or keeping food down for twenty-four hours Signs of dehydration Bloating or pain before an episode of vomiting
		Discuss whether alterations in treatment schedule might be useful	
		Ask for help in controlling pain	
		Take antacids if useful	
		Drink liquids frequently	
		Avoid solid foods	
		Avoid hot foods	
		Avoid cooking odors	
		Use a thorough oral hygiene plan and clean mouth before meals and brush teeth after eating	
		Rinse mouth with nonalcohol mouthwash after vomiting	
		Eat slowly, chew food well	
		Use "seasickness bands" on wrists	

Table 13.4: Radiation Side Effects and Self-Care (Cont'd.)

Side Effect	Occurs When:	Self-Care Intervention	Notify Doctor or Nurse If You Get:
Cystitis (bladder irritation)	Treatment Field Includes: Pelvis	Drink at least 2–3 quarts of fluid daily Avoid coffee, tea, alcohol, tobacco products Urinate as often as possible Take Vitamin C (on the advice of doctor or nurse) to increase acid content of urine and decrease chance of infection	Frequent urination Urgent need to urinate Burning sensation when urinating Spasm pain when urinating Mucus in the urine Blood in the urine
Diarrhea	Treatment Field Includes: Abdomen Pelvis Rectum Perineum	Count the number of bowel movements each day Watch for signs of dehydration—dry skin and mouth, decreased urinary output, fatigue, sunken eyes Drink at least three quarts of fluuids daily Drink fluids at room temperature Design a nutritious liquid diet if diarrhea is severe Try cottage cheese, applesauce, rice, bananas; gradually add foods low in roughage Avoid drinking beverages with meals Avoid foods or drinks that produce gas or cause cramps Avoid caffeinated beverages Check with the doctor or nurse before applying topical pain medicines such as Desitin or vitamin A and D ointment to the anal area	Severe diarrhea (more than four bowel movments —liquid or formed —in a day) Over-the-counter drugs such as Pepto-Bismol, Kaopectate, or Imodium are not effective
Sleepiness, changes in level of consciousness	Treatment Field Includes: Head (brain) Spinal cord	Ask doctor or nurse about possibilities for this side effect	Change in level of alertness, increased sleepiness, confusion
Irritation of lung tissues (pneumonitis) Difficulty breathing (fibrosis)	Treatment Field Includes: Chest Breast	Pace activities to avoid becoming short of breath Humidify air with a vaporizer or through central heating system Drink warm fluids Suck on a cough drop or throat lozenge to quiet cough Drink at least 3 quarts of fluids daily	Shortness of breath Fever Dry cough

Radiation
Therapy

191

Table 13.4: Radiation Side Effects and Self-Care (Cont'd.)

Side Effect	Occurs When:	Self-Care Intervention	Notify Doctor or Nurse If You Get:
Bone marrow depression: *Anemia (decreased red blood cells) *Bleeding or bruising (decreased platelets: thrombocytopenia) *Infection (decreased mature white blood cells: leukopenia, granulocytopenia)	Treatment Field Includes: Large treatment fields and/or a treatment field that covers long bones in legs, arms, or sternum	Rest to conserve energy Stay away from crowds Take temperature every four hours while awake if signs of infection Use antiseptic, nonalcohol mouthwash Discuss diet, especially how much fluids to drink each day Always wear shoes or slippers to prevent injury to feet Wear gloves to do manual labor such as gardening, dishes, where there is a chance of getting small cuts or scrapes Protect against sunburn Use electric razor to avoid accidental cuts Avoid sexual activities that risks tears in the anus or penis; use lubrication	Dizziness Chills Fever (oral temperature greater than 101.5°F) Sore on skin; swelling and redness anywhere on the body Shortness of breath Extreme tiredness Rapid pulse Injury results in bleeding that does not stop within one hour Severe bruise or multiple bruises

14

◆ ◆ ◆

Systemic Therapy: Chemotherapy and Biotherapy

Pamela J. Haylock, R.N., M.A.

Systemic therapies—chemotherapy and biotherapy—function at cellular and even molecular levels to interrupt cell cycle or the cell's surroundings, thereby modifying growth and reproduction of cancer cells. Different chemicals have been used in attempts to modify growth of cancer since the first century A.D., when colchicine—a chemical still used in the treatment of gout—was used to treat tumors. Arsenic was first used against chronic leukemia in 1965. In an ironic twist, events early in World War II brought the use of chemicals into the scientific treatment of cancer. Soldiers who were exposed to mustard gas experienced severe infections, sometimes resulting in death, as a result of damage to bone marrow, where infection-fighting white blood cells are normally produced. Malfunction of the marrow results in decreased white blood cells and subsequent suppression of the immune system. Between 1942, when nitrogen mustard was first used in the treatment of lymphomas, and 1972, when Cisplatin was approved for treatment of testicular cancer, the major arsenal of chemotherapy drugs still in use at the start of the twenty-first century was developed.

Chemotherapy

Chemotherapy is a systemic therapy, targeting cells that are rapidly dividing. Some chemotherapy drugs work on cells only during one specific phase of the cell cycle—these are called *cell-cycle-specific* drugs. Other drugs, called *cell-cycle nonspecific*, work on cells regardless of the phase of the cell cycle.

Cell-cycle-specific agents damage cells that are in a specific phase of the cell cycle. These drugs are *schedule dependent*—the cell must be in a specific phase and the correct concentration of the drug must be achieved for optimum *cell kill* to occur. Usually, damage occurs in the S or M phases. These drugs are most effective on rapidly dividing cells. It is usually necessary to maintain a specific concentration of *cytotoxic* drugs—drugs that are toxic to cells—over a long period of time to allow the cancer cells to reach their most vulnerable phase.

Cell-cycle-nonspecific agents are equally toxic for cells in any phase of the cell cycle. They are dose dependent rather than schedule dependent—optimal cell kill and the toxicity the patient experiences are in proportion to the dose received.

Drug classifications are based on the chemical structures and the ways these cytotoxic drugs damage cells. There are five major classifications of chemotherapy drugs, plus a miscellaneous class in which drugs that don't fit in the other classes are placed. Table 14.1 provides a brief overview of the classifications, their mechanisms of action, and the kinds of cancers each is used to treat.

The ability of cytotoxic drugs to kill cells is based on the principle of *first order kinetics*. First order kinetics incorporates four actions:

1. A certain drug dose will kill a constant *percentage* of cells with each dose, rather than a constant number of cells.

2. Repeated doses are needed to decrease the total number of cells.

3. The number of cells left after each treatment depends upon the results of previous therapy, the time between repeated doses, and the doubling time of the tumor.

4. The tumor is eventually reduced to a number small enough that the immune system is able to kill remaining cells.

Chemotherapy drugs can be used alone, in *single-agent chemotherapy,* or in protocols that use two or more drugs, referred to as *combination chemotherapy.* Most chemotherapy regimens today involve combinations of drugs. The decision about which drugs to include in a treatment plan is based on how each drug affects cancer cells.

Table 14.1: Cytotoxic Chemotherapy, Mechanisms of Action, and Common Uses

Classification	Mechanism of Action	Uses	Drug Name	Major Toxicity
Alkylating agents (alkylators)	Cell-cycle nonspecific. Interfere with DNA synthesis and directly damage existing DNA.	Lymphoma Breast cancer Testicular cancer Pediatric cancers Brain tumors	Busulfan Chlorambucil Cyclosphamide Ifosfamide Carmustine (BCNU) Lomustine (CCNU) Streptozocin Carboplatin Cisplatin Dacarbazine (DTIC)	Possibly cause cancer Suppress bone marrow Broken down (metabolized) by the liver Eliminated from the body through the urinary tract
Anti-metabolites	Cell-cycle specific. Act in the S phase and block the production of DNA and RNA	Most effective against tumors that are growing rapidly: Breast cancer Testicular cancer Gastrointestinal system Lung cancer Head and neck cancer Skin cancer	5-Azacytadine 6-Mercaptopurine Cytarabine Fludarabine Fluorouracil Methotrexate Thioguanine	Suppress bone marrow Nausea and vomiting Mucositis Photosensitivity Broken down (metabolized) by the liver Eliminated from the body through the urinary tract
Antitumor antibiotics	Cell-cycle nonspecific. React with DNA and block production of RNA	Lymphoma Testicular cancer Leukemia Sarcoma Wilms' tumor Head and neck cancer Lung cancer Breast cancer Stomach cancer Pancreatic cancer Bladder cancer	Daunorubicin Doxorubicin Bleomycin Dactinomycin Mithramycin Mitomycin	Suppress bone marrow Damage muscle in the heart Broken down (metabolized) by the liver Eliminated from the body through the urinary tract
Plant Alkaloids: vinca alkaloids and podophyllo-toxins	Cell-cycle specific. Interfere with mitosis and block production of DNA and RNA	*Vinca alkaloids:* Lymphoma Acute leukemia Myeloma Breast cancer Testicular cancer Melanoma (Vindesine) Colon Lung	Vinblastine Vincristine Vindesine	Broken down in the body by the liver Eliminated from the body through bile, feces, and urine

Table 14.1: Cytotoxic Chemotherapy, Mechanisms of Action, and Common Uses (Cont'd.)

Classification	Mechanism of Action	Uses	Drug Name	Major Toxicity
Plant Alkaloids (cont'd)		*Podophyllotoxins:* Lymphoma Acute leukemia Pediatric sarcoma Neuroblastoma Testicular cancer Brain tumors Breast cancer	Etoposide (VP 16) Teniposide Taxol Taxotere	Podophyllotoxins are eliminated from the body through the urinary system and to some extent through bile
Hormones	Change the environment by blocking essential hormones and substituting similar chemical agents that can't be used by the cancer cells	Tumors that are sensitive to hormones: Breast cancer Prostate cancer	Adrenocortical agents: Hydrocortisone Prednisone Dexamethasone Androgens Dromostanolone Halotestin Testosterone Antiandrogen Flutamide Progestational agents Medroxyprogesterone (Depo-Provera) Megestrol (Megace) Antiestrogens Tamoxifen Estrogens Gonadotropin releasing Leuprolide (Lupron)	Specific metabolic changes are associated with each hormone
Miscellaneous	Can't be categorized		Procarbazine Hydroxyurea Mitotane Suramin Topotecan Aminoglutethamide Asparaginase	Most are broken down in the liver and elimnated through he urinary system

Drug selection is based on three factors:

1. The drug must be effective even when it is used alone.

2. The drugs selected must have different actions during the cell cycle.

3. The toxicity caused by each drug must be different than the toxicity caused by the other drugs in the combination.

Combination therapy takes advantage of cancer cells' traits of continuous division to trap the cells in the phase or phases when they are most vulnerable. The sequence of drug administration can be very important to the overall success of combination therapy. For example, one type of chemotherapy is given to increase the percentage of cells in a specific phase. This is called *synchronization*. The cell kill that occurs as a result of the first drug sort stimulates other cancer cells to enter cell division, where they will be vulnerable to the next drug. Another mechanism—called *recruitment*— transforms resting cells into dividing cells. As a result of cell kill, cells in resting phases are *recruited* back into the cell cycle and are more vulnerable to drugs that work on dividing cells.

When Chemotherapy Fails

Why is it that cancer cells seem to survive despite cancer treatment? The question of *treatment failure* has been a source of concern for decades. (An aside: Some doctors and nurses say, "The patient failed therapy." I suggest it was the treatment that failed the patient.) Only recently has the concept of multidrug resistance (MDR) been recognized. It seems that instead of being killed outright, some cancer cells mutate, giving rise to new cells resistant to drugs that have been used. It is thought that these mutant cells contain a pump that flushes out the cytotoxic agents, causing cancer chemotherapy to fail. MDR is the rationale for the use of combination chemotherapy; cells might become resistant to one drug, but not to a second or third drug that is used in the protocol.

Strategies to minimize the likelihood of MDR include using cytotoxic agents from different drug groups, using combination therapy, using the largest chemotherapy doses possible to achieve maximum cell kill, maximizing the concentration of drugs that are right at the tumor site through use of different administration routes, and using specific schedules or *sequencing* to promote recruitment and synchronization of tumor cells.

To achieve the desired effect of a chemotherapy protocol, the prescribed drug sequence and dosing schedule must be maintained. There is a known *dose-response relationship*—a specific dose must be given for the desired response to occur. Most people are at least somewhat familiar with some of the toxic side effects of chemotherapy. Over the years, ways of reducing the distressing side effects without risking the maximum benefit of the drugs have been refined. The best cell kill is achieved when the cancer cells are exposed to a specific concentration of the drug for the longest period of time; there is a fine line between the dose that kills the cancer cells and a dose that is beyond *host* tolerance—what the patient can tolerate. To minimize the toxicity patients experience and maximize cell kill, protocols are designed around one of three administration plans:

1. high-dose intermittent therapy (high doses of drug are given intermittently at specified intervals)

2. low-dose intermittent therapy (low doses of drug are given at specified intervals)

3. low-dose continuous therapy (low doses of drugs are given continuously throughout a scheduled protocol)

Routes of Administration

Chemotherapy is given by several different *routes of administration*:

- oral: by mouth

- intramuscular: injected into muscle

- intravenous: injected into a vein

- intra-arterial: injected into an artery

- intraperitoneal: injected into the peritoneum (the abdominal cavity)

- intrapleural: injected into the space between the layers of tissue surrounding the lungs (the pleural space)

- intrathecal: injected into the fluid surrounding the brain or spinal cord

Side-Effects of Chemotherapy

Although great efforts have been made to minimize problems, all current forms of cancer treatment have some unpleasant side effects. Some treatments have more side effects than others; some side effects are more serious than others. Not every chemotherapy drug causes every side effect. Talking to the medical oncologist and the oncology nurse about which drugs will be used in a planned protocol—knowing what to expect, what you're up against—is an important part of making an informed decision and planning the right kind of self-care activities. Table 14.2 lists the most common side effects of the most common chemotherapy drugs in use today and what can be done to prevent or minimize them.

The most well-known and notorious side effects of chemotherapy are nausea and vomiting, followed closely by hair loss and fatigue. Bone marrow depression is one of the most consequential of all known side effects. Painful mouth sores and taste changes can be caused by some kinds of chemotherapy, and can interfere with appetite and ability to eat and swallow.

Table 14.2: Common Chemotherapy Side Effects

Side Effect & What Happens	Some Chemo-therapy Drugs That Cause It	Other Complicating Factors	Why It's Important	What You Can Do To Prevent or Minimize Side Effects
Bone marrow suppression Good bone marrow function depends on rapidly dividing cells that will be damaged by chemotherapy. The lowest point in bone marrow function—called the nadir—usually occurs within 7 to 14 days after treatment	*Alkylating agents* *Busulfan *Carboplatin *Chlorambucil *Cisplatin *Ifosfamide *Thiotepa *Plant Alkaloids* *CPT-11 (Irinotecan) *Etoposide (VP-16) *Paclitaxel (Taxol) *Taxotere *Teniposide (VM-26) *Topotecan (Hycampta-mine) *Antimetabolites* *Chlorodeoxyade nosine (2-CdA) *Cytarabine (Ara-C) *Floxuridine (FUDR) *Fluorouracil (5-FU) *Methotrexate *Antibiotics* *Dactinomycin (Actinomycin) *Daunorubicin (Daunomycin) *Doxorubicin (Adriamycin) *Epirubicin (4,Epidoxorubicin) *Idarubicin (Idamycin) *Mitomycin (Mutamycin) *Mitxantrone (Novantrone)	Other problems and medications can cause decreased bone marrow function, too: infection, anemia, malnutrition, alcoholism, and cirrhosis of the liver. Medications that can interfere with bone marrow function include phenothiazines (a class of antidepressants), indomethacin, sulfonamides, anticonvulsants such as phenytoin (Dilantin), tranquilizers, and antibiotics.	The bone marrow produces white blood cells that fight infection, red blood cells that carry oxygen throughout the body, and platelets that help form blood clots and prevent bleeding problems. When the bone marrow is damaged, as it is with many chemotherapy drugs, the formation of these important blood cells is impaired.	*Create a list of all medicines—both prescribed and over-the-counter—being used. Take this list to each doctor or nurse appointment, and discuss possible effects and interactions of these medicines with chemotherapy drugs. *Learn about ways to minimize the potential for infection or injury that could cause bleeding, and take the needed precautions. *Discuss the possible use of hematopoietic growth factors (Granulocyte colony-stimulating factor or Granulocyte-macrophage colony-stimulating factor) with the medical oncologist. *Learn to recognize the early signs and symptoms of fever and infection. Report these signs and symptoms to the doctor or nurse immediately. *Report problems with easy bruising or undue bleeding from seemingly slight injuries to the doctor or nurse. *Report problems with breathing, shortness of breath, or dizziness to the doctor or nurse right away. *Monitor and regularly report levels of fatigue.

Systemic Therapy: Chemotherapy & Biotherapy

Table 14.2: Common Chemotherapy Side Effects (Cont'd.)

Side Effect & What Happens	Some Chemotherapy Drugs That Cause It	Other Complicating Factors	Why It's Important	What You Can Do To Prevent or Minimize Side Effects
	Nitrosureas *Carmustine (BCNU) *Lomustine (CCNU)			
Nausea and/or vomiting Nausea and vomiting often occur within 24 hours after the administration of chemotherapy. They can also occur before chemotherapy ("anticipatory" nausea and/or vomiting) or can be delayed, occurring after 24 hours and lasting several days after therapy.	This is not a complete list, but it does include the drugs most associated with this side effect. With some drugs, the higher the dose, the more likely nausea and vomiting will be a problem. *Cisplatin *Nitrogen mustard *Streptozotocin *Dacarbazine *Cyclophosphamide *Cytarabine *Carmustine *Melphalan *Lomustin *Fluorouracil *Doxorubicin *Daunorubicin	Radiation therapy fields that involve the esophagus, stomach, and small bowel can cause nausea. Infection, obstruction of the bowel, and electrolyte imbalance can cause nausea with or without vomiting. Spread of cancer to the brain or liver or pain can cause nausea and vomiting. All factors should enter into the equation when looking for the exact cause—and therefore the right treatment strategies—for preventing or minimizing.	Not only is nausea an unpleasant feeling, but nausea and vomiting can make it difficult if not impossible to maintain the good nutritional status needed for healing and repair of normal tissues.	*Discuss the likelihood of nausea or vomiting that is associated with the drugs being used. *Ask about taking an antianxiety drug the day of or evening before therapy. *Ask for instructions in using relaxation or guided imagery exercises before, during, and after treatment. *Use a portable tape or CD player to listen to music during chemotherapy administration. *Discuss medicines that prevent or minimize nausea and vomiting. *Eat a light meal before treatment. *Discuss ways to prevent dehydration or electrolyte imbalance. *Learn the signs and symptoms of dehydration and electrolyte imbalance, and report their development right away. *Eat a clear liquid diet, advancing to other foods and beverages. *Maintain a regular, moderate exercise schedule.
Sores in the digestive system The mucous	Bleomycin Busulfan Carboplatin Cyclophosphamide	Radiation therapy to the head and neck and infection can also cause	Any open sore is a source of infection. In an already vulnerable person,	*Visit a dentist before beginning treatments. Dental caries and gum problems should be managed before starting

Side Effect & What Happens	Some Chemotherapy Drugs That Cause It	Other Complicating Factors	Why It's Important	What You Can Do To Prevent or Minimize Side Effects
membranes that make up the lips and line the mouth, esophagus, and the entire digestive tract are composed of rapidly dividing cells that, like rapidly dividing cancer cells, will be damaged by some kinds of chemotherapy. As cells are damaged, sores form.	Cytosine arabinoside Dactinomycin Doxorubicin Etoposide Floxuridine 5-Fluorouracil (5-FU) Idarubicin Mitomycin Plicamycin 6-Thioguanine Vinblastine	sores to develop.	infection can be a very serious problem. In addition, the pain of these sores can interfere with a person's appetite, leading to nutritional problems.	chemotherapy. *A good oral care plan is used every 2 to 3 hours while awake and includes use of a nonalcohol mouthwash, regular, gentle flossing and brushing. *Notify the doctor or nurse immediately if sores develop. *Oral pain medicines, including those that are applied directly onto the sore, should be prescribed. *Avoid smoking and use of alcohol: both tend to dry out the mouth and promote the development of sores. *Avoid eating foods that are very hot, cold, spicy, salty, or that have sharp edges (such as corn chips): any of these can damage the lining of the mouth. *Avoid the lemon-glycerin swabs that are frequently offered in the hospital: they are drying and can increase discomfort and burning.
Fatigue Though not life-threatening, fatigue can cause stress and fear and affect quality of life. Exactly why it occurs is not known; fatigue is probably	Fatigue is the most common side effect of all cancer treatment modalities and is associated with all kinds of chemotherapy.	Because of its multiple causes, a full history and physical, along with evaluation of other data including laboratory tests, will be important in devising plans for managing	Fatigue can be debilitating and has sometimes led people to consider discontinuing potentially curative treatment. There are many self-care interventions and other measures that	*Establish a routine: go to bed at a regular time. *Take short naps during the day. *With the doctor's approval, perform low-intensity exercises such as walking, swimming, during the good times of the day. *Make sure other symptoms and side effects are well managed.

Table 14.2: Common Chemotherapy Side Effects(Cont'd.)

Side Effect & What Happens	Some Chemo-therapy Drugs That Cause It	Other Complicating Factors	Why It's Important	What You Can Do To Prevent or Minimize Side Effects
caused by the sum of many events in the life of a person with cancer.		or minimizing fatigue.	can help in limiting the impact of fatigue.	*Make sure diet and hydration are the best they can be. *Get help in meal preparation if needed (*Meals on Wheels* is a good resource). *Talk with a mental health professional to minimize anxiety.
Hair Loss (alopecia) Hair follicles are composed of rapidly dividing cells that will be damaged by some forms of chemotherapy, causing the hairs to fall out. Hair loss usually begins within two weeks after chemotherapy is started. In most cases, hair will grow back once treatment stops and often begins to grow between treatment cycles. Hair loss can occur on the eyebrows, eyelashes, chest, and pubic areas.	The most likely drugs to cause hair loss are: Cyclophospha-mide Daunorubicin Doxorubicin Etoposide Ifosfamide Taxol Actinomycin-D Cisplatin 5-Fluorouracil Idarubicin Methotrexate Mithramycin	High doses of radiation therapy to the affected body-parts can also result in alopecia.	Hair loss can impact physical appearance and affect one's body image, sexuality, and self-esteem.	*Discuss the chances of alopecia with the medical oncologist and/or nurse. *Consider purchasing a wig or hair piece before the hair loss begins. This offers the best chance for a good match of color and style. *Use sunscreen on the scalp during any exposure to sun. *Use head coverings to protect from sun and extreme temperatures. *If changes in self-esteem or self-image limit normal activities and social outings, talk to the doctor, nurse, social worker, or other counselor.

Table 14.2: Common Chemotherapy Side Effects

Side Effect & What Happens	Some Chemotherapy Drugs That Cause It	Other Complicating Factors	Why It's Important	What You Can Do To Prevent or Minimize Side Effects
Neuropathy Nerve injury is caused by inflammation or degeneration of nerves and can result in weakness, difficulty walking, balance problems, hearing loss, and changes in touch and temperature sensations.	Carboplatin Cisplatin Docetaxel Cytarabine Etoposide Methotrexate Paclitaxel Procarbazine Tenoposide 6-Thioguanine Vincristine Vinblatine Vindesine Vinorelbine	Preexisting health problems such as diabetes, vitamin B12 deficiency and other states of malnutrition, and alcoholism can increase the chances of nerve injury. Radiation therapy to the brain or spinal cord can cause nerve changes that might mimic those from other causes. Other medicines can cause similar nerve damage.	Nerve damage can increase the chances of accidental injuries from burns or falls, or increase sensitivity to painful stimuli. Reducing the dose or changing the administration schedule can limit the long-term effects or the development of permanent damage.	*Discuss the chances of nerve damage associated with any of the chemotherapy drugs being used. *Learn the early signs and symptoms of nerve damage. *Report early signs. *Review the list of other medicines being used—prescription and over-the-counter—with the doctor or nurse. *Inspect feet daily for sores, cuts, or other breaks. *Discuss the use of assistive and protective devices; develop a plan for energy-conserving strategies.

Biotherapy

After surgery, radiation therapy, and chemotherapy, the fourth major form of cancer therapy—a systemic approach like chemotherapy—is *biotherapy*. The idea of biotherapy goes back as far as ancient China and Egypt, where the disease-fighting potential of the immune system was recognized. Modern immunology is considered to have had its beginning in the late 1950s with the recognition of antigens and antibodies. The last two decades of the twentieth century saw the development of techniques to isolate genes and create many of the products that genes normally produce. At the start of the twenty-first century, many *biologic agents* are being tested and developed for use in the treatment of many diseases, including cancer.

How It Works

Biotherapy uses drugs or chemicals to alter or modify biological responses, hence the term *biologic response modifier,* or BRM. The National Cancer Institute defines BRMs as "agents or approaches that modify the relationship between tumor and [the person with cancer] by modifying the person's biologic response to tumor cells, with resultant therapeutic benefit." Biotherapy is based on the idea that cancer cells have substances—distinct protein antigens—on their surface that are potential targets for antibodies, similar to the way bacteria are targeted by antibiotics. Some approaches to biotherapy attempt to stimulate the person's immune response, and other methods involve giving the person antibodies, such as *monoclonal antibodies*, that have been produced in the laboratory.

The way biologicals work in many forms of cancer is not yet known. They can stimulate immune response and cause other biologic actions. There are three major ways in which biologics affect tumor growth. First, they change a person's immune response to the tumor. Second, they can directly act against tumor, suppress tumor growth, or kill the tumor cell outright. And last, they can alter other biological activities that affect the viability of the tumor.

The biological agents most often used in the treatment of cancer are *cytokines* and *monoclonal antibodies*. Cytokines are proteins that regulate immune system function. Cytokines have multiple effects on body systems; one cytokine can influence production and response to other cytokines. Cytokines are given to stimulate the production of certain blood cells and to enhance immunity. Interferon and interleukin are cytokines that are used in the treatment of many forms of cancer as well as chronic hepatitis and multiple sclerosis.

Monoclonal antibodies (MAbs) are tumor-specific factors that are developed from cloned cells. They attach themselves, or *bind,* to target antigens on tumors and signal the body's immune cells to attack and destroy the tumor. In 1998, the first MAbs were approved by the FDA for the treatment of breast cancer. This is just the beginning of what many experts believe will be an explosion in the use of MAbs for other forms of cancer.

Other biologics have found great use in the management of the toxic effects of chemotherapy and radiation. Scientists have cloned and produced factors that affect the body's blood-forming capability. Known as *hematopoietic growth factors*, they stimulate blood cell formation. *Colony-stimulating factors* (CSFs) control the production of a specific cellular component of blood. For example, erythropoietin is a hormone produced by the kidneys that controls red blood cell production and growth. *Epoetin alfa* (Epogen and Procrit) was approved by the FDA in 1989 for use with patients with chronic kidney disease who are on dialysis and later approved for the treatment of AIDS-related and chemotherapy-induced anemia. The granulocyte-macrophage colony-stimulating factor (GM-CSF) Leukine, and a granulocyte colony-stimulating factor (G-CSF) Neupogen, were both approved in 1991 and are both directed at the production of white blood cells to enhance bone marrow recovery after use of chemotherapy drugs that damage bone marrow.

Side Effects of Biotherapy

The most common side effects of biotherapy are often grouped into what is collectively referred to as *flu-like symptoms* or the *flu-like syndrome*. These include fever, chills, muscle aches, fatigue, and rigors—severe shaking chills. The side effects associated with the biologics will differ slightly according to the treatment protocol being used and the preferences of the cancer care team. The following symptom management suggestions are used in many settings, though there is ongoing debate about which strategies work best. Also, the actual drugs used and doses will vary according to the patient's characteristics and current clinical status. For example, aspirin and non-steroidal anti-inflammatory drugs (NSAIDs) might be contraindicated for a person who has bleeding problems.

Fever associated with the flu-like syndrome runs around 39° to 40°C (102° to 104°F) and can resemble the fever of severe infection or sepsis. When fever occurs, an evaluation for infection needs to be completed. The fever linked to biologic therapy may be minimized or prevented by taking NSAIDs such as ibuprofin or acetaminophen *before* the administration of the biologic agent starts. A cooling *hypothermia blanket* can be used to treat chills. Severe, shaking rigors are frightening and should be managed with IV meperedine (Demoral) or morphine. Fever and chills can increase fatigue. High levels of fatigue can lead to diminished intake of food and fluids: for this reason, energy conservation is an important self-care strategy.

Headache associated with the flu-like syndrome could occur as a result of fever and muscle tension. Often, the person is also very sensitive to light. The headache generally begins within a few hours of the start of therapy, but since headaches can be linked to other very serious problems the cause should be carefully explored. Analgesics are appropriate for pain relief. A dark and quiet setting, combined with a cool cloth on the forehead, can be soothing. Massage, acupressure, or reflexology have helped many people get relief from this form of pain.

Muscle and joint pain, called *myalgias* and *arthralgias*, are common side effects of the biologics. Benzodiazepines or other muscle relaxants can be used, and NSAIDs or other pain medicines might work to manage bone and joint pain. Rest, diversional activities, the application of heat or cold, and relaxation techniques might also provide a measure of relief for these uncomfortable side effects.

Cough and congestion and a stuffy nose are common symptoms. Lung congestion, sore throat, and a productive cough, however, are indicative of infection and warrant careful assessment and additional diagnostic tests. Antihistamines and cough suppressants may provide relief of symptoms, but should be used with caution and only on the advice of the doctor.

Nausea, vomiting, and diarrhea can be expected as side effects of biotherapy. They can be treated with antinausea and antianxiety medications.

Mental status can be affected with the use of some biologic agents. The most common of these changes are depression, anxiety, insomnia, and, rarely, psychosis and coma. Astute monitoring for early changes in mental status should result in discontinuation of the agent and reversal of the problem.

Cardiac and vascular problems can be caused by Interleukin-2. Careful monitoring of blood pressure, heart, and lung functions, and quick interventions should a problem occur, minimize the chances of serious, lasting effects.

Other less common side effects of some of the biologic agents, particularly Interleukin-2, include irregular heart beat (arrhythmia), decreased oxygen to the heart muscle, heart attack, and inflammation of the heart itself. Vascular changes can affect the amount of blood being filtered through the kidneys, causing decreased urine output and changes in the blood chemistry—increased nitrogen and creatinine and decreased sodium. Once early signs and symptoms of cardiovascular problems occur, administration of the agent should be stopped immediately. Usually, reversal of the problem begins within twenty-four hours after the agent has been stopped.

To summarize, the use of biotherapy is a valuable component of modern cancer care. Biotherapy is quickly evolving, with new agents being developed and introduced for general use at an astonishing rate. For now, no form of biotherapy is without side effects. When biologic therapy is suggested, it will be important to clarify exactly which agent is to be used, side effects that can be anticipated, appropriate monitoring plans, and how these side effects will be managed should they occur.

Future Directions in Systemic Therapy

"After more than fifteen years of trying, researchers have managed to convert normal human cells into tumor cells in a culture dish. This achievement should help identify new players in tumor formation, and develop treatments that target them."

Jonathan B. Weitzman and Moshe Yaniv, Nature, *Volume 400, July 29, 1999*

"We are at an amazing time in science."

Richard Klausner, M.D., Director, National Cancer Institute, speaking to the National Coalition for Cancer Research, February 26, 1998

Research findings reported in the scientific journal *Nature* describe a great leap forward in the understanding of the molecular events that turn a normal cell into a cancer cell. There is also a growing understanding of cancer biology, the factors that make it possible for cancer cells to break away from a primary tumor site, migrate throughout the body, and set up deadly new sites of metastatic disease. This is crucial knowledge; over half of all patients already have metastatic cancer at the time their cancer is diagnosed.

These scientific directions can't help but lead, ultimately, to cancer treatments that will potentially cure cancers or at least control them more effectively. The cancer treatments of the future will target the molecular structures and functions of cancer cells, rather than targeting any and all cells—normal and abnormal—that happen to be vulnerable at the time treatment is administered. What we currently know is akin to using a cannon to blast away an entire tree. The new treatment modalities, with increased levels of precision, can be compared to hitting a tiny target on the tree with an arrow.

The advances in the understanding of cancer biology have ushered in other new strategies for treating cancer that are sure to be refined as the science moves forward. For example, it is now understood that cancer cells stimulate the formation of new blood vessels—a process called *angiogenesis*—that bring nutrients and oxygen to the newly created cancer cells. This knowledge led to the introduction of new classes of drugs—*antiangiogenesis factors*—that counter the vessel-forming stimuli.

An old drug, Thalidomide (used in the late 1940s and early 1950s to prevent miscarriage and resulting in terrible birth defects in children whose mothers took the drug), is one such antiangiogenesis drug.

Traditional anticancer drugs interfere at one of the stages of the cell cycle. Newly developed anticancer drugs stop the cell cycle at even more precise time frames, adding yet another anticancer target.

It is widely acknowledged that cancer is, at its most basic, the result of accumulated genetic damage. Gene therapy techniques allow damaged genes to be exchanged with normal genes, thereby stopping cancer's lethal sequence of events.

In short, research has exploded in the past five years, and the future of systemic cancer treatment looks exciting. The completion of the National Institutes of Health's Human Genome Project guarantees that great strides are due in the so-called War on Cancer.

Truly, we are at an "amazing time in science," one that offers people who are worried about cancer—those with cancer and the people in their lives—realistic hope for more effective, less toxic control, and possibly even cure, for the diseases we know as cancer.

15

◆ ◆ ◆

Clinical Trials

Jamie S. Myers, R.N., M.N., A.O.C.N.

A clinical trial is "the actual clinical evaluation in which new interventions
against disease are tested prospectively in people."

National Cancer Institute's Definition of Clinical Trials

Clinical trials represent hope for the future and have produced treatments
or cancer that are more effective now than ever before. Successes in our
ability to fight and cure cancer in the future depend on clinical trials being
done today. The precise processes used to conduct clinical trials ensure that
the research is good, scientifically sound, and will be useful in deciding the
value of the protocol being studied. The Oncology Nursing Society (ONS),
the national organization for oncology nurses, asks that clinical trials be
available to all people with cancer. Figure 15.1 summarizes the ONS position statement on cancer research and cancer clinical trials.

People react to being diagnosed with cancer in many ways. Some are
information seekers—they look for any and all information about their
kind of cancer and available treatments. Many are interested in finding out
about treatments for cancer that are still being researched and not yet available to the general public. This type of research is called a clinical trial.
Clinical trials ensure that the new treatments are proven both safe and
effective for people with specific kinds of cancers.

Some people learn about a clinical trial from the oncologist or oncology
nurse. Talking about this option may be frightening because they fear
"being a guinea pig" or "being experimented on." However, the permission

Figure 15.1: ONS Position on Cancer Research and Cancer Clinical Trials

It is the position of ONS that

Federal funding for all levels of cancer research must be greatly increased.

An institutional review board (IRB) process must approve all clinical trials.

All clinical trials must include informed consent.

All people with cancer must have the right to participate in a clinical trial when one is available.

There must be no barriers to clinical trial participation.

Laws must be made to ensure that health insurance plans include coverage for clinical trials and all related care.

Education about clinical trials must be included in both medical and nursing school programs, as well as continuing education programs for health care workers.

Better ways of educating the public about clinical trials must be developed.

Better ways of making sure people in underserved groups have access to clinical trials must be developed.

Concepts of quality cancer care (as defined by the ONS Position on Quality Cancer Care) must be included in all clinical trials.

Coordination of clinical trials must be done by oncology certified nurses (OCNs).

Costs of clinical trials to clinics, doctors' offices, and hospitals must be decreased.

Adapted from the Oncology Nursing Society Position on Cancer Research and Cancer Clinical Trials, Oncology Nursing Forum *25(6), 1998*

process that is the first step to taking part in a clinical trial—called *informed consent*—is very thorough. This process will be described in detail later in this chapter.

Most hospitals, clinics, and office practices insist on an approval process before any clinical trial is offered to patients in that setting. This process includes review and approval by an institutional review board (IRB) that is made up of doctors, nurses, and a representative from the general public. The IRB reviews the clinical trial plan, also called the *protocol*, and consent form for safety, clarity, and ethical implications.

Types of Clinical Trials

Many clinical trials study new cancer treatments; others are designed to study and improve the *quality of life* of people being treated for cancer. Quality-of-life studies may be done along with treatment-related clinical trials. Such studies quite often involve a survey—either an interview or a written form—that is completed at specific times before, during, and after cancer treatment. These surveys look at many aspects of having cancer, such as treatment-related side effects, emotional aspects of diagnosis and treatment, changes taking place in the family or the workplace, and issues about insurance or finances.

A clinical trial might study new ways of reducing side effects of cancer treatment. Some study ways to prevent cancer. People known to be at high risk for developing a specific kind of cancer may be eligible to take part in this kind of study. Prevention studies are being conducted for prostate, breast, and other types of cancers.

There are four levels or phases of clinical trials:

Phase I trials determine the safety of new treatments in humans and identify side effects and toxicities. They also determine the highest dose of the treatment that is safe and well tolerated by the patient. Because Phase I trials are an early stage of research, they are usually done in very large cancer centers on small numbers of patients. Phase I trials are most often used for people whose cancer has not responded to standard treatment.

Phase II trials study the new treatment for a variety of different types of cancer. These trials determine what forms of cancer respond to the new treatment and also identify side effects and toxicities. Like Phase I trials, Phase II trials are used for people whose cancer has not responded to standard treatments. Phase II studies are still an early stage of research and are most often conducted in large cancer centers or university settings.

Phase III trials compare the new treatment to standard treatment. Some Phase III trials compare groups of people receiving standard treatment with groups of people who get the new treatment. Other Phase III trials compare groups of people receiving the standard treatment alone with groups of people getting the standard treatment *and* the new treatment. These trials are usually conducted by many different cancer centers, clinics, and office practices across the United States and include large numbers of patients. Phase III trials may be for people who are newly diagnosed with cancer and have not yet received any kind of treatment or for those whose cancer has recurred or spread.

Phase IV trials determine the best way to use the new treatment as part of standard therapy. These trials may involve slight adjustments in the dose or timing of the new treatment and involve large numbers of patients.

The National Cancer Institute (NCI) is a part of the National Institutes of Health (NIH). The NCI was developed to conduct research, promote research in other institutions, and coordinate cancer-related activities throughout the United States. Since the 1950s, the NCI has been the world's largest sponsor of clinical trials for cancer. The NCI funds twelve cooperative groups that develop and conduct research on treatments for many different kinds of cancer; these groups are listed in the Resources section at the end of this book. All study groups that deal specifically with children's cancers are part of one large group called the Children's Oncology Group (COG). The NCI also supports fifty-eight cancer centers that are recognized as "centers of excellence" for cancer care. A complete listing can be found on the Internet through the NCI home page (www.nci.nih.gov/cancercenters/centerslist.html).

Not all people with cancer can receive cancer treatment at the NCI or one of its cancer center research bases. In order to make clinical trials available to people in many communities, Community Clinical Oncology Programs (CCOPs) were formed. There are currently fifty-seven CCOPs in thirty-six states. Seven of these are Minority Based CCOPs, formed to make sure that people in minority populations have equal access to clinical trials. Community oncologists and hospitals belonging to a CCOP can offer many NCI approved clinical trials. A complete listing of the research groups, CCOPs, and their locations, can be found on the NCI Community Oncology and Rehabilitation Branch website (dcp.nci.nih.gov/CORB/).

Pharmaceutical Companies also develop clinical trials for new cancer therapies. Most hospitals, clinics, and office practices require these trials to be approved by the individual facility's IRB in order to be offered to patients. Like NCI trials, these commercially sponsored studies may provide a level of payment to the facility where the trial is conducted, which helps to cover the costs of staff time to complete necessary paperwork for patient registration and data collection.

Some major cancer centers and office practices develop their own clinical trials. These trials would be available only to patients being treated in those specific facilities. However, the cancer center may apply for NCI approval for the trial, which would make the protocol available to patients through participating CCOPs.

Participating in a Clinical Trial

Participation in a clinical trial is a process that involves several coordinated steps. Each step in the process is important to the scientific validity of the clinical trial. Strict controls imposed throughout the clinical trial process assure that the results can be expected to be the same when the same treatment is used in other treatment settings with other patients who have the same cancer and the same characteristics as patients who participated in the trial. Eventually, use of the experimental treatment is expanded to other groups of patients with perhaps other characteristics or even other forms of cancer. When the treatment is repeatedly demonstrated to be safe and effective in several controlled clinical trials, the Food and Drug Administration (FDA) approval process begins. Study data is reviewed, including the protocol's effects on the size and growth of the tumor, side effects and toxicities of the new protocol, and survival rates of study participants. Comparisons are made between existing "standard" treatment and the new treatment or protocol. The FDA can deny approval and ask that additional data be provided before the treatment is reviewed again. Or, the new treatment is "approved" for use with people in the general public who also have the type and stage of cancer that was studied in the clinical trial.

Eligibility

Every clinical trial has a list of eligibility criteria as well as ineligibility criteria. Eligibility criteria are the characteristics or traits a person must have in order to be included in a trial; ineligibility criteria are traits that a person must *not* have. The oncologist and oncology nurse will review the criteria to determine if you are eligible for participation. This process very often involves additional testing, such as X-rays, scans, or laboratory work. The oncologist or oncology nurse will provide you with a consent form and talk with you about the clinical trial to determine if you wish to go ahead. Table 15.1 lists some examples of typical eligibility and ineligibility criteria.

Table 15.1: Typical Eligibility and Ineligibility Criteria

Eligibility Criteria	Ineligibility Criteria
Patients with a proven diagnosis of cancer	Patients who have previously received chemotherapy or radiation therapy
Patients who have had appropriate surgery	Patients with hepatitis, infection in the blood, or bleeding in the gastrointestinal tract
Patients with healthy bone marrow, kidneys, and liver	Patients with more than one kind of cancer
Patients who are able to be up and around and perform usual activities	Patients who are pregnant or breast feeding
Patients who have signed the informed consent form	Patients who are unwilling to sign the informed consent form

Informed Consent

The informed consent process ensures that people thinking about taking part in a clinical trial are fully aware of exactly what the treatment plan will involve. You will be provided with a very detailed consent form, which describes the purpose of the clinical trial, the treatment that is planned, the randomization process (if any), and any tests that will be performed as part of the trial. The consent form also describes in detail any expected side effects or toxicities of the treatment, outlines whether any or all of the treatment is to be provided at no cost, and discusses how confidentiality is assured or to what level confidentiality is assured while you participate in the trial. Federally funded trials may be subject to FDA review. The consent form explains whether compensation and reimbursement for medical treatments are available to you if you have any *adverse events*, unexpected side effects or toxicities, that must be treated. Finally, the consent form will emphasize that you have the right to withdraw from the trial at any time. You will be required to sign the consent form before any further steps are taken.

Registration

Once all the necessary tests have been completed to determine eligibility for the trial and the consent form has been signed, you will be registered as a participant. This registration assigns you a clinical trial identification number. This number is used to collect and organize data—without using your name—related to the type of treatment you receive, any tests that are done as a regular part of the clinical trial, and any adverse events that occur during your participation in the trial.

Randomization

Many clinical trials involve a process called *randomization*. This is the process used to decide whether the person receives the new treatment being studied or something else. When the randomization process is used, people who are eligible for a particular trial and who choose to participate are randomized to one of two or more groups, sometimes referred to as *arms of the study*. For example, someone who is participating in a Phase III trial may be randomized to the group or arm that will get the standard treatment, or the group or arm that is to receive the new treatment. The randomization process—deciding which patient receives which treatment plan—is done by a computer and is completely random, similar to making a choice by flipping a coin. This process makes sure that everyone is given an equal chance to be in either group; no favoritism is used based on a person's age, sex, race, income, place of residence, or—in the case of cooperative trials—treatment facility.

Treatment

Treatment is administered and closely monitored by the oncologist and oncology nurse. It is generally recommended that oncologists complete a board certification in oncology. Oncology nurses are encouraged to become certified as an oncology certified nurse (OCN). These credentials are one way to determine that your doctor and nurse have special knowledge and expertise in the treatment and management of cancer.

Tests

Most treatment-related clinical trials outline the timing of certain tests that are done to monitor the cancer's response or the patient's tolerance of the treatment being studied. For example, many clinical trials involving chemotherapy require blood tests at certain times throughout the treatment period to check the white blood cell, red blood cell, and platelet counts. Blood may also be drawn to measure the level of the chemotherapy in the blood at specific times after a dose of the treatment. Computerized axial tomography (CAT scan) or other X-ray-type studies may be required after a certain number of treatment cycles to measure the success of the treatment. Some clinical trials require that tissue samples taken at the time of surgery be sent to one designated laboratory for special evaluation. Testing during clinical trials may be done more frequently than with standard treatments. These extra tests may or may not be provided without cost to you.

Costs

Some clinical trial treatments are provided at no cost to study participants. Once treatments are approved by the FDA and become commercially available, they are no longer provided without cost. Costs of additional testing such as blood work, scans, or X-rays will be charged to the patient or the patient's insurance.

Insurance companies may or may not approve payment for tests and patient care related to clinical trials. Many insurance companies do not recognize a responsibility to pay for anything that is *investigational* or not yet *standard of care*. This can include very traditional treatments that have received FDA approval for only one type of cancer but are commonly used successfully in the treatment of other types of cancer. This is called *off-label* use (meaning that this particular use of the drug is not specified on the drug's label). It is important that you know if you will be responsible for any costs related to the clinical trial. Discuss this aspect of the trial with the oncologist, oncology nurse, oncology social worker, and/or the benefits manager of your insurance plan.

Insurance companies' denial of payment for drugs, particularly for off-label use, is an important political issue. Clinical trials are very important to progress toward cures for cancers. Without insurance coverage for clinical trials, many people will not or can not participate and some facilities may not offer participation. Clinical trials are the only proven method for finding new treatments for cancer. Doctors, nurses, and people with cancer are lobbying legislators to demand support for cancer research.

Finding Information

There are a number of ways to find information about what clinical trials are available. A first step may be talking with your oncologist and your oncology nurse. They should be aware of clinical trials that are available in your community and through a local CCOP. The doctor or nurse may also be able to help you by looking into clinical trials at major cancer centers throughout the United States that may apply to your kind of cancer. Gaining entry at a major cancer center is much easier if your doctor makes the referral and talks to a doctor at the center. Arrangements can be made for your medical record (history, X-rays, lab work, pathology) to be sent for review.

The Internet is also a resource. You must use this resource carefully, because not all websites provide scientifically accurate information. Helpful websites are listed in the Resources section at the end of this book.

Making a Decision

It is very important to know that the clinical trial is scientifically sound and has been reviewed for potential benefits, risks, and safety. You might want to ask the following questions before making a decision to participate:

What is the purpose of the clinical trial?

The purpose of the clinical trial should be described in the first section of the consent form and will tell you what the trial has been designed to learn. Most consent forms are very specific about the treatment you will receive. Your oncologist or oncology nurse can describe for you how the new treatment is different from the standard treatment.

What phase (I–IV) is the clinical trial?

The phase of the trial discussed earlier in this chapter will indicate how far along the new treatment is in the research process.

Who is the sponsor and who has reviewed and approved the clinical trial?

By knowing who is sponsoring the trial you will know if it is supported by the NCI, a cancer center, an office practice, or a pharmaceutical company. All trials should be reviewed and approved by an institutional review board (IRB).

What are the expected side effects and toxicities?

Symptoms that you may have because of the cancer and/or the treatment should be explained in detail in the consent form. Be sure to ask your oncologist or oncology nurse about anything you do not understand. The doctor or nurse should also tell you about what symptoms you should report to them so that you can receive the appropriate treatment.

How long will the clinical trial last?

Many clinical trials have a specific time period for providing the treatment. This is then followed by a time period in which you will be seen regularly by your oncologist and oncology nurse for further tests and checkups.

Will I need to be in the hospital for any of the treatment?

It is important to know about any and all tests that are considered part of the trial so you will know what to expect. You will want to know if any of the testing or treatment must be done in the hospital.

Will I be responsible for any of the costs?

The consent form will tell you about any of the treatment that is provided free of charge. All other treatment associated with the clinical trial will be paid for by you or your insurance company.

Will my insurance company approve reimbursement for all related treatments?

Many insurance companies do not pay for any care that is linked to a clinical trial. It is best to talk with your insurance company's benefits manager up front before beginning the trial to find out what is and is not covered by your insurance.

The Future of NCI-Sponsored Clinical Trials

The value of clinical trials research to improving cancer treatment cannot be stated too strongly. The NCI is concerned about problems that keep people with cancer from taking part in clinical trials. Some of these problems relate to costs. Many insurance companies do not pay for care that is linked to any kind of investigation or research. Some clinics, hospitals, and doctors' offices are reluctant to participate in research because of the added expense for staff and data collection. Not all oncologists, clinics, and hospitals are members of a CCOP or cooperative group. To date, the CCOPs have not had access to all clinical trials. The approval process for new clinical trials has been slow due to the number of individual institutional review boards (IRBs) involved. Other barriers to participation have been the time-consuming paperwork required for patient registration and ongoing data collection.

The NCI is working to do away with as many barriers to trial participation as possible. Many changes are being implemented as the NCI Clinical Trials process evolves. The approval process for clinical trials is being streamlined. Phase III trials that have been approved will be available to all participating cooperative groups and CCOPs. Oncologists will apply for credentialing or approval as an NCI investigator. This credential will allow participating physicians to have Internet access to the entire list of NCI-approved Phase III trials. The patient registration process will eventually be done completely online. Forms and data collection requirements will become more standardized to reduce the amount of time and energy spent on unnecessary and expensive information management.

The NCI is working with managed care organizations so that reimbursement for care related to clinical trial participation is covered by insurance plans. Currently, a pilot agreement is in place with the Department of Defense TRICARE/CHAMPUS system and with the Department of Veterans Affairs, involving managed care organizations for people who have retired from the military.

These changes are exciting. However, it will take time to put all of them into effect. Many of the strategies will be piloted before they are widely available. A pilot of the new system was initiated in 2000, using genitourinary, lung, breast, gastrointestinal cancers and adult leukemia studies. The new system will be available first to oncologists and facilities that are current cooperative group and CCOP members. Gradually, the new processes will expand to include new members who have successfully completed the online application for credentialing.

Final Thoughts

The decision to take part in a clinical trial is an important one. There are many questions to ask and many things to consider. Your oncologist and oncology nurse will be important resources for you as you learn about the treatments available for your cancer. As an experienced oncology nurse, I am grateful for the difference clinical trials research has made in the lives of the patients and families with whom I work. Over the past twenty years, I have seen cure rates for many cancers improve dramatically. I have also watched the quality of life improve for people receiving treatment for cancer. I believe that clinical trials research is the only way we will develop the tools to win the war against cancer.

16

◆ ◆ ◆

Complementary and Alternative Therapies for Cancer

Lynn M. Collins, R.N., M.N., A.O.C.N.

Complementary and alternative therapies, sometimes referred to as unorthodox, unproven, or questionable therapies, are a major topic today and provoke strong feelings, positive and negative. These forms of treatment have been around for hundreds of years, and there is an increased trend toward using them. A recent study published in the *Journal of the American Medical Association* (*JAMA*) documents an increase from 427 million visits to alternative practitioners in 1990 to 629 million visits in 1997 in the United States alone. These visits to alternative practitioners account for $21.2 billion spent, with at least $12.2 billion paid out-of-pocket. *Integrative care*—the integration of the best of conventional and alternative therapies under one roof—is now the trend, with major medical centers creating specialized integrative care clinics. Despite these changes, controversy about the use of alternative and complementary therapies still exists.

Critics of alternative treatments fear that patients and their families will be swayed toward fraudulent and potentially harmful treatments, that they will delay conventional forms of treatment and use only alternatives, lured by the promise of a cure versus a long-term chronic or recurrent illness. The critics point out that these cures—or even claims of success—have never been scientifically proven and therefore mislead consumers.

As proponents and critics of these alternatives meet, complementary therapies have unfolded. With the growing acceptance of these therapies, other alternatives are being explored and tested. Many resources on complementary and alternative therapies are available; this chapter provides a general introduction to the topic that will hopefully help consumers make informed and wise choices.

Many organizations attempt to define and delineate acceptable alternative therapy. The U.S. Office of Technology Assessment (OAT) created a panel to analyze methods of alternative treatment and create a directory of these therapies. This directory is a good reference tool, but is simply a reference tool and does not provide specific information on all forms of therapy. In 1992, the Office of Alternative Medicine (OAM) was created as part of the U.S. National Institutes of Health (NIH) to evaluate and provide information about commonly used alternatives. A major goal of this new department is to facilitate the legitimate, scientific evaluation of alternative therapies. More recently, governmental funding was given to four regional areas to study alternatives commonly used in these distinct areas. In 1999, the National Cancer Institute (NCI) established the Office of Cancer Complementary and Alternative Medicine (NCCAM) specifically to study complementary and alternative therapies used for people affected by cancer.

Defining and Differentiating Conventional, Alternative, and Complementary Therapies

Conventional medical practices are easily defined as services and medicine provided by physicians trained in accredited medical schools. Conventional practices are also referred to as *Western medicine* and *allopathic medicine*. Alternative medical practices are more difficult to define because they are offered by a variety of practitioners who have been educated and trained in a number of ways. To help differentiate between the various therapies, this chapter is divided into three major sections:

- Complementary Practices

- Known Alternative Practices

- Less Known Alternative Practices

Complementary practices are those treatment modalities used along with conventional medicine. They complement medical treatments and improve well-being by addressing spiritual, psychological, social, and physical concerns.

Jeffery White, M.D., director of the NCCAM, defines *alternatives* as practices used as a *sole approach*, or in place of conventional medicine. Dividing alternatives into *known* and *unknown* leads the consumer to a better understanding of what risks may be linked to these therapies. *Known alternative practices* may involve a health philosophy; the treatments and side effects are known and understood. *Less known alternatives* include practices offered in other countries or modalities in which the specifics of treatment and side effects are uncertain. In these alternatives, risk is difficult to assess because specifics of the therapy are not known.

Many health care consumers today choose to use complementary therapies as a way to have the best of both worlds. Complementary practices have been increasingly accepted in the past decade, with the medical community showing a growing readiness to recommend and even use these practices to improve the quality of life of people who undergo conventional medical treatment. According to Dr. Jonas of the Office of Alternative Medicine in a *JAMA* paper, the growing use of complementary therapy has to do with the increase in chronic diseases, interest in spiritualism, wariness of physicians as decision makers, and desire for quality of life. There has also been an enormous societal shift to the information age. Personal computers, the World Wide Web, and the media bring medical information into our homes. Healthy lifestyles and a focus on living longer and better are now the norm.

Alternatives are gaining in use, too. Many patients try alternatives before seeking help in the conventional medical community. In diseases such as cancer, this can decrease the chance of success with conventional treatment. Some people add alternatives to their conventional therapy without disclosing these adjustments to their health care team. This can be hazardous if there are serious side effects, as both therapies may have to be discontinued while causes of the side effects are explored. According to a November 1998 report in *JAMA*, communication between patients and conventional doctors about alternatives has remained about the same since 1990. Only about 40 percent of people inform their conventional medicine physician about using alternatives.

There are some risks involved in seeking alternatives. No quality standards have been established for alternative practices. No special training or license to practice is required of many alternative practitioners. Lack of monitoring could lead to poor care. The so-called "natural" products often used in alternatives are unmonitored and vary greatly in the way they are manufactured and stored. Contamination and inconsistent dosing could lead to complications, drug interactions, and toxicity. Conventional medicine uses randomized, controlled clinical trials to assure safety and quality of the treatment modality being used. Alternative practitioners quite often rely only on anecdotal evidence—unpublished and unscientific success stories that are difficult to duplicate.

Social factors also influence the interest in and use of alternative practices. American health care and the health care systems in many industrialized countries evolved around the idea of *illness care*, in which medical attention is sought only for episodes of illness. Once the problem is managed, the patient resumes his normal lifestyle, whether that lifestyle is healthy or not. Alternative practitioners focus on the prevention of disease through diet and other quality-of-life boosting methods. They emphasize healing, and the teaching of healing practices often translates to practitioners who spend more time with their patients. A 1998 *Life Magazine* story reports that the average time a patient gets to speak, uninterrupted, to his conventional medicine physician is twenty seconds. Payment and insurance plans have also altered communication between patient and physician. High-tech advances are wonderful, but are only a part of what a person needs for quality medical care.

Who uses these treatments? The picture of a poor, uneducated person being duped into alternative treatments is not an accurate reflection of the people using alternatives. Educated, motivated, and affluent people tend to look for and use alternative and complementary practices. Both men and women use these practices, but women tend to use more than one at a time whereas men tend to use only one therapy. Some people fear conventional treatments, especially for cancer, and turn immediately to alternatives, hoping for a fast, simple cure. Others believe they cannot be helped by conventional medicine and turn to the solace seemingly offered by alternatives. Then there are the miracle seekers—people looking for an end to emotional and physical distress, who search out anyone offering a cure. On the whole, however, people using alternative and complementary therapies need to recognize both the advantages and limitations of these practices.

Complementary Practices and Cancer

Numerous complementary therapies can be useful to people facing cancer. For convenience, they will be categorized as:

- diet therapies
- ancient Chinese practices
- massage
- mind-body approaches

Diet Therapies

A good diet is important whether a person is healthy or ill. When a diagnosis of cancer is made, many people look for ways to improve their health, and one of the easiest ways to do this is through the diet. It is not surprising, then, that a common complementary practice used by people with cancer is a change in diet. Eating is a primary family and social time and if it becomes stressful due to imposed dietary restrictions, quality of life is decreased. Finding a diet that suits one's lifestyle is important.

In the 1970s, an Eastern diet known as the *macrobiotic diet* became popular. The macrobiotic diet is a multiple-step vegetarian diet plan made up of unprocessed foods, whole grains, fruits, and vegetables. The original macrobiotic diet was structured so that a person would become more spiritual and less of the material world as he descended the steps of the diet. Theoretically, less food was consumed and an increased spirituality was achieved with each step. In the past, a macrobiotic diet regime was difficult because ingredients were not widely available. The growing popularity of health food stores has increased access to macrobiotic dietary selections, and packaged macrobiotic foods are now available. Many hospital kitchens also provide macrobiotic selections. The key to a macrobiotic diet is following a plan that provides a balance of foods and enough calories to maintain the body's healthy metabolism. Most other diets that are considered to be "cancer fighting" tend to follow a similar vegetarian, whole-grain philosophy. Limiting intake of processed foods and eating more whole grains is also important in a balanced diet.

Organic foods are grown without pesticides, chemicals, or hormones. Health food markets and many grocery store chains now offer organic fruits and vegetables, although free-range chicken and beef without hormones are typically available only in health food markets. Proponents of organic foods believe that eliminating chemicals and hormones reduces promotion of cancer by reducing carcinogens in the body, and they also contend that the vitamin content is superior in foods that have not been treated with dyes or preservatives. Organic foods usually cost more than food produced for general consumption.

Nutritional supplements come in many different forms and usually are touted as ways to improve energy, mood, and well-being. Most nutritional supplements contain a mixture of herbs and vitamins. Herbs will be discussed in detail later in this chapter. Many experts suggest that nutritional supplements can ease the side effects of conventional therapies such as chemotherapy and radiation therapy, although the claim is not proven. Examples of supplements are Barley Green, Juice Plus, and Coenzyme Q. It is important to check the ingredients to make sure they do not interact with conventional therapies.

Vitamin therapy has long been thought to enhance the nutritional status of people with cancer. Controversy exists about whether additional vitamins or normal food sources of vitamins—fresh fruits and vegetables—provide true antioxidant coverage. In general, people get most of the necessary vitamins by eating a balanced diet and regular meals. Even so, Dr. Joe Jacobs in *A Guide to Alternative Medicine* says that most people with cancer are probably somewhat deficient in important nutrients and supplements are appropriate. In the 1970s, some megavitamin plans were promoted as a cure for cancer and a number of other chronic illnesses. However, the current thought is that large doses of vitamins can often be more harmful than good.

Vitamins now believed to be cancer fighters are vitamins A, C, E, and D. Of these, vitamins A, E, and D are *fat soluble*—what is not used immediately is stored by the body. Vitamin C is *water soluble*—what is not used immediately is excreted or taken out of the body in the urine.

Dr. Linus Pauling did much of the early research on *Vitamin C* and cancer. In Asia, Vitamin C is linked to prevention of gastric (stomach) and bladder cancers. Vitamin C enhances collagen growth, is useful in fighting infection and trauma, and appears to break down nitrites. Large doses of Vitamin C are not toxic but may cause gastric upset or flatulence (gas), and possibly kidney stones. As much as ten grams of Vitamin C per day have been well tolerated over a long period, but it is recommended that the daily dose be divided evenly throughout a twenty-four-hour period.

Derivatives of *Vitamin A*, called *retinoids*, are proving very useful in reversing some cancers. Large doses of Vitamin A do not provide the same benefit. Retinoids are thought to boost the immune system, maintain the integrity of skin and mucous membranes, and bind to carcinogens in lungs. Retinoids are recommended for people at high risk for lung cancer, such as ex-smokers. People who are current smokers should check with a physician before taking Vitamin A or its derivatives; at least one study indicates that Vitamin A may actually promote the development of lung cancer in people at high risk. Too much Vitamin A can cause drowsiness, headaches, vomiting, and increased blood cholesterol and triglyceride levels.

Vitamin E has long been thought to have special healing properties. Inhibition of cancer, reduction of low density lipids and cholesterol, and protection against free radicals that may play roles in cancer development are just a few of the benefits attributed to Vitamin E. There are no side effects reported at higher doses; even so, high doses of Vitamin E are not recommended.

Vitamin D is thought to be useful for inhibiting cancer cell growth, enhancing the immune system, and decreasing colon cancer risk. Vitamin D needs ultraviolet light to the skin and proper kidney function to be activated. High doses may cause anorexia, diarrhea alternating with constipation, and nausea and vomiting.

Many doctors now recommend that people with cancer take these specific vitamins in their daily recommended doses. Because the vitamin industry is not under the control of the Food and Drug Administration (FDA), packaging and dosing of vitamins may vary greatly; check recommended dosages and find supplements that are easy to swallow and are not costly. Supplements packaged together can be a good option.

Ancient Chinese Practices

An old Chinese prayer says, "When you have a disease, do not try to cure it. Find your chi and you will be healed." Chinese healing practices are now widely available in the United States and Europe. They are based on the theory that an energy system called *chi* or *ki* flows through the body. Altering or aligning the flow of energy by balancing the *yin* (deficiency; contraction or hypoactivity) with the *yang* (the excesses in the body; swelling or hyperactivity) is the primary focus of these practices. Herbs, exercise (to increase chi), and energy alignments are used to achieve and maintain balance. Acupuncture, acupressure, tai chi, and herbs are the Chinese practices most commonly used by people with cancer.

Acupuncture Acupuncture involves placing small needles under the skin along twelve *meridians*, the energy pathways that link organ systems. There are over one thousand places within a meridian where needles can be placed to restore health by realigning energy flow. Acupuncture was introduced into the United States in the early 1800s but began being more widely used in the early 1970s. Since that time, schools and clinics have been established to teach and provide acupuncture. In 1998, the National Cancer Institute performed a number of clinical trials studying acupuncture in people with cancer-related pain and nausea and vomiting associated with chemotherapy. Both studies validated the value of acupuncture, and the practice was subsequently approved by the FDA for the management of cancer-related pain, nausea, and vomiting. There are differences between acupuncturists trained in traditional practice and those trained in more modern acupuncture. Organizations that validate the practice of acupuncture are listed in the Resources section at the end of this book.

Acupressure Acupressure is based on the same principles as acupuncture, but is applied by the practitioner's hands instead of needles. It is the older of the two practices and includes the Japanese techniques of *shiatsu* and *reflexology*. Acupressure focuses on relieving pain and preventing disease by relieving tensions before they develop into illness. *Acupressure points* or *tsubos* are thought to be areas of decreased electrical resistance along the meridian. The practitioner presses these points for approximately one minute, altering the energy flow. Massage is used to redirect the energy to its correct path. The practice of acupressure has been expanded to self-administration and has also been adapted and used in therapeutic massage. *Reflexology* and *shiatsu* are similar in that pressure is applied to specific points on the body to control organ systems. Mapping is done and pressure is applied according to the desired effect.

Tai Chi Tai chi is an ancient Chinese martial art consisting of 108 slow, fluid movements meant to calm the mind and increase agility. It tones muscles and tissues, thereby supplying energy that must be kept circulating through the meridians. Finding one's center or *chi* is the most important aspect of tai chi. When used by people with cancer, the movements are thought to focus the energy and expel the negative. Tai chi's benefits include increased muscle tone, blood flow, and oxygenation of tissues in a safe, slow, calm manner. In the United States, tai chi is an increasingly popular form of exercise. Specially trained instructors often offer special classes for people with cancer at integrative centers.

Massage

Massage is a scientific series of manipulation techniques in which a therapist uses his or her hands and sometimes elbows, forearms, or feet to apply moving or fixed pressure to the body. The philosophy of massage therapy is *vis medicatrix naturae*, or helping the body to heal itself. It is aimed at healing or increasing well-being. The two basic massage styles are *traditional European* and *contemporary Western*.

Traditional European methods of massage, including *Swedish massage*, are based on concepts of anatomy and physiology and use five categories of soft tissue manipulation:

- *effleurage* (gliding strokes)

- *petrissage* (kneading)

- *friction* (rubbing)

*Complementary
and Alternative
Therapies*

227

- *tapotement* (percussion)

- *vibration*

Contemporary Western methods of massage, based on concepts of human function, target personal growth, including emotional release and balance of mind, body, and spirit, in addition to the traditional applications. From here, massage has evolved into *neuromuscular massage, sports massage, deep-tissue massage, myofacial release, myotherapy*, and *manual lymph drainage*.

A Guide to Alternative Medicine says that massage therapy is the most commonly used complementary therapy, indicating that twenty million Americans have received a massage. Massage therapists are now accredited by a number of national organizations. Standardization of techniques is gaining in acceptance and facilitates research in uses of therapeutic massage.

The benefits of massage are obvious. Most people report a sense of well-being, better mobility, release of tension, and decrease in pain following a massage session. Touch is a potent form of communication, and people continue massage therapy as much for the therapeutic relationship as for the physical rewards. Through touch, a sensitive massage therapist can gain information about pain, tenseness, and strain in the body. Many people report emotional releases such as crying or clarity in thinking about problems during and after massage. Clearly, the relationship and touch combine for positive outcomes.

As important as touch is, using the wrong kind of touch, or *toxic touch*, increases tension as the body guards itself. A massage performed by an inexperienced or nonaccredited massage therapist can create negative feelings.

Can people with cancer have massage therapy? A number of massage therapists will not perform massage on someone with an active cancer, for fear of causing the cancer to metastasize if lymph flow is increased. Although this question has not been addressed with solid research, many people with cancer use any number of massage techniques in combination with relaxation and reflexology. Michael Lerner, in his book *Choices in Healing*, recommends open communication with the therapist about where metastatic sites are located and the presence of any pain. A good massage therapist will work with a person with cancer to optimize the benefits of massage. The benefit certainly seems to outweigh the risk, but it is wise to check with one's doctor before starting a massage program.

Mind-Body Approaches

The link between the mind and body in healing remains a mystery in the medical community, although almost everyone believes that a positive attitude helps, exercise and diet make a difference, and emotional support is valuable. It is impossible to establish a single plan that can be useful to every person with cancer. Mental imagery, psychoneuroimmunology, journaling, music therapy, meditation, hypnosis, and art therapy are all ways to connect the mind and body in healing disease.

Mental Imagery Imagery can be useful for stress reduction, relaxation, or—at least according to some proponents—actively treating cancer. A passive form of imagery transports the person with cancer to a calm, serene place. For some men, the image may be early morning fishing or hiking in the mountains. *Guided imagery* is more active: a facilitator helps the man visualize his cancer and then imagine ways to destroy the cancer cells. The mental picture can be real or symbolic; for some men, it is important to get a clear picture of the cells while others prefer a cartoon image. One man receiving radiation therapy for Hodgkin's disease claimed he saw a Star Wars–like video game in his head as he tried to imagine what the radiation was doing. Another man visualized his cancer cells being attacked by video-game-like soldiers that represented his chemotherapy.

The study of *psychoneuroimmunology* (PNI) in the conventional medical community legitimizes many mind-body techniques. PNI studies the effects of mental processes on measurable data in the body such as hormonal levels and immune function. As the study of PNI evolves, the link between the mind and body is becoming more clear, encouraging skeptics in the conventional medical community to recognize the value of and perhaps even use these techniques. Whether or not imagery prolongs life is unclear; that it improves the quality of that life is crystal clear.

Journaling and Art Therapy Writing and creating art are physical extensions of imagery. Writing feelings and thoughts about cancer is often easier than speaking about it. Daily journaling provides a memoir of the experience that may be useful in the future. Art therapy techniques range from representational drawings of cancer to visual representations of feelings. Art has been useful with children and adults in crisis and illness situations. It is a safe expression of feelings that promotes relaxation.

Music Therapy Since the days when David sang psalms to King Saul to ease his anxiety and sleeplessness, music has helped to soothe and relax. The tempo of music induces varied responses in the central nervous system. An increased tempo creates happiness and energy, while slower, methodical tempos create relaxation. Music therapy is used in the treatment of pain, sleep disorders, anxiety, and stress disorders.

Hypnosis Hypnosis alters perception and so is a valuable therapy for pain relief and reducing anxiety in people with cancer. *Hypnotherapy* uses hypnosis as its base to seek answers to emotional blockages. Hypnotherapists often theorize that disease is a direct cause of unresolved issues; hypnosis uncovers these issues, allowing the therapist to aid the patient in resolution.

Meditation Meditation is a mental exercise that clears the mind, helping the person focus on the present. The desired result is that the person can control his mind and increase his self-awareness. Meditation can be done by focusing on and repeating a phrase or mantra, or by simply clearing one's thoughts. Advocates of meditation believe it recharges the immune system; decreased stress and improved relaxation are possible additional benefits of meditation. Being able to clear the mind of the issues surrounding cancer can be a helpful exercise. Meditating during radiation and chemotherapy treatments makes the time pass faster, perhaps reduces stress and anxiety, and, some believe, is a way to diminish physical side effects of cancer and cancer therapy such as nausea, vomiting, and fatigue.

Spiritual Approaches Spirituality goes far beyond religion. When a man gets a diagnosis of cancer, there is often a break in his spirit. It may be triggered by his fear or an image of his own mortality; regardless, he can be temporarily wounded. Spiritual healing encompasses any number of techniques that can help revive the spirit. Spiritual health incorporates the body, the psyche, the rational mind, and the intuitive spirit.

Health and spirituality have been linked since early human history. Native American healers called on their gods to help treat the sick; priests and shamans have been involved in healing for centuries. Meditating, energy healing, and using crystals for spiritual cleansing are all used in many cultures and settings to realign one's spirit. Some healers use psychic energy to heal, claiming they can feel where the energy is blocked in a person and ask questions to verify their conclusion. Spiritualists use a variety of techniques to unblock and realign energy in a person who is ill and teach strategies that help the person open himself to spiritual energy.

Religion can play a part in spiritual healing. Some people use prayer as a mantra for meditation, and many physicians incorporate prayer into their treatment plan, actively praying with and for their patients. All this can be somewhat intimidating for someone who does not see himself as religious or feels very private about that aspect of his life. More than a few researchers are exploring the potential healing benefits of having others pray for a patient. In 1998, a controlled, blind study was done to determine if having others pray on the patient's behalf helps with recovery from surgery. Those in the experimental group—those being prayed for—had fewer side effects and recovered faster after open-heart surgery. Although one study does not prove something conclusively, it opened the door to a more spiritual focus in health care and validated an idea that many people believe works.

There are many paths to spiritual health. As Michael Lerner in *Choices in Healing* reveals, people with cancer have an extra motivation to seek spiritual health due to their sudden life-threatening circumstances. He compares having cancer to being in a battle trench that is being shelled by the enemy. According to Lerner, the cancer diagnosis can provide an awakening to something that is beyond the moment, opening a person to the ultimate questions:

— What is the meaning of my life?

— What do I truly value?

— What happens when I die?

— How should I live my life now?

Each man must find his own path to spiritual awakening and health, whether in an organized way or by a path he creates for himself.

Known Alternative Practices

Known alternatives are remedies or treatments used to treat cancer and other diseases *in place of* conventional medicine. Side effects of the treatments are well documented. At times these treatments will be used to complement conventional therapy, but most often they represent a lifestyle and a health philosophy, and a choice must be made to use them exclusively. Known alternatives are best categorized as

- pharmacologic therapies

- health philosophies

- programs

Pharmacologic Therapies

Antineoplastins Antineoplastins are pharmocologic agents created and produced by Stanislaw Burzynski, M.D., at the Burzynski Research Institute near Houston, Texas. Dr. Burzynski first isolated antineoplastins from urine. Today, antineoplastins are made in his laboratory, and this form of treatment is only available at his clinic. Burzynski believes antineoplastin is part of the *parallel biochemical defense system* (BDS) that is independent of the immune system. This BDS reprograms defective cells such as cancer cells and allows them to function normally.

According to Burzynski, BDS is made up of many polypeptides, which he named antineoplastins. With cancer, there is a lower amount of antineoplastins which, Dr. Burzynski says, is the reason cancer grows and new cancers develop.

Antineoplastin treatment is given intravenously or orally in capsules and can only be used in Dr. Burzynski's own clinic. Most advanced cancers are treated with the IV drug. There are ten different types of antineoplastins, costing from $135 to $685 per day for treatment. Additional costs include room, diagnostic tests, pumps, and catheters. Treatment can cost tens of thousands of dollars per year, and insurance does not usually pay for this form of treatment. Dr. Burzynski has thus far not allowed antineoplastins to be used with any form of conventional treatment.

In 1991, the NCI evaluated patients' responses to antineoplastins by evaluating Dr. Burzynski's clinic files. After this initial study, a clinical trial to examine an antineoplastin's dose, side effects, and antitumor activity in people with brain tumors was conducted at Memorial Sloan-Kettering Cancer Center in New York City, the Mayo Clinic in Rochester, Minnesota, and the NIH Clinical Center. As a result of the many disagreements about patient accrual and conduct of the study, a full study was never completed. Since then, no other trials of antineoplastins have been conducted. Dr. Burzynski has published hundreds of articles touting his claims for antineoplastins, but few are published in peer-reviewed journals. In these articles, Burzynski claims a 46 percent cure rate for colon cancer, and an 80 percent cure rate for brain tumors and prostate cancer.

In 1997 Dr. Burzynski was tried in a federal court for transporting antineoplastins across the Texas border—an illegal action—and numerous other charges. In the back of the courtroom, patients and even family members of deceased patients were prepared to testify on Dr. Burzynski's behalf. The trial ended in a hung jury. After it was over, many observers believed that it was the drug's effectiveness that was on trial.

Shark Cartilage The use of shark cartilage as a cancer treatment is based on some scientific fact. Tumors often grow because they are able to build their own blood supply systems. A component of shark cartilage is an *antiangiogenesis factor,* or *angiogenesis inhibitor*, an agent that works against cancer and, more important, its metastases, by breaking down or preventing the development of blood vessels that carry nutrients to the tumor. The premise of shark cartilage is *Sharks Don't Get Cancer*, the title of I. William Lane's book on the subject. (Actually, sharks *do* get cancer.) Even though the use of shark cartilage to fight cancer elicits hot debate, the development of antiangiogenesis factors is seen as a monumental step forward in cancer research, offering great hope for eventual effective treatment applications.

Testimonials of cancer regression without side effects among people who have used shark cartilage exist, but to date no published clinical trials have validated this treatment. Because the rectum absorbs medications very effectively, the method of administration is a retention enema—an enema that the patient holds in for thirty minutes. In the NIH studies, shark cartilage in powder and liquid forms were not absorbed by the human body. Since those NIH studies, Dr. Lane has written several rebuttals describing the molecule's real size and how it is absorbed. Dr. Lane has a clinic in the Bahamas where he administers shark cartilage.

Despite questions about the absorption of oral formulations, shark cartilage is available in capsule form at many health food stores. Dosing varies widely, depending on the company that produces the product. Some companies mix additives with shark cartilage; some products contain only a small percentage of shark cartilage. No side effects have been described in the literature, though there are at least anecdotal reports of indigestion and nausea after taking the oral form. Since cartilage contains a lot of calcium, anyone who has a condition in which calcium should be restricted should avoid shark cartilage.

Should people take shark cartilage? Can it work? I know a seventy-five-year-old man with prostate cancer who religiously takes shark cartilage capsules. He is not a surgical candidate and he sees his oncologist every six months. He feels safe and is convinced that the shark cartilage is keeping his tumor at bay. The capsules are within his budget, and he is actively doing something nontoxic instead of just worrying. He explored the information fully, and this was his decision.

Hydrazine Sulfate Hydrazine sulfate, a chemical compound originally developed to fight the cancer-related wasting syndrome called *cachexia*, has been found to have some ability to shrink some kinds of tumors. Its advocates claim hydrazine sulfate affects cancers of the prostate, rectum, colon, and lung. Even though hydrazine sulfate has not been approved by the FDA as being an effective cancer-fighting drug, its value in reversing, to some extent, the extreme loss of weight and muscle mass that many people with cancer experience has been recognized by many cancer experts. A normal dosage for hydrazine sulfate is one 60 mg tablet three times per day. While taking hydrazine sulfate, some people with cancer are able to gain weight and feel stronger. Hydrazine sulfate can be toxic when used in very high doses, although ability to tolerate high doses varies from person to person. Side effects include nausea, dizziness, drowsiness, itching, and, occasionally, numbness in fingers and toes. Although hydrazine sulfate is not used as a cancer treatment in the U.S., many foreign clinics offer it as part of a regular, anti-cancer protocol.

Herbal Therapies Herbal therapies utilize over 500,000 different types of plant life. Herbs are also known as *botanical medicine* and, in Europe, as *phytotherapy* or *phytomedicine*. An herb can be a leaf, flower, root, stem, seed, bark, fruit, or any other plant part used for medicinal purposes. In conventional medicine, 121 prescription drugs come from plants, and three-fourths of those were first used as folk medicine. Information is gained each day about different herbs, but as yet only five thousand herbs have been studied for their medicinal properties.

The practice of using herbs to treat illness began in the earliest days of civilization and spans cultures from China to Native America. Herbs are combined into specific therapies or used by herbalists and naturopaths to treat specific symptoms or diseases. Herbs have not been approved by the FDA, and most have not been studied, so there is very little clinical evidence on which to base actual use.

Table 16.1 is a short list of herbs commonly used by people with cancer, with information provided by proponents of these herbal therapies, unless otherwise stated. There are thousands of other herbs about which very little is known. As is obvious from the information presented in Table 16.1, just because a substance comes from nature does not mean it is totally safe.

Health Philosophies

Homeopathy Homeopathy is a system of medicine founded by Samuel Hahnemann. It is based on three major principles, which Hahnemann and his followers referred to as "laws":

1. Like cures like (*law of similars*).

2. The more a remedy is diluted, the greater its potency (*law of the infinitesimal dose*).

3. An illness is specific to the individual (*a holistic medical model*).

Approximately 500 million people throughout the world use homeo-

Table 16.1: Herbs Used in Cancer Treatment

Herb	Uses	Rationale	Side Effects	Considerations
Saw Palmetto	Used to reduce symptoms of prostate enlargement. The herb should be used in an oil-based preparation or berries; dried or tea forms have little effect.	A chemical in the berries is thought to counteract androgens, the hormones responsible for prostate enlargement. In an initial study reported in *JAMA*, blood flow and recovery were better when taking the herb.	May influence the results of blood tests done in prostate cancer screening.	Men should check with their physician if they are on a conventional medicine for enlarged prostate, as Saw Palmetto may reduce the effectiveness of both. Using this herb does not replace prostate screening.
Echinacea	This herb is used to fight infection and stimulate the immune system. Most commonly taken as a tea, using 2–3 teaspoons and letting the mixture steep for 5 minutes. Drink the tea every 8 hours.		May interfere with blood pressure medications	Self-medicating to prevent infection after taking chemotherapy may be counterproductive. Men who have had bone marrow transplantation should not take this herb to boost immunity. Echinacea should not be used for more than 2 weeks or it begins to suppress the immune system.
Astragalus (milk vetch)	Used in cancer patients to boost the immune system and often recommended for people taking chemotherapy. Packaged as a capsule, tincture, or tea.	Not described.	Unknown	Unknown.
Buckthorn	Thought to have antitumor activity. Buckthorn is one of the natural products being tested at this time.	Not described.	A potent laxative, considered much stronger than psyllium-based products.	This herb should not be taken for more than two weeks as it can create a "lazy bowel"—dependence on chemicals for stimulation. Check with your physician if you are taking chemotherapy.

Table 16.1: Herbs Used in Cancer Treatment

Herb	Uses	Rationale	Side Effects	Considerations
Ginseng	Ginseng is thought to stimulate white blood cells and increase production of human interferons that fight viruses and cancer. Chinese medicine practitioners use it to treat stomach cancer and claim success. It appears to boost energy.	Not described.	Unknown.	Ginseng is very costly, so buying from a reputable company is important. Often, preparations that claim to have Ginseng do not.
Rosemary	A potent antioxidant. To achieve any benefit, rosemary oil must be used.	May inhibit the growth and development of cancers.	Larger doses of rosemary oil can cause intestinal cramping and may be poisonous. Smaller amounts are also linked to intestinal, kidney, and stomach problems.	The herb used as a food seasoning has none of these side effects.
Tea	Tea, whether green, black, or prepackaged for a quick cup at home, is thought to have anticancer properties.	Thought to be an antioxidant. Has been weakly linked to tumor regression. Whether everyone derives these benefits is unclear.	None.	Large doses of green tea are loosely linked with esophageal cancer.
Chaparral	Used by Native Americans in the Southwest and in South America. It comes from the leaves and twigs on the bark of the creosote bush.	Some regression of lymphoma and lymphosarcoma, leukemia, and lung cancer has been anecdotally noted.	Unusual, debilitating fever has been noted after taking this herb for a period of time.	Liver damage has been reported.

Table 16.1: Herbs Used in Cancer Treatment

Herb	Uses	Rationale	Side Effects	Considerations
Essiac	A combination of herbs—sheep sorrel, Indian rhubarb, slippery elm, and burdock root. Claims that it cures cancer have not been substantiated.	Not described.	Contains pollen that can trigger allergic reactions.	Was given to nurse Rene Caisse by an Ojibway healer. She labeled it with her name spelled backwards and began giving it to people with cancer. Memorial Sloan-Kettering Cancer Center attempted an investigation, but it was halted when Ms. Caisse refused to share ingredient information with the lab. The leaves may be poisonous if ingested.
Iscador (mistletoe)	Used more in Germany and Switzerland, this herb cannot be sold in the United States. A number of different preparations can be taken orally or injected into the fat layer of the abdomen.	Has shown antitumor activity in animal studies.	Unknown.	Very large doses may cause liver problems and anemia.
Pau d'Arco (taheebo, lapacho, ipes ipe roxo, or trumpet bush)	Used for cancer and malaria. Sold in health food stores.	Lapachol, the most potent ingredient, has been studied the most as an anticancer agent.	In the doses that are recommended for cancer, this herb can cause nausea and bleeding.	Considered extremely toxic, this herb has been banned in Canada.
Aloe vera	This natural product has been thought to have magical properties ranging from healing wounds to curing cancer.	Not described.	May cause diarrhea when ingested. Bleeding and alteration of clotting factors have also been seen.	Testing its ability to cure cancer by drinking large doses has shown minimal results.

pathic medicine. Homeopathy has been used to ease the side effects of conventional therapy, and some people see only homeopathic doctors to manage their cancers.

According to the *law of similars*, what causes a symptom will relieve that symptom when given in a smaller dose. Homeopathic treatments are developed by giving disease-free individuals certain substances, and then monitoring these people for side effects. The substance is then used to treat whatever side effect occurred. For example, if an herb caused nausea in a normal person, that herb, in a much smaller concentration, would be used to treat nausea.

Homeopathy practitioners believe that the more diluted the medicine, the more potent it becomes—the *law of the infinitesimal dose*. Remedies are prepared by diluting a substance with pure water or alcohol, then vigorously shaking. Homeopathic solutions are so dilute that no molecules of the original substance remain. Practitioners believe the energy from the original substance remains and treats the problem.

In accordance with the last principle—that illness is specific to the individual—a homeopathic practitioner, before prescribing remedies, will interview the patient thoroughly to determine a profile for his disease. This one-on-one communication is a primary reason why homeopathy is popular.

Homeopathy is very controversial because of the inconsistencies. How can something that is not there be helpful? Also, some practitioners do not believe that homeopathy should be used as a complement to conventional medicine, because homeopathy is a natural healing philosophy. For many people, it comes down to a choice between conventional or alternative.

Ayurvedic Medicine Ayurveda, which means *science of life*, has been practiced in India for five thousand years. Popularized in the United States by Deepak Chopra, M.D., ayurvedic medicine is gaining in acceptance. According to this philosophy, *constitution* is the most important aspect in treating a person. There are three body types (or *doshas*): the *vata* (thin), the *pitta* (muscular), and the *kapha* (fat). The body type is a blueprint to a person's innate tendencies. Most people are a mixture of body types, with one being dominant.

Each body type has specific sensitivities and tendencies. Vata body types tend to be slender, with prominent features, veins, and joints. They have cool dry skin. They seem to initiate projects but are poor at completion, tend to be moody and erratic but are articulate and imaginative. Pitta body types are of medium build, strength, and endurance. They are fair with blonde or red hair and have quick, biting tempers but are usually very intelligent. Pittas sleep and eat regularly, tend to perspire, and are often warm and thirsty. Kapha body types are heavy, solid, and strong, with a tendency to be overweight. They are relaxed, slow to anger, and slow to react. They love to sleep long hours but tend to procrastinate. Each body type has an area in the body where individuals express reactions when they are out of balance, although each cell in the body carries tendencies for each body type.

Seven factors are thought to disrupt physiological harmony and create disease: genetic, congenital, internal, external trauma, seasonal, natural tendencies or habits, and magnetic and electrical influences. Evaluation of a patient is done through the pulse, tongue, eyes, and nails.

Ayurvedic treatment includes *detoxification and cleansing* through massage, steam saunas, removal of blood, and herbal treatments. The next step is *palliation*, which balances and pacifies the doshas through yoga, spiritual healing, ingestion of herbs, breathing exercises, meditation, and lying in the sun. *Rejuvenation* then enhances the body's own ability to function and is accomplished through special herbal preparations, powders, jellies, and tablets, plus physical and breathing exercises and yoga.

Ayurvedic medicine has been used by people with cancer, though not in a controlled, scientific study. Many people like to incorporate the holistic aspects as a complement to conventional medicine. Because of its strong herbal base, there needs to be excellent communication among the ayurvedic practitioner, the conventional doctor, and the patient to make sure that no drug interactions occur. Many times, the patient must make a choice between conventional and ayurvedic medicine.

Residential and Walk-in Programs

There are many programs available in which to receive complementary and alternative therapies. Many of these programs have been developed to provide a number of services. Diet, nutrition, massage, guided imagery, aromatherapy, and support groups are components of several more common programs. Most residential programs are used when people have completed conventional therapy, while the walk-in programs are used in a complementary way during and after conventional therapy.

The Wellness Community started in Santa Monica, California, in 1982 and became a haven for Gilda Radner, who was one of its biggest supporters. The Wellness Community now has centers all over the United States. Its focus is to teach positive ways to cope with cancer, such as mutual aid groups, imagery, and self-help strategies. The Wellness Community concepts gave rise to Gilda's House, which follows similar philosophies while operating on corporate and community grants and donations. Both women and men are welcome at Gilda's House facilities, and services are free to the person with cancer.

Commonweal was founded in 1976 by Michael Lerner, Ph.D., author of *Choices in Healing*. Located north of San Francisco in Bolinas, California, its three major program components are serving high-risk young people, helping people with cancer, and ecology. They also focus on families and professionals who work in these areas. The cancer programs at Commonweal are (1) the Commonweal Cancer Project, promoting informed choice in combining complementary and conventional medicines; (2) the Commonweal Cancer Help Program, an intense week of psychosocial support, spiritual guidance, yoga and relaxation techniques, and nutritional counseling for people with cancer; and (3) the Institute for the Study of Health and Illness, a training program for health professionals interested in understanding alternatives and their history. The Commonweal staff is well trained and respected in their fields of study. The program costs over a thousand dollars to attend; there is some financial help available on a limited basis.

The Wellspring Center in Watertown, Massachusetts, provides services for people with life-threatening illnesses and their loved ones. It provides resources, support, guidance and programs.

Exceptional Cancer Patients is an organization started by Bernie Siegel, M.D., author of *Love, Medicine and Miracles*, in New Haven, Connecticut. The program offers group sessions and individual psychotherapy. Cancer patients are instructed in ways to make spiritual and emotional changes to improve their quality of life and extend their lives.

The University of Arizona Clinic of Andrew Weil, M.D., is probably the most famous of the integrative medicine clinics being formed in many major medical centers in the United States. Dr. Weil sees patients for alternatives and integrates conventional care with herbs, nutrition, relaxation techniques, and other complementary therapies. His website on the Internet, called "Ask Dr. Weil" (cgi.pathfinder.com/drweil), attracts thousands of visitors every day.

Less Known Alternative Practices

The category of *less known alternatives* includes many treatments that are not generally offered in the United States. Many were developed in this country but moved, either because they were unaccepted or their methods were banned by the FDA. These practices are considered less known because many of the original creators of the therapies are no longer living and/or the therapies have changed. Most of these therapies are not given to people being treated with conventional cancer therapy.

Laetrile

The value of Laetrile, also known as *amygdalin* or *vitamin B17*, has been widely debated. It is derived from the pits of apricots that are dried and crushed. In the mid-1970s, laetrile was the new hope in cancer treatment, but it fell out of favor after a Mayo Clinic study showed it offered no benefit to people with cancer. In addition, laetrile contains at least 6 percent naturally occurring cyanide, and it has been responsible for a few deaths among patients who used very large doses. Laetrile is rarely given alone to treat cancer, but is administered along with a proteolytic enzymes diet, vitamins, and minerals. Many clinics in Mexico supplement nutritional or enzyme therapies with laetrile.

Immuno-Augmentative Therapy

Immuno-Augmentative Therapy (IAT) was developed in the 1970s as an immune booster that supposedly aids in destroying tumor cells. Lawrence Burton, Ph.D., isolated four blood protein components used in IAT. According to his theory, deficiency in any of these four protein components could lead to cancer. The four components were identified as (1) the tumor antibody (destroys cancer cells); (2) the tumor complement (activates the tumor); (3) the blocking protein (inhibits the tumor antibody); and (4) the de-blocking protein (neutralizes the blocking protein). Dr. Burton published his methods and results in newspapers and magazines, but never in scientific journals. The NCI evaluated IAT and found that the components are indeed proteins that occur normally in blood, but have no antitumor activity. IAT is considered unproven, but a clinic in the Bahamas continues to offer Dr. Burton's IAT.

Gerson Therapy

The Gerson Therapy is a nutritional therapy developed by Max Gerson, M.D. He believed that cancer would not occur in bodies that have a balanced and functional liver, pancreas, immune system, and thyroid gland. He created a low-salt vegetarian or vegan diet with crushed fruit and vegetables supplemented ten times per day. A detoxification process includes three or four coffee ground enemas daily. Dietary supplements include electrolytes and pancreatic enzymes. Dr. Gerson treated many famous people in the 1930s who had cancer and other diseases. His daughter currently runs the Gerson Clinic in Tijuana, Mexico. Although the diet has stayed very similar to the original, there are new additions to the treatment.

Kelly's Nutritional-Metabolic Therapy

Kelly's Nutritional-Metabolic Therapy was created by William Kelly, D.D.S, in the late 1960s to treat his own pancreatic cancer. Dr. Kelly theorized that cancer occurred as a response to ineffective protein metabolism. He believed that protein-digesting pancreatic enzymes were the body's first defense against cancer and that a deficiency left a person vulnerable to disease. Kelly created a diet plan that was high in whole grains, fruit, and vegetables, and restricted protein. He supplemented the diet with proteolytic enzymes and raw juices and recommended coffee enemas for detoxification. The diet was geared to the metabolism of each patient. Nicholas Gonzalez, M.D., has adopted the diet and now treats patients in a similar way. Dr. Gonzalez claims approximately 80 percent of his patients are doing well on the diet. In order to be treated with the diet, a patient must be willing to adhere to it 100 percent of the time. No other therapy can be used. The NCI is currently reviewing case files and may propose a clinical trial.

The Hoxey Therapy

This therapy has its roots in the folk medicine of the American southwest. Legend has it that a horse with a cancer on its leg was put out to pasture to die. After the horse grazed on the grasses, the tumor went away and the horse was cured. Dr. Hoxey later created a cancer treatment from those same herbs, and the mixture has been used ever since. Some of the herbs are listed in Table I, including cascara, potassium iodine, buckthorn, and burdock root. The Hoxey method is on the unproven therapy list of the American Cancer Society (ACS), but the treatment is available at the Hoxey Clinic in Tijuana, Mexico.

Live Cell Therapy

Live Cell Therapy involves the injection of cellular material from organs, fetuses, or embryos of animals, theoretically to stimulate healing and treat illness. The theory of live cell therapy is that cells injected into the body find their way into damaged organ systems and stimulate the body to heal itself. Cells from the pituitary gland, male and female gonads, liver, and connective tissue are used. Ted Allen, M.D., who performs cell therapy in a clinic in the Bahamas, believes cell therapy revitalizes and stimulates the immune system to prevent or fight disease. He believes that cell therapy enhances the entire body of a cancer patient and helps him during chemotherapy or radiation treatments. The clinic is also working with injecting the cells of cancer-resistant animals to prevent and treat cancer. The major side effect of this therapy is allergic reaction to the cells. In cases of allergic reaction, cellular therapy must be stopped.

Oxygen Therapy

Oxygen therapy is based on the theory that lack of oxygen at the cellular level may be a primary cause of cancer. The therapy consists of reoxygenating cells in a number of ways: patients may drink water infused with ionized oxygen; oxygen may be given through the rectum, veins, arteries, or under the skin; high concentrations of oxygen can be inhaled through masks or oxygen tents; hydrogen peroxide (H_2O_2) can be injected into the vein, breaking down in the body into two molecules of oxygen. In addition, ozone is used in combination with diet, vitamins, and herbs to treat cancer. There are numerous side effects associated with oxygen therapy. It is not currently available in the United States.

Evaluating Complementary and Alternative Therapies

Because complementary and alternative therapies are so popular today, many people with cancer feel pressured to try one or more of these treatments. Using complements is a personal choice. For example, during a support group discussion on complementary therapy, everyone in the group began discussing dietary changes. A young, single father of two, recovering from testicular cancer treatment, sat quietly. When pushed regarding his dietary regime, he blurted out, "Fast food!" Getting fast food two days a week helped him cope with his job, his children, and his recovery from therapy. Certainly, his plan was to change his diet, but for the time being taking advantage of fast food was his coping strategy. Trying to adhere to a strict dietary plan with two school-aged children would have increased his stress level. Complementary therapies should complement not only conventional therapy, but also a person's lifestyle.

The FDA holds conventional medicine practitioners to a strict set of guidelines to prove a drug or other form of treatment is safe. The clinical trials process described in Chapter 15 is the accepted scientific method of proving safety and effectiveness of new forms of therapy. To protect consumers, the dose as well as the method and schedule of administration are described on the package insert and label recommended by the FDA. Any side effects that have been noted are documented. Have you ever read the package insert for Tylenol? The list of potential side effects is huge! Effectiveness is also defined for consumers on the package insert. The Shirley Amendment, passed by the U.S. Congress in the early 1900s, countered the rampant use of harmful alternatives available at the time by mandating "truth in labeling," meaning that every single additive to a medication—including coloring and preservatives—must be listed on the label. Another section of the Shirley Amendment mandated that no boastful claims be made about the drug. So, for instance, if the drug was used for fevers, the company could not claim that the drug also cured male pattern baldness unless this second claim was verified. Today, the FDA holds companies to this standard.

When evaluating complementary and alternative therapies for cancer, it is important to realize that a diagnosis of cancer creates a sense of fear and vulnerability. Remember that:

- There is not one cause, nor is there one cure, for cancer.

- One test done once cannot diagnose cancer.

- Testimonials promising a fast, painless cure are too good to be true.

- Secret formulas you can only buy through the mail are likely to be fraudulent.

- It is illegal to sell drugs and formulas over the Internet.

- You should be wary of treatments that have only testimonials as proof of effectiveness.

- There is no cure for cancer that is being suppressed by the medical community.

- If you must use a password to talk to the practitioner, the practitioner may be hiding something.

- You should always check out any drug, formula, or practice with good sources.

After researching any potential treatment option, it is important to determine, perhaps with the help of a loved one or a health care professional, if this is a viable option. The National Cancer Institute recommends that patients ask themselves the following questions when deciding on cancer treatment:

- Has the treatment gone through clinical trials? This information can be found at any reference library if it has been published in a scientific journal.

- Do the practitioners of a therapy say the medical community is suppressing their cure from the public?

- Does the treatment contain a "secret formula" that only a small group can use? Reputable physicians publish their data, making it useable by any physician.

- Is the treatment said to be harmless, painless, and without side effects? Because of the kind of disease cancer is, treatments are very powerful and have side effects.

- Is the treatment based only on a nutritional or diet therapy? To date, there is no known dietary cure for cancer.

In addition, some other questions may help in decision-making:

- What does my doctor say? It is vital to ask the advice of your oncologist and make sure the treatment will not interfere with conventional therapy.

- How much does this cost? Since many complementary and alternative therapies are not covered by insurance, the financial impact of the therapies can be great. It is also important to check on insurance coverage, since grass-roots organizations are being formed to demand insurance reform that will include consideration of complementary therapies.

- Do I have to stop or avoid conventional therapy? Unless your medical philosophy is to use only alternatives, it is important to find out if you are expected to continue conventional cancer therapies.

- Does the person offering the treatment have credentials? Untrained personnel may not perform the treatment at the level of someone with training.

- Do I know what the therapy entails? Am I aware of all the parts of this treatment? A good decision cannot be made unless it is an informed one.

- Can I physically do these therapies? Complementary therapies take time, energy and often involve shifts in the normal, day-to-day routines. Starting something and then having to stop for any reason can be debilitating.

Whether to use complementary or alternative therapies is still a confusing issue for people who are fighting cancer and the side effects of conventional cancer treatment. Using these therapies is a highly personal choice that each man must make for himself. It is important to support men who choose to use conventional medicine as well as those who try complementary therapies.

In a consensus conference held by the National Cancer Institute, it was unanimously agreed that alternative practices and practitioners must be held to the same standards as practices and practitioners of conventional medicine. The position that alternatives simply cannot be studied in the same way as conventional treatment was rejected. Instead, benefit to patients must be proven through systematic investigation and reports in scientific journals that can be reproduced and critiqued by other physicians.

With new ideas comes controversy, and as the paths of complementary medicine and conventional medicine converge, controversy is certain to occur. If, in the end, a joint venture helps one person with cancer improve his quality of life, it is worth it.

Part IV

•••

Quality of Life Issues

17

♦♦♦

Taking Control of Cancer Pain

Carol P. Curtiss, R.N., M.S.N.

Cancer and pain *do not* have to go hand-in-hand. Not everyone with cancer has pain. For those who do, something can always be done. Still, many people fear cancer-related pain more than cancer itself and worry they won't be able to control it.

There are many reasons why people are not provided with adequate comfort measures. Most of these are easy to overcome. This chapter will tell you about cancer pain, discuss barriers to finding relief, and describe ways you can become a pain management partner with your doctor and nurse. For those who want more information than can be provided in this one chapter, our book, *Cancer Doesn't Have to Hurt*, by Haylock and Curtiss (Hunter House, 1997) can be a useful resource.

Sources of Pain

Pain can be an issue at any time during a course of cancer. It can be of short duration, such as that caused by a needle stick or an uncomfortable position during a physical examination, or a long-term, chronic problem. *Nociceptive pain* arises from sources in muscles, organs, or bones. It's usually easy to describe and locate. *Neuropathic pain* involves nerves and is often described with words like "burning," "shooting," "electric-shock-like," or "numbness." Its location can be difficult to pinpoint. Both neuropathic and nociceptive pain can be managed.

Cancer treatment is sometimes the source of pain or at least discomfort. Surgery can cause or aggravate pain, as can side effects of chemotherapy and radiation therapy, such as mouth sores, skin reactions, constipation, or infection. Having cancer does not provide an exemption from normal stresses and strains that go with living. The wear and tear of getting to treatments and trying to keep up with things at home or work can contribute to pain. Problems that are totally unrelated to cancer, such as arthritis, stress headaches, or aches from exercise might also cause pain.

Removing the cause of pain—for example, relieving pressure on nerves or organs by shrinking the tumor—is the best way to relieve it. Even when the cause can't be removed, the pain can be managed. Your doctor and nurse can help sort out the kinds of pain being experienced and design appropriate management strategies.

Barriers to Appropriate Pain Management

More than 90 percent of all cancer pain can be managed with simple methods, and health care professionals have the knowledge, skills, medicines, and technology to manage it appropriately. Still, studies continue to show that cancer pain is undertreated. Barriers to appropriate pain management are complex; doctors, nurses, the person with pain, the public, insurance underwriters, and, last but not least, regulators and legislators are all involved.

Laws, Regulations, Insurance, and Cost

Outdated laws or regulations that interfere with cancer pain management persist. Handling, storage, prescription, and distribution of controlled substances used for pain—also called *analgesics, analgesic opiates,* and *narcotic analgesics*—are controlled by state and federal laws and regulations. Many state regulators and lawmakers are working to update these laws so that they prevent abuse of drugs but still offer easy access to persons who need analgesic medicines.

A study published in the *New England Journal of Medicine* documents that limited access to narcotic or opiate analgesics—pharmacies refusing to stock these drugs or physicians neglecting to prescribe them—is common in urban areas populated by people of lower socioeconomic status. The authors of this study as well as editorial reviewers speculate that racial stereotypes such as the myth that "black people don't experience pain in the same way as whites" also play a factor in limiting access to these medications. Evidence suggests that access to strong analgesics is also limited in rural settings.

Limits by some insurers on the number of refills or the number of pills per refill can impede access to appropriate prescription medicines. For many people, the cost and availability of medicines are also barriers. The doctor, nurse, social worker, or pharmacist can intervene to help if cost or availability are problems.

Health Care Professionals

Many health care professionals do not know how to manage pain adequately. In general, they receive very little education about pain management as part of their basic educational preparation. Some are reluctant to change outdated ideas, prescribing patterns, or interventions in spite of new information; others—thankfully, a shrinking number—still believe that little can be done for cancer pain. Nothing could be further from the truth! Because a person's pain is invisible, it can be easy for friends, family, or doctors and nurses to forget or ignore. Some people with cancer tend to be stoic or believe that getting pain under control will mean trading comfort for clear thinking. Others, incorrectly, believe that nothing can be done anyway, or that the doctor or nurse will know when pain is present. Many people, especially men, don't tell others about their pain because they think talking about it is a sign of weakness, while enduring it is a sign of strength. These beliefs cause people to suffer needlessly.

Unrelieved pain causes important physical, psychological, and social changes. Pain decreases immune response and interferes with the body's ability to heal. It sometimes prevents people from moving about, increasing the risks of complications like pneumonia, blood clots, and other serious problems. Ignoring pain is ignoring the body's call for help.

Pain that persists over time causes anxiety and depression in even the strongest person. It prevents concentration and interferes with relationships, work, and play. Unrelieved pain takes away energy that could be used to deal with cancer and cancer therapy. Enduring pain needlessly saps strength.

Reporting comfort levels—or lack of comfort—to health care professionals routinely and accurately is an important part of dealing with cancer and promoting quality of life. Mild to moderate pain is far easier to control than severe pain. The goal is to prevent pain rather than waiting for it to return or get worse.

Fear of Addiction

The myth that people who use strong analgesics become addicts is one of the greatest barriers to cancer pain control. Doctors, nurses, pharmacists, people who have pain, families, and the public worry about addiction. In reality, studies continue to show that addiction is very rare when an individual, with no history of substance abuse, uses medicines for pain. In fact, the incidence of addiction is no greater than 0.1 percent!

Addiction is a psychological problem, and it's unusual in people with cancer pain. The addicted person seeks and uses drugs for reasons other than pain relief and continues using drugs in spite of a decrease in overall function, negative mood changes, and an overall decrease in quality of life. This is referred to as "use despite harm." Behaviors focused on getting and using drugs are *extremely* rare in people with cancer-related pain. People with cancer use analgesics to get around better, enjoy family and friends, return to work, and improve quality of life. Fear of addiction should never prevent anyone from using medicines for pain relief.

Misunderstanding of Physical Dependence and Tolerance

Physical dependence and *physical tolerance* are two important terms often confused with addiction. Addiction is a psychological problem. Dependence and tolerance are biological symptoms and are easy to manage. *Physical dependence* is an expected effect in all people who take strong medicines such as morphine, oxycodone, and hydromorphone. The only important thing to remember about physical dependence is that these medicines should never be stopped abruptly. Anyone who takes strong pain medicines for more than a few weeks will be physically dependent on that medicine. Abrupt cessation of the drug causes signs of physical withdrawal within twenty-four hours. This is not addiction and is easily managed by gradually decreasing the dose over a few days.

Tolerance is also a physical problem, although not a very important one. Tolerance means that, over time, more medicine may be needed to control the same amount of pain. Tolerance is rarely a problem for people with cancer-related pain. Increases in the amount of medicine needed are usually related to new sources of pain. Tolerance is not addiction either. If concerns about addiction or tolerance prevent you or someone you know from getting relief, talk to a doctor, nurse, or pharmacist who has expertise in pain management, or get additional information from other reliable sources.

Pain Assessment

Pain management is a team effort, and the person with pain should expect to be the team captain: only he knows about his pain and what relieves it. There is no blood test or X-ray that depicts a person's level of pain. In fact, self-report—what the person says about his pain—is the most important information for experts to consider in devising a pain management plan. Holding back this information impedes effective pain control. Expect doctors and nurses to ask about comfort levels at every office visit or routinely if during an acute hospital stay. If they don't ask, tell them anyway.

A rating scale is important for measuring changes in pain and pain relief. A common rating scale is a zero-to-ten scale, with zero meaning "no pain" and ten "the worse possible pain you can imagine." Ratings for one person cannot be compared to those of another person. The rating scale helps doctors and nurses understand pain more clearly and determine whether the pain management strategies being used are working.

Questions about pain and pain relief are called *assessment*. A good assessment includes a physical exam, questions about pain, and a review of the analgesic plans being used.

Assessment questions should include:

- Do you have pain or discomfort anywhere right now?

- Have you had pain or discomfort in the last twenty-four hours? Since your last visit?

- Where is the pain? Do you have more than one spot that hurts? Does the pain move from one spot to another?

- When did the pain start? How long does it last?

- What makes it better? What makes it worse?

- Have you had this pain before? What relieved it? What have you tried so far?

- What do you think is causing the pain?

A zero-to-ten scale can also be used to rate relief. Rating pain before taking medicine and one hour later helps to find out how well the medicine works. This is important information to use when adjusting the plan. Questions about relief include:

- How much relief do you get?

- How long does the relief last?

- What level of relief would let you do the things you'd like?

- Does the pain completely disappear? Does it return before the next dose of medicine is due?

- Exactly how are you using medicines and other therapies to relieve pain?

- How often are you taking each medicine? What is the dose each time?

- What else helps to achieve comfort?

Expect questions about the ways pain interferes with life, such as:

- Does pain affect sleep, appetite, mood, concentration, work, or ability to move around, socialize, or play?

- What does the pain prevent you from doing?

Questions about side effects are also an important part of a complete assessment. Expect questions about how often bowels move and how difficult it is to have a bowel movement, since constipation is a common side effect of strong analgesics and preventing constipation is an important part of the pain plan. If you aren't offered information about preventing constipation, ask for it. Report other problems such as nausea, sleepiness, or anything that concerns you.

Keep a written record of pain and pain relief ratings. In this record, describe side effects as well as any concerns and new problems. Bring the record of pain scores to appointments with doctors or nurses so they can get an accurate picture of what the pain has been like since the last visit. When you're in the hospital, report pain using the rating scales and expect your reports to be taken seriously. Pain ratings are important vital signs just like blood pressure, pulse, temperature, and respiration. Many hospitals, including the entire U.S. Veteran's Administration hospital system, use "pain as the fifth vital sign," a mandate that requires the routine assessment of pain in each patient.

Pain Management

The best pain management plan is put together by care providers and the person with pain and uses a variety of approaches. Everyone involved in a person's care must understand the pain management plan. Medicines often are combined with nondrug strategies to improve comfort. Be sure to know to whom to report unrelieved pain, what to report, and where to get help outside of routine office hours. Bring pain reports along for each health care visit and include the names of all medicines, the doses, the schedule for their uses, and other important information. Don't hesitate to ask questions.

Using Medicines for Pain Relief

The goal of cancer pain control is to give the greatest amount of relief, with the fewest side effects possible, in the simplest way. Analgesic drugs are the mainstays of cancer pain treatment. Each person responds to medicines in different ways. What works for one person may not work at all for another, even if the pain seems similar and the medicine is the same.

Non-opioids and *opioids* are the two main families of analgesics. Non-opioid analgesics include acetaminophen (Tylenol and others) and non-steroidal anti-inflammatory drugs (NSAIDs) such as ibuprofen (Advil, Nuprin, Motrin, and others), ketoprofen (Orudis and others), naproxin sodium (Aleve and others), choline magnesium trisalicylate (Trilisate), celecoxib (Celebrex), rofecoxib (Vioxx), and others. All of these except Trilisate, Celebrex, and Vioxx are available without a prescription. These medicines work for mild to moderate pain only, but can be used along with stronger analgesics to manage severe pain. Each has a limit—sometimes referred to as a *ceiling*—on the dosage. Exceeding the recommended dose will not relieve pain more effectively, but will cause more side effects. Read labels and follow instructions carefully, and include these medicines in the list of medicines that are reported to the doctor or nurse.

Severe pain requires strong analgesics—opioids, sometimes called narcotics—for relief. These strong opioids include morphine, oxycodone, hydromorphone, hydrocodone, and fentanyl. Table 17.1 lists common opioid analgesics used to manage cancer pain. Meperidine (Demerol), a familiar analgesic to most physicians and nurses, should *not* be used to manage cancer pain. Its effects are very short lived, and normeperidine, a chemical by-product produced when the drug is broken down by the body, causes important side effects when used for more than several days. Meperidine should *never* be used regularly for long-term or "chronic" pain problems such as the pain caused by cancer.

Finding the Right Dose

People respond to medicines in different ways. When using opioids, the "right" dose is the dose that relieves pain with the fewest side effects. Unlike NSAIDs and acetaminophen, opioids do not have a limit, or ceiling,

Table 17.1: Medicines for Treating Severe Cancer Pain

Generic name	Trade names	Comments
Morphine sulfate: Short acting form	MSIR Roxanol OMS Concentrate MS/L RMS suppositories MS/S suppositories	Available in pills, liquids, suppositories, and for injection Each dose lasts 3 to 4 hours
Morphine sulfate: Long acting form	MSContin Oramorph SR Kadian	Available in tablets Except for Kadian, cannot be opened, crushed or changed in any way Medicine is released slowly over 8 to 12 hours for MSContin and Oramorph SR, 12 to 24 hours for Kadian
Oxycodone: Short acting form in combination with acetaminophen or aspirin	OxyIR OxyFast (concentrated dose) Roxicodone Roxicodone Intensol (concentrated solution) Percocet, Tylox Percodan	Available in tablets, liquid, suppositories Each dose lasts 3 to 4 hours Daily dose limit because of acetaminophen or aspirin; not to exceed 4 gm of either per day
Oxycodone: Long acting form	OxyContin	Do not crush, chew, split or change the tablet in any way Each dose lasts about 12 hours
Hydromorphone: Short acting form	Dilaudid Dilaudid HP (concentrated dose)	Available in tablets, liquid, and for injection Each dose lasts 3 to 4 hours
Hydromorphone: Long acting form	Palladone XL	Each dose lasts about 24 hours Do not chew, crush, or split tablet
Fentanyl: Skin patch Oral lozenge	 Duragesic Actiq	Available as patch (Duragesic), for injection, and in oral lozenge (Actiq) Each patch dose lasts about three days; do not alter patch Lozenge on a stick is dissolved by "painting" on the inside of the cheek; use in fifteen minutes, or less if pain is relieved; used for breakthrough pain in people who are tolerant to opioids
Methadone	Dolophine Methadose	Needs occasional dose adjustment even if pain remains the same; do not skip follow-up appointments

on the dose that can be used to relieve pain. With the doctor, nurse, or pharmacist's help, doses can be gradually adjusted, or *titrated,* as high as necessary to provide pain relief. There is never a need to "save the strong medicine until the pain is really bad." That's a myth, a very harmful myth. With the cancer pain expert's help (you should never change the dose on your own), opioids can be adjusted to control nearly all kinds of cancer-related pain.

In nursing school, student nurses all learned about the "Five Rs" of giving medicines safely:

- the right patient

- the right drug

- the right dose

- the right route of administration

- the right time

Sometimes, one or more of these Five Rs can be modified so that using pain medicines does not totally rule the person's life. Strong medicines like morphine, oxycodone, and hydromorphone come in *long acting* tablets made so that their analgesic effect lasts for twelve to twenty-four hours. The drug fentanyl is available in a *transdermal* (through the skin) preparation. It is made especially for people who have severe, constant pain, have difficulty swallowing, have a gastrointestinal tract that doesn't work, or are not conscious. Long acting medicines, taken routinely, help prevent pain from returning. Short acting medicines are used in case *breakthrough pain* occurs—the pain comes back between doses. The person takes the long acting medicine to prevent pain whether or not pain is present, and the short acting medicine only if pain comes back between doses. The doctor, nurse, or pharmacist can teach you how to use the different medicines and different formulations correctly and effectively.

Most pain—specifically, the nociceptive variety—responds to opioids and non-opioids quite well. Pain caused by pressure or irritation of nerves (neuropathic pain) may persist even when opioids and non-opioids pain plans are used. Adding other medicines to the plan may help. Tricyclic antidepressants such as amitriptyline and nortriptyline, and anticonvulsants such as gabapentin and phenytoin, are sometimes effective for managing neuropathic pain. These medicines are not analgesics, but they seem to enhance the analgesic effects of other medications used and are often referred to as *adjuvant* medications. Everyone responds differently to these medicines; some people get excellent relief, others none.

Nondrug Pain Relief

Most nondrug methods will not relieve severe pain by themselves, but can be used along with medicines in the management of severe pain. Be sure to tell your doctor or nurse about everything you are using to relieve pain.

Some of the therapies in the following list are discussed in more detail in Chapter 16:

- acupressure

- acupuncture

- cold

- distraction

- exercise

- heat

- hypnosis

- laughter therapy

- massage

- music therapy

- physical therapy

- reike therapy

- relaxation and guided imagery

- transcutaneous electric nerve stimulation (TENS)

Many of these therapies have been used for years; others are fairly new to pain relief plans. Different therapies work for different people. For the most part, nondrug strategies are fairly inexpensive, easy to take along wherever you go, easily used whenever and wherever the need occurs, and quite effective for some kinds of pain. Most nondrug measures take some practice to really experience the benefits.

The National Institutes of Health recently published a Technology Assessment Report that identifies the pain-relieving benefits of behavioral therapies like relaxation, imagery, hypnosis, and methods such as acupuncture to reduce certain types of pain. Some people who use these therapies report an increased sense of control and an improved sense of overall well-being. Most nondrug methods have few if any side effects.

Technological Approaches to Pain Control

Technology is sometimes helpful for the very few people—1 to 2 percent of people with cancer pain—who don't respond to analgesic medications or nondrug interventions. Medicine injected directly into or around a nerve (nerve block), pain medicine placed directly around the spinal cord through a thin tube called a catheter (epidural or intrathecal pain control), or surgery to interrupt a nerve (ablation) are options. Although not frequently needed for cancer pain, these treatments may offer relief when pain does not respond to other methods.

Dispelling Myths about Pain Medicines

Myth   Only weak people take strong medicines for pain. Trying to bear the pain as long as possible and using medicines only when the pain is really bad is the best plan.

Fact   Preventing pain from returning by using medicines on a schedule makes good sense and is an important part of treating cancer. It also takes more medicine to manage severe pain than mild to moderate pain.

Myth   Strong medicines can only be used for a short time and should be saved in case the pain gets really bad.

Fact   Strong medicines are safe to use, even for a very long time, as long as pain is present. The dose of strong analgesics can be raised as high as necessary to manage pain. There is never a point when the medicine must be stopped because the dose is "too much." "Saving" these medicines causes unnecessary pain and suffering.

Myth   When strong medicines such as morphine are prescribed, death must be near.

Fact   Strong medicines such as morphine are now used for all kinds of pain, at all stages of treatment, for people with and without cancer. These medicines are used for pain after surgery, pain from procedures, some kinds of chronic pain from problems other than cancer, and cancer pain. They are the medicines of choice for most severe pain.

Myth Injections of medicines work better than medicines by mouth and should be used for severe pain.

Fact Approximately 90 percent of all cancer pain can be relieved using pills or liquids taken by mouth as long as the person is conscious, can swallow, and his gastrointestinal system works. In fact, injections of medicines into the muscle (intramuscular or IM) are discouraged for cancer pain because injections cause pain themselves. The key to successful pain control using pills or liquids is to find the right dose. Medicines taken by mouth are partially destroyed and eliminated through the liver, kidney, and gut before they have a chance to relieve pain. More medication is needed to relieve pain when the drug is given orally than when it is given by injection. This is called *equianalgesic dosing*. For example, if 10 mg of morphine given by intravenous injection relieves pain, 30 mg might be needed to get the same level of relief when the drug is taken orally. The doctor or nurse should consult an equianalgesic chart, readily available in most books and references about pain, when switching from one medicine to another or changing the route of administration. Failure to make this adjustment is a common reason that pain relief is not achieved.

Final Thoughts

The man with cancer pain plays an important role in finding a plan that works for him. He must be able to tell doctors and nurses exactly how his pain feels and what, if anything, has provided some relief. This is key to taking control of pain. Look for a health care provider who knows how to manage cancer pain, and get a second opinion if you are told nothing can be done. There is always something that can be done. Having cancer and going through treatment is hard enough without having to deal with pain. Cancer doesn't have to hurt. Work with your doctor or nurse to achieve comfort that allows you to get the most from life.

*Taking
Control of
Cancer Pain*

18

◆◆◆

Cancer, Sexuality, and Sex

Debra Thaler-DeMers, B.S.N., R.N., O.C.N.

Cancer impacts a person's whole being, not just the body part affected by the disease. Cancer can have physical, emotional, spiritual, and sexual effects. Quite often, sexuality is overlooked by a man and his health care team when treatment needs are being considered. Still, sexuality is a very real concern. All forms of cancer and cancer treatment have the potential to interfere with sexual health. Any possible changes that cancer treatment can have on a man's sexuality may affect his choice about a particular treatment. Some men might pursue alternatives to surgery and chemotherapy, or even reject treatment, instead of taking the risk of changing sexual function or sexuality. Yet sexual issues are often not discussed with the oncologist, the oncology nurse, or any other member of the health care team.

For the sake of this discussion, *sexuality* is a part of a person's identity, his self-image: how he sees himself physically (body image), how he thinks of himself as a person (mental image), how he feels about himself (psychological and emotional self-image), and how he believes other people see him. Sexuality combines identity—body and mental image—with preferences for intimacy, including both physical and emotional closeness. *Sex* refers to actual sexual activity.

Even though most men find that talking about sex and sexuality is at least slightly uncomfortable, they discover that it is extremely helpful to openly discuss the effects on sexuality and sexual function of the cancer itself and the available treatment options. Testicular and prostate cancers are the cancers that most people think of when considering an impact on sexuality, but all cancers can affect sexuality. While a cancer that affects the sex organs—penis, testes, prostate—will trigger a more immediate response to the potential for a change in sexual function or feelings relating to intimacy, any cancer or cancer treatment that affects the way a man's body works or the way he thinks about himself as a person could also affect his sexuality. It is important to remember that these changes may be only temporary and that by talking about the potential changes, the health care team has a better chance of helping you find ways to work around them. If sexuality has been an important part of your life before cancer, there is no reason you cannot continue to have an active sex life after a diagnosis.

People have varied comfort levels in talking about sexuality. This is important to remember in the context of a cancer diagnosis. You may not feel comfortable bringing up the subject of your sex life, and your doctor may not feel comfortable talking about it either. There is no course in medical school called "How to Talk to Your Patients about Sex Without Feeling Uncomfortable." When you ask members of your health care team questions about sexual issues, be aware of their reactions. If they don't seem comfortable talking about this topic, or if they avoid the discussion entirely, tell them your needs. You might say, "I'm not exactly comfortable talking about this, so I imagine you might feel the same way. Still, I need to know this before I make any decision about my treatment." This will let your doctor, nurse, or social worker know that it's okay if you're both a little uncomfortable. At the same time, you're telling them how important it is for you to get this information.

If you think you are not getting the information you need, ask for a referral to someone who can help you with these issues. Your physician may refer you to another physician, a psychologist, a nurse with expertise in this area, or an oncology social worker. If you aren't comfortable talking about sexuality, educational materials are available in written, video, and audiotape format. Remember to check the date on any material you receive about cancer or the treatment for cancer. Advances in research change the way cancer is treated almost on a daily basis, and information that is even a year old may be out of date. New treatments are being developed that attack the cancer but minimize damage to other parts of the body, including damage to sexual function and fertility.

A brief review of the body's normal sexual functions and sexual response will help clarify questions and concerns, and hopefully make talking with health care team members a little easier.

The Sexual Response

Sexual response is the term used by the renowned sexologists Masters and Johnson to describe the changes that occur from the time of sexual arousal (becoming excited) to the period of resting after sexual activity. Since no two people are exactly alike, or behave in exactly the same manner, your response may be different from any described in this or any other book. Still, the basic physical changes are the same for all people.

The sexual response begins, quite literally, in the mind. Something triggers a physical response—an erotic thought, something you see that excites you, a smell, a touch, or something that you read. It can be one thing or a combination of things. The brain releases chemicals that begin a series of physical changes. Blood builds up in certain parts of the body, notably the shaft of the penis. This causes the penis to enlarge in both length and width and to become hard and erect. Men often experience a feeling of warmth when this happens. It is normal for the penis to change its shape during sexual activity. It may become softer at some point and then become hard again. The degree of erection is different for each man.

Blood also collects in the testes, which enlarge and are pulled up toward the abdomen, a normal response that should not be painful. Some men describe this as having "blue balls," because of the change in color caused by the collection of blood. At the same time that the penis and the testes are filling with blood, the heart beats faster, breathing may be faster, muscles may become tense or have involuntary twitches or spasms, and there can be a feeling of anxiety or tension.

The prostate gland and a gland behind it, the *seminal vesicle*, make the fluid called *semen*. Semen mixes with sperm as it travels toward the penis from the testes. Before ejaculation occurs, a message is sent to a muscle between the bladder and a gland near the prostate that closes the opening to the bladder, so that the semen and sperm move down the penis, rather than into the bladder. When ejaculation occurs, semen and sperm are released from the penis. The amount of force behind this release is different for each man. Semen can ooze out of the penis or it can squirt several inches or more. The amount of force can be different each time a man ejaculates.

During the relaxation phase of the sexual response, the body starts to return to the way it was before arousal. The heart rate, breathing, and blood pressure return to normal levels. Muscles relax. The penis returns to its normal size and shape, loses its hardness, and is no longer erect. Many men feel tired or so relaxed that they fall asleep. The amount of time this process takes is different for each man. It is *not* normal for the penis to remain hard and erect for several hours after sexual activity; if this happens, you should seek immediate medical help. The penis can be damaged if it remains erect for more than three hours after sexual activity.

Many parts of the body must work together for the sexual response to take place. Messages travel from the brain to muscles and blood vessels though the nervous system. Nerves help control the muscles as they either become tense or relax. Blood must flow to the penis and testes and collect there for the penis to become hard and change size, and for the testes to enlarge and move up toward the abdomen. Chemicals called *hormones* must be released at certain times during the process for these body changes to take place. The heart beats faster. The lungs need to take in more oxygen to help the body during this time of increased physical activity. A change in any of these parts of the body may change sexual response. A change may be due to illness, surgery, radiation, chemotherapy, or biologic therapy. It may also be due to emotional stress. The excitement or arousal experienced in the mind triggers the release of chemicals that start the sexual response cycle in motion. If a man is depressed, it will be difficult for him to become sexually aroused.

If cancer or the treatment for cancer has caused changes that interfere with your sexuality, your doctor or other members of your health care team can help you deal with these issues. Medications and other treatments are available to help you maintain sexual activity at whatever level you choose.

Sexuality and Fertility

Some forms of cancer affect the number and quality of sperm that a man produces. Both the number of sperm and their ability to move up the vagina toward a partner's egg (called *motility*) determine a man's ability to father children, or *fertility*. If cancer treatment affects a man's ability to produce sperm, he can choose to store his sperm to preserve his options for having children later.

Sperm Banking

It is better to store sperm—called *sperm banking*—before starting cancer treatment. Some insurance companies will pay for this procedure as a part of cancer treatment, although the doctor may need to write a letter to the insurance company stating that sperm banking is "medically necessary." There is a fee for analyzing the sperm to see if there are enough to make sperm banking useful, as well as a processing fee and an annual fee for storing frozen sperm. When you later decide to use the sperm, it will be returned to you, to your doctor, or to the fertility clinic you choose.

The procedure for collecting sperm is fairly simple and can be done in a medical setting or in the privacy of your own home, using the sperm collection kit provided by the sperm bank. Sperm for sperm banking is collected by masturbation. In a medical office or clinic, a private room is provided. The clinic may have magazines and videotapes available to help you "get in the mood." You can also bring your partner into the room with you. A special type of condom is used to collect the sperm.

At least three separate sperm samples should be collected at least twenty-four hours apart so that the number of sperm in each sample will be as large as possible. The more often you have sex, the fewer sperm are available in each ejaculate. When time is a critical factor for starting cancer treatment, the samples can be collected over three consecutive days. Time may be a critical factor if your cancer is growing very quickly or the tumor is crowding a critical organ, such as your heart or your lungs. Other instances when time is an important factor include cases of acute leukemia, a large tumor located near the brain or a blood vessel called the superior vena cava, or when the tumor is preventing an organ such as the kidneys from working effectively.

Anyone who has reached puberty can bank sperm. If you are young, single, or think you do not ever want children, you may still want to consider banking your sperm. The sperm bank should ask what you would like done with your sperm if you decide later not to use it. You have the option of having the sperm destroyed, donating it to an infertility clinic or a research facility, or donating it to another couple or a family member who agrees to have your child. The important thing to remember is that you control what happens to your sperm. If you are in a relationship, you should discuss all options with your partner, including what you want done with your sperm if you die. Your partner may still want to have your child under these circumstances. She may feel that having your child will be a way for you to "live on" in the family. Inform the sperm bank in writing as to whether anyone has the right to use your sperm after your death. Keep a copy of this letter for your records.

Sperm Retrieval

Some types of cancer treatment affect a man's ability to ejaculate sperm. Sperm may be produced, but are prevented from being ejaculated in the usual manner. A fertility specialist may be able to retrieve sperm either from the testicle or from that part of the body where the normal ejaculation process has been diverted. Men with prostate cancer may experience retrograde ejaculation, where the sperm moves back toward the bladder rather than forward toward the penis. Through medications and/or surgical procedures, sperm from retrograde ejaculation can be retrieved and used immediately or stored in a sperm bank.

Low Sperm Count

If you have never had a sperm count done before your cancer diagnosis, there is no way to tell if a low sperm count is directly related to the cancer. You may have always had a low sperm count; cancer may have nothing to do with it. The important thing is that when you are diagnosed with cancer, you have the option of finding out what your sperm count is and having your sperm stored in case you want to have children sometime in the future.

Sexual Function

The ability—or inability—to produce active, healthy sperm in sufficient numbers to father a child does not physically affect your ability to achieve or maintain an erection. It also does not affect your ability to produce semen, the fluid that is ejaculated from the penis. Semen and sperm are made in two different parts of the body. If you find that you are infertile or have a low sperm count at the time you are diagnosed with cancer, it could be that you have been infertile for some time without knowing it. During that time, your ability to have or maintain an erection was not affected. If you are now having trouble becoming sexually aroused or obtaining or maintaining an erection, and you believe this is related to your infertility, you should discuss this with your doctor. The only thing that has changed is that your mind has now processed an additional piece of information. The ability to have and maintain an erection is *completely different* from the ability to produce sperm. A urologist, fertility specialist, sex educator, or sex counselor can help you understand and work through this concern.

Problems with Erection

One of the things many men worry about after having cancer is that they will be unable to have an erection. The problem, labeled *erectile dysfunction* or ED, is now discussed openly even in television advertisements.

The ability to have an erection depends on several things. The message must come from the brain to release certain hormones that start the sexual response cycle. Many things can interfere with the message from the brain.

The most common is worrying about whether or not you will be able to get an erection, sometimes called "performance anxiety." One way to assess a problem with erection is to check if you have them while you sleep. If you have an erection when you wake up, the physical parts that cause an erection are probably in good working order. To test if you had an erection while you were asleep, put a paper band around your penis at night and see if the band is ripped in the morning. This test should be done with your doctor's knowledge and advice. The paper must rip easily; using something that is too tight might cause permanent damage to the penis.

Once the message has been sent from the brain, chemicals are released that tell the body to make the hormones needed for sexual activity. If the body is not able to make these hormones, or if the hormones are being intentionally inactivated because they are feeding the cancer—as is the case in treatment for prostate cancer—the response cycle must be started in another way. There are treatments that will accomplish this. You will want to evaluate all available treatments for prostate cancer, as well as their possible side effects, before deciding which treatment you and your doctor want to pursue. See Chapter 4 for more information about hormones and the treatment of prostate cancer.

The message travels from the brain to the body through nerves. If the nerve pathway from the brain to the penis has been interrupted at any point along the way, the message never arrives. New *nerve sparing* surgical methods are more successful in preserving the nerves that help a man achieve and maintain an erection. Ask your surgeon if he or she performs this type of surgery. If not, or the hospital where you are to have surgery does not have the equipment to do this type of surgery, ask for a referral to a surgeon and a hospital that provide this type of surgery AND have a good record of success in its use. In situations where the insurance company or the HMO will not pay for this type of surgery, some men opt to pay for access to it out of their own pocket. If the nerve pathway has been interrupted because of damage to the spinal cord, there are methods that can be used to stimulate the body into starting the sexual response cycle. Nerve pathways in the face, nipples, scrotum, and inner thigh can stimulate erogenous feelings and trigger the sexual response cycle.

In order for the penis to enlarge and become erect, there must be good blood flow to the penis. If you have a medical problem other than cancer that disturbs circulation, such as diabetes or hypertension (high blood pressure), that condition (rather than the cancer) may be causing erectile problems. Be sure to tell your cancer doctor about all of your health conditions when you talk to him about any erectile problems.

Several forms of medicines may be useful in treating erectile dysfunction. Some are taken by mouth. Others are rubbed on the penis to relax blood vessels or inserted or injected into the penis to cause an erection. If erectile dysfunction exists because of a problem with blood flow to the penis, you may be able to take the medication called Viagra. Viagra relaxes muscles so that blood can flow into the penis. It can be taken thirty minutes to four hours, with the most common recommendation being one hour, before sexual activity. Viagra requires a written prescription from your doctor, with good reason.

Some men should not use Viagra. Men with leukemia, multiple myeloma, or cardiac problems should not take Viagra. Because Viagra changes the effect of some other medicines, the doctor who prescribes it must be aware of all medicines including over-the-counter drugs and cancer treatments you are taking.

Other treatments aside from medicines can help you obtain an erection. The simplest is a vacuum device that causes an erection by creating a partial vacuum around the penis. This pulls blood into the penis. An elastic ring fits over the base of the penis and traps the blood so that the erection is maintained.

Men who are unable to take Viagra may be candidates for other forms of treatment to help them have and maintain an erection. In some cases, a surgical procedure can correct problems with arteries or veins. Your doctor can order a test—a Doppler ultrasound study, venogram, or arteriogram— that will show whether there is a blockage or other problem that might be corrected with surgery.

Surgery can also be done to place a device—a *penile implant* or *penile prosthesis*—inside you that will allow you to have an erection when you want one. A prosthesis is either a replacement for a part that is missing or something that will help a part of you work better, such as a hearing aid. The difference between a hearing aid and a penile prosthesis is that no one will be able to tell that you have a penile prosthesis, since all of the parts are located inside your body.

One type of penile implant, a *semirigid* implant, makes the penis hard and somewhat erect all of the time and allows you to have sexual intercourse. A fully erect penis is not necessary for intercourse. The disadvantage is that the penis will always look semierect and may be seen through tight clothing. Another type of device lets you get an erection by pressing on a small pump. The pump moves fluid into one or more tubes implanted in the penis. The fluid serves the same purpose as the blood that would normally flow into the penis when you are aroused and causes the penis to become hard and erect. The erection stays until the fluid is released. The way fluid is released varies according to the kind of device that is implanted.

Recently, much attention has focused on erectile dysfunction. Celebrity spokesmen have made it acceptable to talk about this common problem, and research continues to offer new ways to treat it. Be sure to ask your doctor to tell you about all the treatment methods available to help you, or ask for a referral to a physician who specializes in erectile problems.

Problems with Ejaculation

Ejaculation is the release of fluid from the penis during sexual activity. Most men think that ejaculation should happen at the same time they reach orgasm, or at the time of greatest pleasure sensation during sexual activity. This happens in the movies and romance novels and sometimes in real life, but not always. Many men reach orgasm just before or after ejaculation. The situation can be problematic when the time between orgasm and the release of fluid is too long, or when the fluid is released before the man has satisfied himself or his partner. Some time after the fluid is released, the penis returns to its normal, relaxed state.

Cancer surgery may remove some of the body parts that produce semen or help cause semen and sperm to move into the penis. If the prostate and seminal vesicles are removed, or nerves that control the movement of semen and sperm into the penis are damaged, it is possible to have an orgasm with little or no fluid being released from the penis. The fact that there is no fluid will not affect the ability to have an orgasm. If you are concerned about fertility, a fertility specialist can advise you on ways to retrieve sperm without ejaculation.

In some cases, semen is being produced, but instead of moving into the penis it moves backward into the bladder. This is called *retrograde ejaculation*, a fancy term for semen and sperm going in the wrong direction. Normally, there is an opening between the bladder and the prostate that connects both to the *ureter*, the tube through which both urine and semen pass down the penis and are pushed out of the body. When the sexual response cycle is started, the opening closes so that urine is kept in the bladder and semen is allowed to travel down the penis. If the muscles or nerves that control this opening are damaged, it could stay open during sexual activity and the semen and sperm would move into the bladder instead of down the penis. The sensation of ejaculation will not be affected, but no fluid is released. Your doctor can help you decide whether you want to try a treatment to correct this problem. The semen and sperm going into your bladder will not hurt you; they will be washed out of the bladder with the urine, which might look cloudy.

Sexuality and Intimacy

Intimacy involves sharing oneself with another person, in far more ways than through sexuality. Sharing feelings, hopes, dreams, fears, emotions, religious values, touching, hugging, caring deeply about another person— these are all aspects of an intimate relationship.

The Importance of Communication

If you are involved in a relationship at the time of your cancer diagnosis, your partner may have concerns that you will need to talk about together and may also want to discuss these concerns with your doctor. It is important that you both know that cancer is not contagious. You cannot get cancer from kissing, hugging, or from most forms of sexual contact. The only possible link between sexual activity and cancer has to do with human papillomavirus (HPV), the virus that causes genital warts; this virus may cause changes in a woman's cervix that can lead to cervical cancer. If you have an active case of genital warts, using a condom during intercourse will protect your partner from the virus. The virus that causes AIDS (HIV) can also be spread through sexual contact. While AIDS is not a form of cancer, people with AIDS can develop certain forms of cancer such as Kaposi's sarcoma, central nervous system (CNS) lymphoma, and non-Hodgkin's lymphoma. Practicing safe sex will protect you and your partner from getting or passing on HIV.

Talking with your partner about any fears, worries, or beliefs about how cancer will affect your relationship is very important. If you don't share thoughts and feelings, your relationship can suffer; you may think that you are "protecting" one another, but it is better to talk about these things than to keep silent and worry about them alone. When you talk about feelings, use the words "I feel" to start your sentences. This way, your partner will understand that you are talking about the reaction the cancer diagnosis or the treatment has had on you. You are the only person who knows what it feels like to live in your body. Don't assume your partner is feeling something without checking with him or her first.

John and Beverly offer a clear example of how communication can help resolve problems. Beverly believed that all kinds of cancer were extremely painful. Even though John's cancer had been diagnosed from a painless lump in his testicle, and he had never experienced pain except for the first week after his surgery, Beverly was afraid to touch him or to have any sexual activity. She believed that sexual arousal would cause him severe pain. When John tried to interest Beverly in sexual activity, she avoided him,

Cancer, Sexuality, and Sex

truly believing she was doing this to protect him. John felt rejected. He wondered if Beverly was no longer attracted to him because he had testicular cancer. Their relationship began to suffer until John finally decided to ask Beverly why she no longer wanted to be sexually intimate with him. When Beverly was able to say, "I'm afraid I'll hurt you," it was a great relief to both of them. They were able to talk about their feelings and agreed that if anything they did was painful for John, he would let Beverly know right away. He was also sure to tell her when something she did felt good. This helped Beverly to relax and begin to enjoy their physical relationship again.

New Relationships

If you are not involved in a relationship at the time of diagnosis, you may become involved with someone during or after treatment and should think about when you will share the fact that you have had cancer. You might want to tell your partner up front, before or during the first date. This way, if she or he has any concerns about having a relationship with someone who has cancer, you will find out about it early in the relationship. The way you approach the subject of your cancer diagnosis is important. If you are defensive or confrontational you may frighten your partner. Remember that this person has expressed an interest in getting to know you, in beginning a new relationship. If you decide to tell your partner about your cancer early in the relationship, be sure to let her or him know to what extent you want to discuss it. One man might want to put the whole thing behind him and never talk about it again. Another man will think the experience is important in shaping who he has become as a person and want to talk about the impact cancer has had on his life.

Good communication has two parts: talking and listening. Listen to what your partner tells you when you discuss the cancer experience. If he or she has experienced the death of a loved one due to cancer (with cancer affecting one of every two people in the United States in some way, it will be difficult to meet someone who has not been touched in some way), your partner may be fearful and may also be unaware that more than half of the people diagnosed today will be alive five years after their diagnosis. Keep in mind that cancer is many different diseases. Two people with the same exact kind of cancer will not respond in the same way to their disease or their treatment. You could possibly reassure your partner (as well as other loved ones) by letting him or her know that there are currently over eight million cancer survivors in the United States.

An unfortunate but normal response to hearing the word "cancer" is to be afraid and to believe that the person with cancer is going to die in a short period of time. If you are entering a new relationship, you might consider waiting until you and your partner have had a chance to get to know one another and feel comfortable with each other before discussing your cancer experience in depth. One other thought about telling others about your cancer experience: Cancer, through the drama of television specials, movies, and feature articles, has a reputation as a painful, traumatic, and fatal disease. Once you have established good communication skills and feel comfortable being with and talking with each other, it may be easier to share feelings about the cancer experience.

Intimacy in the Hospital Setting

The fact that you are an inpatient in a hospital will not prevent you from having erotic thoughts about your partner. You should feel free to invite your partner to share your bed for hugging, cuddling, or just to be physically close to each other. If you feel that you want to engage in more intimate activities and if your partner is available and willing, there is no reason you cannot be intimate while you are in the hospital, provided you take a few simple precautions.

Talk to your nurse about having some private time with your partner. Post a "Do Not Disturb" sign on the door and make sure all members of the staff know not to interrupt you to check your vital signs or give you medications. You might remind your nurse to inform the nursing assistants and orderlies, the unit secretary, and any nurses that may cover for her while she is on break or at lunch. If you need to take some pain or nausea medication before any sexual activity, ask your nurse to give it to you at least thirty minutes before your private time. If you receive medication according to a set schedule, plan your activity for the time between doses. You might want to put something in front of the door that will make a noise if someone should try to enter without knocking first. This will give you some warning so you can yell, "Wait!" or "Don't come in!" Don't put anything in front of the door that will prevent the medical staff from entering should you need immediate help.

If you want to use lubricant, your nurse can provide you with a tube of KY Jelly. Your partner may obtain condoms or other methods of birth control for you. The nurse or a nursing assistant may be able to provide you with extra pillows to provide comfort and support. If there are not enough pillows available, a rolled or bunched-up blanket can serve the same purpose.

Make sure you know where the nurse call light is and put it close to you. If there is an emergency call light in the room, be sure your partner knows how to use it. This way, if you become short of breath or experience any other problems, someone can come to help you immediately.

Be aware that not all people who work in a hospital are comfortable with sexual intimacy. If you find that your nurse or nursing assistant is not willing to help you arrange for some intimate time with your partner, whether that partner is a man or a woman, ask for someone who is at ease with this issue to be assigned your care. A simple change in staff assignments can help everyone feel more comfortable.

If you do not have a partner, or your partner is not available, you may still have erotic thoughts and desire some form of sexual activity. If you take steps to ensure your privacy, you can engage in masturbation in the hospital setting.

Reconnecting with Yourself

Having cancer is only a part of who you are. While you go through treatment, your attention can be so focused on getting well that you forget about all the things you did and enjoyed before your diagnosis. Give yourself permission to take a vacation from the cancer experience and enjoy yourself. Remember that the sexual response cycle begins in your mind, which is also the source of memories of things that made you feel happy, relaxed, and safe. You had a life before cancer and you have a life after the diagnosis. Think about the things that gave you pleasure before you had cancer. Where was your favorite place? What was your favorite music? Your favorite place to eat? Your favorite food? Who did you enjoy being with? What did you enjoy doing? Thinking about things that brought you joy and living them again in your mind can help you focus on things other than your illness or the effects of your treatment. It can help build a mood that you can use to increase your interest in intimacy.

Changes in Sexuality Related to Cancer

Usually the first reaction to a diagnosis of cancer is to think about survival. At some point in the treatment process, thoughts may turn to how the cancer will affect your sexuality. If you do not think about your sexuality at all, and this was an important part of your life before the cancer diagnosis, your lack of interest in sexuality may be related to the cancer itself or the treatment you are receiving.

The word *libido* refers to your sex drive, or your level of interest in sex. Libido is affected by hormones and by emotions. If all of your energy is directed toward getting well, or if surgery, chemotherapy, biologic therapy, or radiation therapy have made you tired, you may not have any energy left over to think about sex. You may not feel sexually attractive. You may feel depressed. Many other things can change your level of interest in and desire for sexual activity or intimacy:

- feeling nauseated from the treatment

- being constipated or having diarrhea

- being in pain

- changes in the way you look (weight gain, weight loss, changes due to surgery, radiation markings, intravenous catheters, bladder catheters)

- medications to control side effects of treatment (sedatives, antinausea drugs, pain medications, hormones)

- feeling anxious or afraid

- feeling angry

- feeling out of control

- feeling tired or exhausted

This list is far from complete. If you notice that you are no longer interested in sexuality or intimacy and this is something you want to change, talk to your doctor or another member of your health care team. Medications and treatments are available to help you regain interest in sexual activity.

Physical Changes

A change in body image—how you see yourself and how you feel about your body—can affect your sexuality. If you have had surgery to create a new path for food, urine, or stool, you may worry about how your change in appearance will affect your partner. You may also worry about odors from a colostomy or urostomy collection pouch. A change in diet or the use of special liquids or powders in the pouch will help eliminate or mask unpleasant odors. Emptying your collection pouch before any planned sexual activity will also help. There are small collection pouches or even simple stoma covers that hide, minimize, or disguise the changes in the body.

Learning to control a colostomy through irrigation procedures helps many men with colostomies have sex without worry about fecal leakage. Feedings tubes can be coiled against the stomach or abdomen and held in place with Velcro to keep the tube out of the way. Use of romantic lighting (dim lights or candles) can set the mood and keep your mind, and your partner's, focused on things of more interest than your collection bag or other changes in your appearance.

Pain or nausea can cause a loss of interest in intimacy. Sexual activity, including cuddling, holding, and touching can be a good distraction from feelings of pain or nausea. Your mind has a hard time concentrating on more than one thing at a time. Taking prescribed medications for pain or nausea thirty minutes to an hour before any sexual activity will help relieve symptoms and leave your mind free to focus on the pleasures of being with your partner. Your favorite music, a romantic atmosphere, or a favorite place will give the mind more things to focus on and distract you from your cancer experience and all that it entails.

Cancer of the penis is very rare but does occur. If caught early, it may be treated with radiation or chemotherapy rather than surgery. When surgery is needed, it is usually possible to save part of the penis. If there is still a penis, it is possible to have an erection and orgasm. The desire for sex is not changed by the surgery although depression and anxiety can affect a man's ability to have an erection or orgasm. If there has been damage to the nerves or blood vessels, a penile prosthesis (discussed earlier in this chapter) can be used.

Some forms of cancer treatment, such as certain chemotherapy drugs or radiation therapy to certain parts of the lower abdomen, may change sensations you experience during sexual activity. These are usually temporary changes. If they happen to you, be sure to let your doctor know about them. If you are receiving radiation therapy, you should tell the radiation oncologist (radiation doctor) as well as the doctor who is in charge of your cancer treatments. If you notice the changes soon after surgery, talk to the surgeon as well as your cancer doctor. Don't assume that these changes are a normal part of cancer treatment. Anything that is different during or after your treatment should be reported to your cancer doctor. It is better to let your doctor tell you that it is normal than for you to assume it is normal and say nothing to your doctor.

Special Things to Consider

Hormones Hormones play a role in your emotional state, so it is perfectly normal to have changes in emotions whenever hormonal levels are affected by cancer and/or cancer treatment. You may feel depressed and might want to withdraw from your partner or from your family and friends. Talk to your doctor, your nurse, or another member of your health care team about the way you are feeling, both physically and emotionally. Medications can help you cope with these changes. Most important, you need to know that your sex life is not over. There are many different ways to express your sexuality. You could think of this as an opportunity to explore new techniques and methods that you would not have known about before.

Low Red Blood Cell Counts It is important to be aware of your red and white blood cell counts and your platelet level while you are going through cancer treatment. Red blood cells carry oxygen throughout your body. If you have a low red blood cell count, you may feel tired much of the time and you may become short of breath. Sometimes people do not notice they are short of breath until it becomes very difficult to breathe. Sexual activity is like any other physical activity—your body will need more oxygen. You will breathe faster to get more oxygen into your lungs and circulating around your body. If your red blood cell count is low, your body may not be able to provide enough oxygen, and you may get short of breath.

One way to compensate for diminished energy or shortness of breath is to use different positions for sexual activity. Any position where you are relaxed and don't require a lot of effort to stay in that position will help conserve your breath and your energy. You might want to sit up or place pillows behind your back to support you in a more upright position. The more upright you are, the more your lungs can expand and take in more oxygen with each breath. Pacing your activity will not only help you breathe but will prolong your sexual pleasure. If you find you are getting short of breath, let your partner know and slow your pace for a time until you are breathing easily and feel ready to change the pace. There are many books and educational videos that can help you explore and discover positions and techniques that allow you to enjoy sexual activity without worrying about becoming short of breath. *The New Joy of Sex* by Dr. Alex Comfort is an example of an illustrated guide to sexual activity.

Low White Blood Cell Counts Your white blood cells help you fight infection. When the white blood cell count is low, your body is not able to fight off bacteria, and your immune system is not able to protect you from infection. This is called being *immunosuppressed*. Sexual activity with your partner will not cause an infection by itself, but you should be careful with all things, including sexual activity, when your white blood cell count is low. The most important way to prevent infection is to wash your hands before and after any activity. Anyone you come in contact with when you are immunosuppressed should also wash his or her hands before touching you.

Anyone with a cold, virus, or other infection should not visit you when your white blood cell count is low. You should not have intimate contact with your partner if he or she has a cold or other infection. If your partner is feeling sick in any way, you should avoid intimate contact. It is better to avoid an infection than to try to cure it later.

One of the ways bacteria enter your body is through breaks in the skin. If you have a cut, it is important to keep it clean and covered with a bandage. Some forms of sexual activity can cause small tears or breaks in the skin or mucous membranes that become an entrance point for bacteria. Anal stimulation or anal intercourse can cause tears too small for the eye to see. Bacteria can enter through these tiny openings. Using lubrication decreases the risk of tears, but it is best to avoid anal intercourse when the white blood cell count is low.

Oral sex adds to the risk of infection when a person has a low white blood cell count and develops small breaks in the mucous membranes that line the mouth. Sexual activity can induce tears, or breaks in the mucous membrane may develop as a result of chemotherapy. The simple act of eating, especially hard or sharp foods like hard crackers, nuts, or candy, can tear the fragile mucous membrane. Many types of bacteria live in a person's mouth. Normally, your body has become used to and recognizes your partner's bacteria just as it recognizes its own bacteria. When you are immunosuppressed, bacteria from your partner's mouth might cause infection. The risk of infection is low, but remember that the best way to treat an infection is to prevent it from happening. It is safer to avoid oral sex, both heterosexual and homosexual, when the white blood cell count is low.

Low Platelets Platelets are blood cells that help with clotting. When you cut yourself, you will bleed until a clot forms. If you bump into something, you will often get a black-and-blue mark—a bruise or *hematoma*—caused by bleeding under the surface of the skin. If your platelet count is low, it takes longer to form a blood clot. Until it forms, you will continue to bleed. You should avoid sexual activity that can cause you to bruise or to tear skin or mucous membranes when your platelet count is low. Anal sex, sadomasochistic practices, bondage, and the use of some "sex toys" are examples of sexual activities that should be avoided when the platelet count is low.

High White Blood Cell Count If you have leukemia, the white blood cell count will probably be higher than normal. This does not mean you have a normally functioning immune system. In leukemia, the white blood cells do not mature properly. They remain in an earlier or "immature" form of development called the *blast phase* and are not able to fight off infection. You have a lot of white blood cells, but they are essentially useless in fighting infection. You have the same risk of infection as someone with a very low white blood cell count and should use the same precautions in your sexual activity.

People with leukemia tend to have high white blood cell counts and low red blood cell and platelet counts. One of the safest forms of sexual intercourse for a heterosexual man in this circumstance is vaginal intercourse using a condom and generous lubrication. A safe form of sexual activity for a homosexual couple would be mutual masturbation using generous lubrication.

Multiple Myeloma One of the effects of multiple myeloma is the risk of stress fractures; your bones break very easily. Any activity, including sexual activity, that involves the use of bones and muscles increases this risk. This does not mean you should live your life in a protective bubble. Choosing positions that provide support and comfort during sexual activity, and making generous use of pillows, decreases your risk of a stress fracture. If you experience pain at any time during sexual activity, let your partner know immediately. Check to be sure you can move that part of your body without pain. If there is redness or swelling, or if the pain does not subside, call your doctor.

Cancer of the Penis If you have had invasive cancer of the penis and the entire penis has been removed, your surgeon may have created an opening for urine that is located behind the testicles and in front of the anus. You will have to sit down to urinate. This does not affect your ability to become sexually aroused, achieve orgasm, or ejaculate. While there is no longer a penis, the ability to have sensation in this area remains. The semen will be released through the same opening as urine.

Rectal Cancer If you have a tumor located low in the colon, near the rectum, removing the tumor may involve closing the rectum and creating a colostomy for elimination of feces. Homosexual men who have enjoyed anal intercourse prior to this surgery will no longer be able to engage in this activity. It is important to talk about this with your partner. There are many other methods of sexual activity you and your partner can explore to enhance your relationship.

Sexually Transmitted Diseases

Whether you have cancer or not, it is important to protect yourself from sexually transmitted diseases. When you have sex with someone, you are essentially taking the same risk as if you were sleeping with every sexual partner of your partner. Most people are not comfortable talking about sexually transmitted diseases, but remember that the best way to treat an infection is to prevent it.

Some sexually transmitted diseases have no symptoms, so it is possible to have a disease without knowing it. Herpes and genital warts can be spread by skin-to-skin contact. People who are being treated for cancer and people with cancers such as lymphoma and leukemia are more at risk for these two viral infections. Parasites can be passed between partners through anal intercourse or anal-oral contact. Hepatitis and HIV are spread through many kinds of sexual contact.

The best protection for sexually transmitted diseases is to use a latex condom and *only* water-based lubricants such as KY Jelly. Condoms should be used any time there is contact between a penis and a mouth or a penis and an anus. If you are performing oral sex on a woman, you should place a dental dam or plastic wrap such as Saran Wrap over the woman's vulva to prevent infection. Using flavored condoms or things like whipped cream can diminish the taste of the barrier.

Final Thoughts

Sexuality is a part of each person's identity—who we are, how we think, and what we feel. Sexuality and intimacy are different for each person. You are the only person who knows what sexuality means to you and how it affects your quality of life. What I hope you have learned from reading this chapter is that sexuality does not end when you are diagnosed with cancer. No matter what type of cancer you have, or what treatment you decide on, there are health care professionals who can help you find a level of sexual activity and intimacy that is comfortable and is what you want and need. If the first doctor or nurse you talk to about this important subject is not able to help you, ask him or her to refer you to someone who can. You have the right to ask questions and get answers about sexual issues.

19

◆◆◆

End-of-Life and Palliative Care

Jerome Koss, R.N., O.C.N.

In contemporary American society and in some other industrialized cultures as well, death is often seen as medical failure rather than a natural end, the way birth is a natural beginning. Although advances in medical technology allow us to extend life, sometimes unwanted consequences create a quality of life that is much less than what most people would knowingly choose. Perhaps a half century ago most people died in their homes. Today, more than half of all people die in hospitals, hospices, or nursing homes. Many people's lives are extended for longer than they wish, in situations that might be viewed as lacking in dignity. Most people, if given a choice, would prefer a peaceful and serene ending to their lives. When suffering caused by pain or other symptoms is unbearable, or if quality of life is diminished or even absent, many people wonder if it is right to hasten death or withhold treatment that seems to prolong anguish. For a person whose cancer cannot be controlled, planning what his life's end will be like is of extreme importance.

End-of-Life Concerns

More attention is paid to end-of-life issues in society today than has been in the past, in part because people have more interest in making their own health care decisions. Information in the media is geared toward helping people with cancer and their loved ones cope with terminal illness. Most people no longer want their physicians, with little discussion with the patient or his family, to make all the decisions; they want to discuss openly and honestly their prognoses and the symptoms and problems they might experience as they near the end of life. They want symptoms such as pain to be minimized. They want more choice as to how and where their deaths should occur.

People want good quality of life, in all of life's stages. Quality of life means different things to different people, especially as life is coming to an end. Most people, when nearing death, want to maintain connections with their family and other significant people in their lives. They want to strengthen relationships with loved ones, maintain their role in the family as much as possible, and feel that their life has had meaning. They want control over the medical decisions that affect them. At the end of life, most people do not want to feel isolated. They want to be free from undue suffering and to preserve their dignity.

These end-of-life concerns can vary depending on age. Younger men generally place more significance on dignity issues such as the ability to carry out personal needs. Symptoms like pain can challenge a younger man's feelings of control. Middle-aged men tend to focus more on issues such as the well-being of their families, whether they were successful in achieving personal goals, and the meaning of their lives. Older men seem to be more concerned about being a burden to caregivers and loved ones.

There is no right way to approach the end of life. Just as in the day-to-day decisions of living, people need to consider their own needs and choices and those of family members and friends. The end of one's life is just as unique as the rest of it. Understanding the challenges of getting matters in order can help the dying person and his loved ones cope effectively.

Nurses and social workers who regularly take care of people with cancer recognize the deficiencies in care at the end of life. A position statement released in 1999 by the Oncology Nursing Society and the Association of Oncology Social Workers identifies specific areas of concern and helps establish the foundation for the ideas presented in the remainder of this chapter. This position is summarized in Figure 19.1 and might assist readers in asking for appropriate end-of-life services wherever care is provided.

Maintaining Control in Life's Concluding Chapter

Dying people tell us that even at life's end, maintaining a sense of control over what happens to them—physically (controlling pain and other dis-

Figure 19.1: ONS and AOSW Joint Position on End-of-Life Care

The position of the ONS and AOSW is that people with catastrophic, potentially fatal illnesses and those close to them should be able to expect and receive reliable, skillful, and supportive care. It is the position of ONS and AOSW that:

*Health care professionals must work to improve care of dying patients, identifying and relieving symptoms relating to the process of dying;

*Health care professionals must recognize the spiritual component of care and make resources available to those who wish them;

*Health care training programs must include content that will help health care professionals change—for the better—the care available to dying patients and their families;

*Health care professionals must be sensitive to the different kinds of suffering patients and families experience throughout the dying process;

*Research efforts must be supported that provide a scientific basis for care provided to dying patients and their family members;

*Health care professionals need to work toward improving the financing of care and to simplify regulations that impede relief of pain and suffering;

*Health care professionals must plan for and give care that takes the patient and family's cultural issues into consideration;

*Patient and family decision making must be supported, and emotional distress minimized, through help in getting and understanding accurate information relating to end-of-life care planning.

Summarized from the position published in Oncology Nursing Forum *26(1): 15, 1999. The position can be downloaded from the ONS website (www.ons.org).*

tressing symptoms) and emotionally (assuring that their needs and desires are met, to the extent possible)—is crucial. Most Americans value *self-determination*, or autonomy. More and more, people are taking charge of their own health care and making profound decisions in order to achieve the kind of death they want. People with advanced disease are often faced with the difficult choice between full and aggressive or limited life-sustaining treatment. Life-sustaining measures—such as tube feedings or mechanical ventilation on a machine that helps with breathing—serve to prolong but not prevent the dying process. Finally, a man and his family members may choose to stop treatment entirely when death seems to be near.

Gathering Information

Information about prognosis and the specifics of treatment can be complex, even overwhelming. As in all kinds of decision making, it is critical that the pros and cons of all possible decisions be understood and weighed. The potential for stress during the dying process is great, so weighing the options before stressors make decision making more difficult is very important. Some patients don't want any information, don't want to participate in decisions about their care. All patients have a right to know what is happening to them; at the same time, health care professionals must be respectful and sensitive to every dying person's wishes and needs.

Advance Directives

Advance directives are specifically designed documents that give the person a voice in his health care decisions should he be unable to communicate. When prepared properly, advance directives are extremely helpful in making one's wishes known. There are two frequently used types: a living will and a durable power of attorney.

The Patient Self-Determination Act of 1991 mandates that health care professionals teach patients and families about advance directives at the time of hospital admission. Hospital staff is usually willing to answer any questions about this subject. All fifty states and the District of Columbia have laws authorizing the use of advance directives. The laws vary from state to state, so it is important to know the law as it applies in the state where care is being provided. For example, Alaska has legislation that provides only for living wills. Laws in Massachusetts, Michigan, and New York only allow for power of attorney—the appointment of a health care agent to make decisions on your behalf. The other forty-six states allow for both. More information about these legal terms can be found at the Choice in Dying website (www.choices.org).

A living will is a document that clearly defines what type of care you would want in certain situations if you are not be able to speak for yourself. It can reflect your end-of-life wishes. You can list every medical intervention you want to avoid, or you can make it clear that you want every possible measure—often referred to as *heroic measures*—taken to extend your life. It is extremely important to use specific language in order to leave no room for misinterpretation. For example, "heroic measures" might be defined differently by different people or in different health care facilities. Some people consider cardiopulmonary resuscitation (CPR) to be a heroic measure; others do not.

A power of attorney is a document that lets you designate a person close to you, someone you trust and who respects your values and wishes, to make decisions about your care. This document can also be referred to as a *health care proxy* or *appointment of a health care agent*. It is very important that you discuss your wishes with the person you have chosen to assume these responsibilities. You should also confirm his or her willingness to act on your behalf. You may use a power of attorney in addition to a living will, thereby using your designated health care agent or proxy to interpret your wishes if needed. Remember that a living will or power of attorney go into effect *only* if you cannot communicate your wishes.

When there is no advance directive and a person is unable to make his wishes known, the next of kin is most often asked to make decisions. This may not be the person you wish to guide your health care, for many reasons. Many men choose not to burden a wife with these responsibilities; relatives may not share one's views about life-sustaining treatment. In any case, communicating your wishes through a living will or choosing someone to make your health care decisions can ease a difficult situation for everyone concerned and avoid a struggle to figure out what you would want to have done. If you don't say what you *do* want, you could get what you *don't* want.

Many sources of assistance are available should you decide to put together a living will or power of attorney. Your doctor or hospital could help. You could use the services of a lawyer, although law does not require it. In addition, there are Internet sources and computer software designed to assist you; you can even download state-specific advance directive packages at websites such as Choice in Dying (www.choices.org). Most importantly, if you do execute an advance directive, make sure that all your health care providers know that it exists and provide them with a copy whenever necessary.

Another helpful resource is a nonprofit organization called Aging with Dignity (www.agingwithdignity.org). Aging with Dignity has produced a document called *Five Wishes*™ that can be used to guide discussions about advance directives, power of attorney, and health care proxy. Figure 19.2 includes the basic elements of *Five Wishes*™.

Crucial Questions and Decisions

Many people, when they consider the issue at all, think that they would like to die very quickly, and to be in reasonably good health until the end. The truth is, this sort of death eludes many of us, and sudden death can be extremely difficult for loved ones. Planning for the end of life, including assuring that distressing symptoms are managed well, allows the dying person and his loved ones time to say good-bye. By learning about and using available resources, it is possible to alter the process of dying from one characterized by pain and suffering to one of serenity and peaceful closure.

An advance directive, when written properly, can be very helpful in limiting the interventions you don't want and help you to shape the kind of

Figure 19.2: *Five Wishes*™

My Wish For:

1. The Person I Want to Make Care Decisions for Me When I Can't
2. The Kind of Medical Treatment I Want or Don't Want
3. How Comfortable I Want to Be
4. How I Want People to Treat Me
5. What I Want My Loved Ones to Know

Five Wishes™ meets the legal requirements under the health decision statutes of 33 states and the District of Columbia. Even in states where it is not legally recognized, *Five Wishes*™ can serve as a guide to help you discuss your end-of-life care choices with your family and doctor.
Individual copies of *Five Wishes*™ are $4; for orders of 10 or more, please send $1 per copy. Check or money orders may be made payable to Aging with Dignity. Send requests to: Aging with Dignity, PO Box 1661, Tallahassee, FL 32302-1661. *Five Wishes*™ can be viewed from www.agingwithdignity.org, and is also available in Spanish and Vietnamese.

death you do want. A good palliative care team can assist the dying person and his family with planning for the end of life and provide the support and comprehensive symptom management needed to make the dying process proceed just that way. Death is an important life process and can resemble an event such as birth. The same kind of planning as for a natural birth can be done to make a more natural kind of death.

Symptom Management

Many people say that they do not fear death as much as they fear the process of dying. Death, particularly in American society, has come to be surrounded by issues of loss of control of body functions, physical pain, and emotional suffering. When the physical symptoms are managed effectively, the patient and his family can then cope with the emotional aspects surrounding the dying process and death.

Table 19.1 provides a list of some of the more common symptoms at the end of life and suggestions for ways to minimize or even eliminate them. This list is far from complete. The Resources section at the end of this book suggests several more comprehensive resources to help dying persons and caregivers cope with the physical dying process. Each dying person will encounter his own set of symptoms, and requires a plan of care devised just for him. The patient and/or his caregivers can make a list of any and all symptoms the patient has and have the nurse or doctor help prepare a plan to alleviate them.

Prolonging Life

It is important to be very clear about one's wishes with regard to common life-prolonging measures such as maintaining or withdrawing food (nutrition) or fluids (hydration) and other life-sustaining interventions such as the use of a ventilator. Not every dying person wants the same thing.

State laws and medical and ethical authorities agree that there is no difference between *withholding* or *withdrawing* life-sustaining treatment such as tube feedings once they have been started. This means in effect that it is not morally or legally any different to stop the ventilator (or "pull the plug") once it has been started than to choose not to accept the use of the ventilator in the first place.

Unless otherwise directed, hospital staff is obligated to use *all means*—the measures included in *cardiopulmonary resuscitation,* or CPR—to revive a person whose heart has stopped or who has stopped breathing. You can indicate in your living will that you do or do not wish cardiopulmonary resuscitation. Directions around CPR should be discussed with your doctor and, if it is your choice to forego resuscitation, the doctor must write a *do not resuscitate* order (DNR)—sometimes called a *no code*—in your medical record. It is very important to remember that once this DNR order is written, ***you can change your mind***—the order can be canceled. You can also make changes to your living will at any time; just make sure that these changes are made known in the living will document and that all those concerned—family, friends, and all health care providers—are also aware of any changes in your end-of-life wishes.

Euthanasia and Assisted Suicide

Many people at the end of their lives have found serenity, peace, and even readiness for death. Others face hopelessness, depression, and fear—fear of the unknown, fear of increased suffering, fear of being left alone. To some, suffering can be caused by intense physical symptoms such as pain; to others, by loss of dignity or feelings of isolation, loneliness, and despair. When physical and emotional pain are not well managed, some people seek death prematurely as a means to escape suffering. The word *euthanasia* is derived from the Greek words "eu" meaning good and "thanatos" meaning death. Nowadays, it has come to mean ending extreme suffering by an act that ends life; to many people, it means "mercy killing."

Table 19.1: Suggested Interventions for Symptoms Common at the End of Life

Symptom	What Causes It	What to Do about It
Pain	Pressure on nerve endings, broken bones, pressure on organs (See Chapter 17 for a more complete review of cancer-related pain and pain management)	Find out exactly what is causing pain. Eliminate the source of pain if at all possible. Ask for the help of a pain specialist nurse or doctor. Use pain medicines as they are prescribed and other kinds of pain management strategies regularly—around the clock.
Confusion, delirium, and dementia	Medicines, bodily changes in fluid and electrolyte levels, pain, infection, severe constipation, sleep deprivation, heart disease, and endocrine problems	Find the reason for the confusion and manage it appropriately if at all possible. When this is not possible, medicines can be used to decrease confusion and agitation. Keep the patient's surroundings as familiar as possible, and avoid too much stimulation such as noise and light.
Seizures	Tumor located in the brain and subsequent pressure inside the skull, sleep deprivation, missed doses of antiseizure medicines, lack of sleep, stress, excess alcohol, and some kinds of medicines	Identify the reason for the seizure and make changes in the plan of care to eliminate or at least minimize the problem.
Spinal cord compression causing partial or complete paralysis	Tumor pressing on the spinal cord causing pain at the site and paralysis below the site; usually due to spread of the cancer to the spinal cord or the area surrounding the spinal cord	Early discovery of this problem and prompt treatment with radiation therapy and steroid medicines can prevent progression of paralysis and sometimes reverse the symptoms.
Breathing difficulties; shortness of breath (dyspnea)	Movement, posture, cough, and even anxiety or stress; tumor blocking the airways or putting pressure on the airways; fluid collection inside the chest, around the diaphragm, or around the heart; infection such as pneumonia; anemia; weakness of the muscles in the chest (respiratory muscles)	First, direct treatment to the cause. Infection can be treated with antibiotics. Blocked airways might be treated with radiation therapy. Next, work to manage symptoms by giving oxygen or medicines (for example, to promote the elimination of fluids). Position changes can help; elevate the head with pillows. Limit activity, and reduce anxiety through relaxation exercises, prayer, medication, resolution of fears and conflicts, and modification of surroundings. If fluid accumulation is a potential cause, limit fluids and alter diet to reduce fluid accumulation. Check and take care of oral hygiene.
Cough	Lung cancers, accumulated fluids and obstructions from other kinds of cancers, medical conditions other than cancer such as congestive heart failure, dry air, envi-	If cause of cough cannot be identified or treated, manage the symptoms: change the patient's position, warm and humidify the air, remove environmental irritants, encourage the patient to breathe deeply and cough

Symptom	What Causes It	What to Do about It
	ronmental irritants such as smoke and pollen	in a way that removes irritants. Cough syrup might help. Medicines can dilate the airways and decrease the thickness of secretions. Morphine and other kinds of opioids can suppress cough. Other medicines can help decrease anxiety.
Hemoptysis (coughing or spitting up blood)	Tumors, especially lung tumors and tumors in the esophagus; infection in the lungs	Medicines and treatment specific to the cause of the bleeding are important. Medicines can also be helpful in reducing anxiety. Change the patient's position and minimize the patient's activity. The amount of blood involved is important; massive amounts of blood is a serious sign while small amounts of blood often indicates a problem that can be managed.
Profuse sputum (phlegm)	Irritation and/or infection in the airways and lungs (thick sputum can block the airway, making it hard for the person to breathe; sputum can also provide bacteria with a good place to multiply and set up a site of infection)	Position changes can help; patient can lie on back or on side with head slightly raised, to prevent sputum from entering airways and lungs. Remove sputum from mouth with simple bulb syringe or suction machine; nurse or doctor should demonstrate correct use to prevent damage to inside of mouth and throat. Medicines—such as scopolamine, given through existing IV line or placed under tongue—can help dry up secretions.
Pressure sores (decubitus ulcers or bedsores)	Pressure on the skin (usually where little fat padding covers bones, such as hip bones, tailbone, ankles, heels, elbows, back of the head) resulting in decreased blood flow to area; friction caused by bed linens rubbing the skin; moisture of sweat, urine, and feces	Assess the skin every few hours. Change position at least every 2 hours. Keep the skin clean and dry; use nonirritating soap, use lotions sparingly, and avoid powder and talcum. Keep sheets and bedclothes free of wrinkles and food crumbs. Use devices like sheepskin pads, alternating pressure mattresses, and special air beds. To the extent possible, make sure the patient has enough water so that he is not dehydrated. Control pain so the patient can remain mobile. If pressure sores develop despite efforts to prevent them, care measures should be used to prevent infection.
Itching (pruritus)	Blockage of the bile duct, kidney failure, infections that affect the skin	Bathe with sodium bicarbonate. Apply moisturizing lotions, calamine lotion, other medicated lotions, and an anesthetic gel every 2 hours. Antihistamine ointments might be

End-of-Life & Palliative Care

Symptom	What Causes It	What to Do about It
		useful, but some patients develop allergies. Keep fingernails trimmed short and free of snags and sharp edges. Patient could wear gloves while sleeping. Patient should avoid drinking coffee and alcohol. Use mild detergent to clean bed linens and clothing.
Mouth infections	Malnutrition, dehydration, and mouth sores caused by some forms of cancer treatment; mouth provides a place for bacteria, fungi, and viruses to multiply	Perform a frequent—perhaps as often as every 2 hours—gentle mouth care process. Use a soft toothbrush, mild toothpaste, and a nonalcohol mouthwash or simple salt-water solution or use a water-pick device on a low setting. Floss gently; floss last in areas where there are sores. Perform mouth care before sleep and before and after meals. Clean the mouth after patient is suctioned. Soothe pain from mouth sores with popsicles or plain ice.
Nausea and vomiting	Certain medicines and various forms of cancer treatment; too much calcium in blood (hypercalcemia) caused by spread of cancer into bones; severe constipation and blockage of the bowel (impaction); swelling of the brain; kidney failure	Treat the cause if it can be determined. Make sure the patient is not constipated. Try diet changes: include soft drinks, soda crackers, and other salty foods; decrease fatty and strong smelling foods; offer more water. Offer smaller than usual meal portions more often. Keep the patient's room cool, his head slightly raised. Encourage patient to use relaxation techniques such as progressive muscle relaxation or listening to music. A number of antinausea medicines are available; try finding a protocol that includes 2 or more types of antinausea medicines.

Compiled from Terminal Illness: A Guide to Nursing Care *by Charles Kemp and* Handbook for Mortals *by Joanne Lynn and Joan Harrold.*

There are different forms of euthanasia. In *active voluntary euthanasia* someone other than the patient, with the patient's consent, acts with the primary intent of ending the patient's life, for example, by giving a lethal injection. *Involuntary euthanasia* is an intervention administered to cause death against the patient's wishes or without his consent. In *nonvoluntary euthanasia*, the patient is unable to consent. *Passive euthanasia* is a term used by some people to refer to the hastening of death by withdrawing or withholding life-sustaining measures such as tube feedings or mechanical ventilation. This is the only type generally regarded by society as ethically or morally acceptable. Passive euthanasia usually occurs in situations in which the benefits of additional treatment are nil or minimal.

In *assisted suicide*, a person provides the means for a patient to end his life, knowing the patient's intention but not acting directly, thereby distinguishing the act from euthanasia. *Physician-assisted suicide* (PAS) is when a physician makes the means or the information necessary for a patient to commit suicide available to him. In the United States, Supreme Court decisions have placed the burden of this hotly debated issue with each state. Physician-assisted suicide is currently permitted only in the state of Oregon, and only under very tightly controlled conditions. It is not mentioned specifically in the laws of North Carolina, Utah, and Wyoming, and it remains illegal in the remaining states. This may change depending on how physician-assisted suicide is used in Oregon.

Euthanasia and physician-assisted suicide continue to be illegal throughout the world. However, under a new law expected to be enacted in the Netherlands in 2001, a physician who helps a patients end his or her life will not be subject to legal prosecution but will be accountable to a panel of medical, legal, and ethical experts. Criteria established by the Royal Dutch Medical Association for deciding whether euthanasia is excusable were used in the new law's language: Was the request voluntary? Is the person competent to make the decision and have all the information he or she needs? Is the situation hopeless? Are there no alternatives that would lessen suffering? Finally, a second physician must also examine the person and endorse the decision. This law will apply only to doctors, not to others who help a patient die, and doctors can still refuse such a request.

In Australia's Northern Territory, voluntary euthanasia was legalized by the Rights of the Terminally Ill Act of May 1995. The Act was reversed by the Australian Federal Parliament in 1997. Although the act allowed for euthanasia, it was allowable only under circumstances in which other effective options were nonexistent.

The issue continues to be widely discussed throughout the world. More discussion around euthanasia can be found in the chapter written by Roy and MacDonald, "Ethical Issues in Palliative Care," in *The Oxford Textbook of Palliative Medicine* (see Resources).

There are compassionate and well-meaning people on both sides of the debate over physician-assisted suicide. Professional organizations such as the American Medical Association, American Nurses Association, and the Oncology Nursing Society have opposed physician or nurse participation in assisted suicide, citing their dedication to life. These organizations advocate instead for improved pain and symptom management and expert palliative care. Many conservative religious groups maintain the view that God gives life and only God should take it. Suicide is considered a crime in the Islamic world. Liberal Christian groups and organizations such as the Hemlock Society feel suicide should be a matter of individual choice.

Stopping Cancer Treatment

Choosing to forego further treatment aimed at curing or controlling cancer is one of life's most difficult decisions, fueled by fear of what will occur when treatment ends. The statement "Nothing else can be done" is one of the most frightening that could ever be uttered to someone with cancer, bringing to mind pain and unavoidable suffering. If we could just wipe out that phrase from human communications, we would make a huge step forward in approaching death and dying in the best possible ways.

The concepts of palliative care provide hope that the dying process is a part of life, while maintaining the dying person's dignity as physical discomforts are eliminated and fears are expelled. The new message should be, "There is always something that can be done," reflecting a new direction in the dying person's feelings of hope. Instead of hoping for a cure, or for control of the cancer for a while longer, the dying person now hopes to reach the end of his life with grace and dignity or perhaps to resolve personal conflicts or to provide for the security of loved ones.

Hospice and Palliative Care

The involvement of a palliative care or hospice team is one way to assure that the best end-of-life care is provided. Palliative care is described in the following ways:

> "Taking care of the whole person—body, mind, spirit—heart and soul. In the palliative care perspective, dying is something natural and personal. The goal of palliative care is that you have the best quality of life you can have during this time." (Last Acts Campaign)

> "The total care of patients with progressive and advanced disease for whom prognosis for survival is limited and the focus for care is on relief of suffering and promotion of the best quality of life for patient and family. Relief of pain and other physical symptoms, as well as attention to psychological, social and spiritual problems are essential. Palliative care is best provided by an interdisciplinary team." (American Academy of Hospice and Palliative Medicine)

Palliative care is also known as *comfort care*, because caregivers work to promote the relief of pain and other kinds of suffering in every possible way. Palliative care is directed at providing comprehensive symptom management. Its goal is the best possible quality of life through providing expert care for all patient and family needs. This includes all physical, psychological, spiritual, social, and existential needs. Palliative care can be provided to people nearing the end of life in the home or in the hospital, nursing home, or inpatient hospice.

The services of a hospice or palliative care team have historically been underused for many reasons, including:

- limited access to facilities and experts, such as in rural areas

- a person or family's lack of awareness that palliative and hospice care exists

- denial that death is nearing or of the need for hospice

- a persistent myth that less than optimal care is given in hospice because curative and life-sustaining measures will be stopped

- cultural barriers such as misperceptions and myths commonly accepted as truth in various cultures and surrounding changes in the focus from cure to caring

- lack of financial resources

Problems or barriers also exist on the health care provider side that make finding a good palliative care team critical. These barriers include:

- Lack of understanding of good pain and symptom management techniques, such as fear of ending a person's life by liberal use of opioids to treat pain.

- Lack of sensitivity to cultural differences. A dying person's attitudes, beliefs, and behaviors are a reflection of their cultural background; lack of understanding of these issues can lead to problems with communication, accurate assessment, and treatment.

- Personal biases as to how death should happen or even where death should occur. The patient and family may need to be assertive with the health care provider to assure that the patient's wishes are respected.

A good palliative care team is essential in providing quality, comprehensive end-of-life care. In palliative care, an integrated approach is put in place to relieve pain and suffering *as defined by the dying person*, with the view that he is a unique individual who has had a variety of experiences that influence the care he needs. The members of the palliative care team should respect the dying person's goals, preferences, and wishes, including withdrawing or withholding treatment. They should treat him in ways that always maintain dignity, relieve suffering, and promote personal growth in preparation for a peaceful death. Settling old disputes, talking about issues that have gone unresolved for years, and being at peace with oneself at life's end may be elements of personal growth for the dying person. For family members, it may also include preparing for loss and facing the bereavement process and the inherent changing roles in the family.

Palliative care teams should be interdisciplinary, a group of varied professional and nonprofessional people bringing a wide range of expertise to the care needs and situation at hand. The dying person should, whenever possible, be included as part of this team, joining in discussions of his dying process. A palliative care team can be assembled regardless of where care is provided and should include, at a minimum, the following members:

The primary care doctor, oncologist, or a specialist in palliative care: This should be a doctor with whom the dying person has a good relationship, and can trust to see that he is treated according to his wishes. He or she must be able to have honest, open, and ongoing discussion with the dying person and his family throughout the final stages of life, and respect all decisions made about ending treatment and managing symptoms. This doctor must be willing and able to provide aggressive symptom management, such as the use of enough and the right kind of pain controlling medicines, to help the dying person decide on and achieve an acceptable level of comfort.

A nurse: Nurses are expert in the coordination of the care rendered by the entire team and can be important communicators. Because of the nurse's close and frequent interaction with the patient and family, she or he is often in a good position to help solve problems and advocate for the assistance of other team members as new needs arise. The nurse should strongly support care that is in line with the patient's wishes and values and maintain the patient's decision-making power.

The family: Who and what his family consists of should be defined by the patient. To minimize confusion surrounding communications and decision making, it may be helpful if one trusted family member or a friend is the designated family representative to this team. The level of family involvement in care and decision making should be determined by the patient first, and then by the family representative, as the patient desires. Family and loved ones can be very helpful in explaining the wishes of the patient who is unable to communicate effectively, especially when there is no advance directive or an advance directive is written in very broad terms. Family members are crucial in providing emotional support, comfort, and reassurance, and may also wish to be active caregivers, depending upon physical and emotional resources.

A social worker or case manager: The social worker or case manager can help locate and coordinate supportive resources such as home health care aides, inpatient hospice services, or financial help. They are especially helpful in dealing with insurance and managed care issues, and renegotiating family and loved ones' caregiving roles.

Pastoral care: The presence of a minister, priest, rabbi, or other spiritual counselor may help the dying person cope with issues such as the meaning of life, the meaning of suffering, and the importance of hope.

A counselor: The counselor might have credentials as a psychologist, psychiatrist, family counselor, or bereavement counselor. Regardless of credentials, the effective counselor can help the patient and family deal with emotional and psychological issues such as dealing with loss, sadness, and depression. He or she can also help provide for closure and help resolve conflicts that arise throughout this stressful time.

A pharmacist: The pharmacist can help the physician and nurse devise plans to use medications to manage pain or other symptoms most effectively. He or she can provide advice about possible alternate medications or routes of medication administration, and make sure that one type of medicine does not interfere with the desired action of another.

The hospice team can also include dieticians, physical and occupational therapists, and even speech therapists. Hospice care and palliative care can take place in a hospice unit of a hospital, a freestanding hospice, or in the dying person's home. Regardless of where care is given, hospice uses a team approach, and the dying person and his family are involved in planning care. Twenty-four-hour access is provided for home care and home health aide assistance, medical equipment and supplies, prescription medicines for symptom management—including pain medicines—and bereavement care for family members.

Paying for End-of-Life Care

Paying for care at the end of life can become an important consideration and source of conflict for many families. The last weeks and days of life are emotionally draining. Fear of becoming a burden to family—especially from a financial perspective—is, according to many dying people, one of their greatest concerns at the end of life. The costs imposed by complex care needs can be a burden that the family will carry even after their loved one dies. The choice to use hospice care, in addition to promoting the quality of life during this time, also can significantly reduce the burden of expenses that concerns many dying persons.

The hospice benefit through Medicare and private insurance: People who are on Medicare and many forms of private insurance have what is called a *hospice benefit* as part of their insurance plans. A patient who opts to use his hospice benefit restricts his care to those measures that offer him comfort and the management of distressing symptoms. Clearly, the hospice benefit is used only when a person knows he has no chance for cure or control of his illness. To qualify to use the hospice benefit, the doctor and medical director of a certified hospice need to state, in the patient's medical record, that the patient is terminally ill—meaning that if nature runs its course, the patient is not expected to survive beyond a few months. The patient also needs to give an informed consent that says it is his choice to use the hospice benefit.

Over three thousand hospice programs provide services in all fifty states, and most are Medicare certified. Many private insurance companies and HMOs have copied Medicare's hospice benefit, so hospice care can often be paid for by private and public insurance payers.

Medicaid: The Medicaid program, jointly run by the Health Care Financing Administration (HCFA) and each state, pays for some services for low-income people who are elderly, blind, disabled, or receive public assistance, and those who have low-paying jobs. Each state decides who is eligible for Medicaid assistance, and must cover inpatient and outpatient hospital care, nursing home and home health care, and care given by doctors and certified nurse practitioners. Medicaid also pays for laboratory and X-ray services, and care given in rural health clinics and other government supported community health centers. Prescription drugs for some low-income and disabled people are also paid for by Medicaid. A social worker can help in making an application for this assistance.

The U.S. Veteran's Administration (VA) is a possible source of assistance for anyone who has served in any of the U.S. Armed Forces. Although qualifications for VA assistance have been tightened in recent years, the VA can still offer assistance and services, particularly if the dying person's illness can be directly related to his military experience. A VA benefits counselor can help veterans determine their eligibility for assistance.

A hospital or clinic's social worker can help a man and his family determine what sort of assistance they could expect from private and public— Medicare, Medicaid, VA—insurance. (For more information on paying for care, see Table 20.1.)

Final Thoughts

Death is something that everyone, someday, will experience. The movement that started with the publication of Elizabeth Kubler-Ross's book *On Death and Dying* over twenty years ago, and the growing acceptance of hospice care, are changing and improving the way we care for people nearing death. To the extent possible, managing distressing symptoms such as pain, nausea and vomiting, confusion, and breathing difficulty goes a long way toward relief of physical suffering. Addressing emotional and spiritual concerns is critical as well. Seeing to the needs of friends and family members, particularly those in caregiving roles, can eliminate the fear of being a burden that troubles so many dying persons. Attention to these details can diminish feelings of regret and guilt, and offer the dying person and his family the opportunity to use the last days of life as they choose.

20

♦ ♦ ♦

Survivorship

Pamela J. Haylock, R.N., M.A.

"From the time of its discovery and for the balance of life, an individual diagnosed with cancer is a survivor."

National Coalition for Cancer Survivorship Organizational Charter

From the time of diagnosis and for the balance of life, a person diagnosed with cancer is a *cancer survivor*. In the early 1980s, when the phrase was first coined, I had a little trouble accepting it. At that time, the word "survivor" was primarily associated with terrible events such as the Holocaust, conjuring up images of survivors of the Nazi death camps, or survivors of the atomic bomb explosions. These societal events were horrendous and affected humanity on such a huge scale. Could they possibly be compared to the experiences of people who've faced cancer? On second thought, however, using the word "survivor" for those who've gone through an experience with cancer does seem fitting.

The diagnosis of cancer is a rite of passage that admits a person to a new way of life, a fellowship based on shared experiences and common feelings. Granted, this isn't a club anyone willingly joins, but a high degree of camaraderie seems to be part of the cancer experience. A person works his way through the physical and emotional hurdles of diagnosis, treatment decisions, and the challenges imposed by treatment. All along, he anticipates the great sense of relief that will come when treatment concludes.

Doctors and nurses at cancer treatment facilities and doctors' offices often acknowledge the completion of this ordeal. Individuals and families celebrate in their own ways. Then comes the realization that it's nearly impossible to put cancer completely behind you. Jobs change, insurance rates or even access to insurance changes; family relationships and sometimes physical appearance and body functions all change.

Cancer survivorship is characterized by the challenges faced daily by the millions of people who have a history of cancer. Survivorship is living with, through, and beyond cancer. Clearly, survivorship involves a transition to a different life.

Needs of Cancer Survivors

There are close to ten million Americans alive today with a history of cancer. Nearly five million of these have lived with cancer for at least five years. In fact, around 60 percent of all people diagnosed with cancer survive long-term. Researchers who focus on survivorship say it involves many aspects of physical, psychological, social, and spiritual well-being, and that all of these needs must be addressed for the person to cope as well as is possible. Physically, many survivors have problems caused by cancer and cancer treatment for months and years, even after treatment ends. Emotionally, a survivor lives with fear of recurrence, doubts, anxiety, depression, and uncertainty about what his future holds. The health care system—or lack of one—forces survivors to struggle to get and keep health insurance as well as their jobs. Sometimes, it is a struggle to keep a family together or the bonds of friendship intact. The lives of survivors and their family members and loved ones can be quite different from their lives before cancer.

Fitzhugh Mullen, a physician, cancer survivor, and a founder of the National Coalition for Cancer Survivorship, says that survivorship runs on a fairly defined course, with three stages: acute, extended, and permanent. The *acute* stage starts with diagnosis and continues through the first courses of treatment. During this first stage, the new survivor focuses on basic physical survival. When the cancer responds to treatment, survivors move to the next stage, a stage that Mullen calls the *extended* or *intermediate* stage. During this time, the survivor might continue on a maintenance form of therapy to control the cancer, or the cancer may appear to be cured. Even so, many survivors describe this as being in limbo—between heaven and hell. The future is uncertain; hope for cure is offset by the fear of recurrence. Despite the emotional turmoil so common to survivors during this time, supportive resources are difficult to come by. Finally, the survivor enters into *permanent* survivorship or long-term survival. Doctors often link this stage to a state of cure: the chances of recurrence diminish as time goes on. Friends and family members might convey the impression that the survivor should just feel lucky to be alive, to have completed cancer treatment, and the survivor is expected to move on with his life.

Two prominent nurse scientists, Karen Hassey Dow at the University of Central Florida School of Nursing and Betty R. Ferrell at City of Hope National Medical Center in California, also suggest that three key themes are common to cancer survivors. First, there is a *quick change*. One day, you are a healthy man, thinking about working and taking care of the business of your life. The next, you are facing a life-threatening illness. Most people agree that the time of initial diagnosis is the one in which cancer survivors feel especially vulnerable.

The second theme identified by Dow and Ferrell is the *transition to a different life*. The transition pathway includes physical hardships, emotional losses, and facing death. During this time, survivors face the loss of the way life used to be, and then enter a recovery process. Finally, survivors learn to live with the *altered life* that comes from the complete change in life's meaning. Dow and Ferrell ask that health care professionals, friends, and family members help survivors find meaning from their cancer experience and to regain a sense of control.

Several studies have confirmed that cancer survivors share a fairly consistent list of needs—many of which go unmet. Generally, needs fall into one of four categories:

- emotional and social needs (including family issues)

- economic needs (financial, insurance, and employment)

- medical staff needs (information and availability)

- community needs (including home care and transportation)

Specifically, cancer survivors need prompt medical attention, emotional support, pain and other symptom management, practical help, attention to employment and financial problems, and information.

Even though these needs are well known, it is distressingly apparent that for many cancer survivors, for a variety of reasons, they go unmet. The consequences of unmet needs range from mild inconvenience, to diminished quality of life, to debilitation or life-threatening crises. In all aspects of life, individuals are expected to assume responsibility for their own well-being. The world of cancer is no different, conferring tremendous importance on the concept of responsibility for self.

Cancer Victim, Cancer Patient, and Cancer Survivor

Look at these phrases and consider their meanings. They tell the story of the evolution of how cancer is viewed in our society. *Cancer victim* was the phrase used in the early part of the century to describe those afflicted with the disease. The word "victim" denotes someone who is powerless to control events around him, and indeed a cancer diagnosis was almost universally viewed as a death sentence. Eventually, the word *patient* was used, as people with cancer more or less passively submitted to the care being ministered to them by health care professionals. With new treatment methods, increased survival time, and relatively good health despite the diagnosis, people with cancer began to assert themselves, to assume control, and to ask and eventually demand that their needs be met. Societal trends including civil rights, women's rights, consumers' rights, human rights, and increased access to medical information have changed passive patients to informed consumers of health care services. These people are no longer victims; they are not just patients: they are empowered.

Survivorship Skills

Generally, when a person prepares for a new experience in life, he tries to learn about whatever this experience might entail. Quite often, learning what to expect leads to learning new skills. For example, a person embarking on a trip to a foreign country might attempt to learn the language and understand the culture of that country. If he decides to view this new country from a bicycle, he will also undertake a training program that helps him gain skills and confidence in his ability to successfully complete his trip. In this way, the man will be *empowered*—in control of meeting his goals. The information the man found, and the skills he mastered, allow him to meet his needs.

Empowerment assumes that a person understands his needs better than others can and should have control over important aspects of his life. The following *self-advocacy skills* help cancer survivors achieve this sense of control, adapt to life after a cancer diagnosis, prevent or overcome limitations, and devise strategies for effective living:

- the ability to find and use information

- the ability to communicate with the health care team, family, and friends

- the ability to make well-reasoned decisions

- the ability to work through and solve problems

- the ability to work through a give-and-take process with the other people in one's life, to negotiate with others

This skill set is the foundation for *The Cancer Survival Toolbox*, a resource developed by the National Coalition for Cancer Survivorship (NCCS), the Oncology Nursing Society (ONS), and the Association of Oncology Social Workers (AOSW). The original *Toolbox* is a set of audiotapes, structured to help the listener learn and gain confidence in using each of these skills. The *Toolbox* is also available in print version on the NCCS website www.cansearch.org.

Finding and Using Information

Good information is critical throughout the cancer experience. Getting it is somewhat like shopping. Most people do a lot of comparison shopping before making a big purchase such as a home or a new car, but many men make little effort to use a similar process when selecting a cancer doctor or deciding on a course of cancer treatment. Shopping offers the consumer the best chance to know what he's buying and to be happy with his purchase. Finding and using good, solid information is critical to successful coping strategies.

Asking questions of reliable sources is a first and easy way to start. But who do you ask? The best place to start is with one's own cancer care team members. The medical oncologist, oncology nurse, oncology clinical pharmacist, social worker, and dietician are just a few of the cancer care team members who can help you find reliable information. Local libraries and bookstores generally have a supply of cancer-related books. The trick is to make sure the books are recent publications. Cancer care is in a constant state of flux, and new information is available almost daily; books published more than three to five years ago may not contain the most up-to-date information.

The Internet has resulted in an absolute explosion of information, some very good, some misleading. Enlisting a trusted guide, such as the oncology nurse, social worker, doctor, health resource center librarian, or public librarian, can help assure the quality of information gathered from Internet-based resources. The American Cancer Society and the National Cancer Institute provide print, telephone, and Internet-based information services.

Finally, a most important source of information will be other men who have had the same kind of cancer or who have gone through the treatment options being considered. The medical oncologist or surgeon might have a listing of former patients who have agreed to talk with newly diagnosed survivors. Community-based cancer support groups are another valuable resource. National advocacy and/or support groups often provide a listing of peer counselors in different locations. The doctor, oncology nurse, or oncology social worker can help you locate other cancer survivors.

Communication

Communication involves listening, talking, body language, understanding, responsibility, and trust. The man with cancer and the involved health care professional need to agree to an open give-and-take of communication, where each contributes his ideas and his opinions, but also listens to and considers the other's perspective. Communication problems between doctors and their patients can include lack of privacy, use of medical terms that the patient does not understand, limited time devoted to talking and listening to each other, and reluctance to bring up sensitive or embarrassing topics like sex, fear of dying, and pain. Experts suggest that a man can foster good communication with the health care team members in several ways:

- Before any visit with the doctor or nurse, write out your questions, with the most important questions at the top of the list.

- Take a family member or friend who can act as a second set of ears.

- Take a small cassette tape recorder to the appointment. Let the doctor, nurse, or other team member know that you want to record the conversation so you can listen to it later when you are not so anxious or pressed for time.

- Ask for explanations in terms or words that you understand.

- Use rephrasing techniques: After listening to an explanation, see if you can explain it back to the other person, in your own terms. "So, let me see if I understand what you mean." "What you're saying is _____." Ask the doctor or nurse to verify whether this is actually what he or she means.

- Use "I" techniques: "When this happens, I feel as if _____." Relate everything back to yourself—how *you* react, what *you* are thinking.

- Try role playing: Ask a friend or family member to act the role of the person with whom you need to communicate, so you can practice communicating your needs.

Making Decisions

One of the most difficult aspects of a new cancer diagnosis is that a person is suddenly forced to decide on things about which he probably knows very little, at a time when anxiety, stress, and fear complicate the decision-making process. The decisions made in these difficult conditions will affect the rest of the man's life, and the lives of everyone around him.

Good decisions are based on having all the facts and can only come as a result of a sound information-seeking process. Unfortunately, a vast amount of information is available. One source of information often conflicts with another. What source do you believe? How do you decide?

In any decision-making process, a man first needs to think about what is important to him. What aspects of his current life and lifestyle matter to him most? How would the alternatives being considered affect this lifestyle? Figure 20.1 illustrates a model for decision making commonly used by counselors to assist people in reaching decisions about complex issues. At the top of a sheet of paper, list things that are important in your life. Then, draw a line down the middle of the paper. If, for example, you are trying to decide about one treatment modality versus another, list the benefits on one side of the page and the drawbacks on the other. This kind of exercise can help you take a good look at the things that matter, and in the end feel comfortable with your decision. It can also highlight gaps in available information and tell you that you need to stop, find additional information, and then resume the decision-making process.

Figure 20.1: Decision-Making Model

Things That Are Important to Me:
My relationship with my family
I want to be able to have normal sexual relations with my wife
Being able to do my job well
I want to have another child
I want to be able to travel to third world countries

Benefits
This treatment offers me a good chance for cure
The doctor who will oversee the treatment is known to have a great deal of expertise
Long-term, there seems to be less chance for recurrence

Drawbacks
The treatment runs a high risk of making me sterile

Solving Problems

Cancer survivorship is a continual process of solving problems. Some problems are small; others are big. Problem-solving skills help a person carefully think through dilemmas, defining what exactly the problem is, determining viable alternatives or solutions, making a decision, and putting the decision into action. Peer support, professionally led support groups, and individual counseling sessions can help a person learn and use problem-solving skills with confidence.

Modeling is a popular method of problem solving in which one person or a group uses or models acceptable ways of working through problems. Groups or individual counseling can provide a setting where individuals practice problem-solving techniques through *role playing*. Role playing helps a man learn to communicate better with the cancer care team members, family members, and others with whom he needs to interact.

Negotiation

A cancer diagnosis often results in significant changes in day-to-day business and family roles. The man who is normally a breadwinner may need to rely on his wife or partner to provide for his family for a time. A friend or family member may need to take over at least a few day-to-day chores. Maybe for the time being someone else will have to walk the dog, or even coach Little League. Some men may need to take time off from work or change their job descriptions, at least temporarily. Most distressing of all, sometimes a cancer diagnosis and treatment results in employment problems or loss of insurance and other benefits, requiring the cancer survivor to be fully aware of and ready to exercise his legal rights. Any and all of these situations require some level of negotiation.

Negotiation is simply a process of give-and-take. A first step is to have a full understanding of what you want to achieve at the end of the negotiation process. What do you want to happen? Where are you willing to step back or compromise? A second step is to understand what the other person might hope to gain. What is this person's history with this kind of situation? What is his or her bottom line? What would past dealings tell you about what that bottom line might be?

In the best-selling book *Getting to Yes: Negotiating Agreement Without Giving* (1991), authors Fisher and Ury say there are generally four points that count in the negotiation process, and they suggest ways to approach each:

People: Separate the people from the problem.

Interests: Focus on interests, not positions.

Options: Generate several possibilities before deciding what to do.

Criteria: Insist that the result be based on some clearly defined or objective standard.

You Are Your Own Best Advocate

While I was preparing this chapter, my daughter relayed a story about her friend Ron's cancer experience. Ron was fifty-four when he had a PSA test. At that time, his PSA level was 10.48 (normal PSA for a man Ron's age is 2–3), and though it was marked "high" on the laboratory's printout, it went unnoticed by his doctor. Three years later, Ron's PSA was over 37. By this time, his doctor told him that he would probably live no more than three years. Through friends, Ron got additional medical opinions, different doctors, and finally some hope. Ron had surgery to remove his prostate; he will receive additional cancer treatment, and he has a good chance at full recovery. That's the good news. The bad news: On top of what his insurance covered, Ron owes $10,000 to hospitals, clinics, and doctors.

Ron's story is not at all unusual. Ron *should* have been diagnosed three years earlier. At that time, it is more than likely that his cancer would have been much smaller and would probably not have spread outside of his prostate. His chances for cure would have been much higher. The lesson to learn from Ron's experience is that we all *must* be more assertive and more prepared to assume the responsibility for our own health. I know it is disappointing to learn that none of us can totally depend on doctors, nurses, or other health care professionals. But given the complexity of modern medical care, and the disorganized way in which some health care services are provided, men (and women, too) must assume active roles in assuring their own health.

The Oncology Nursing Society (ONS), the professional association that represents more than 29,000 registered nurses and other health care professionals specializing in cancer care, released its Patients' Bill of Rights for Quality Cancer Care in 1998. This Bill of Rights is consistent with the ONS position on Quality Cancer Care and outlines what cancer nurses believe people should demand from their health care providers and health care insurance or HMO plans. Inherent in this position, however, is the assumption that patients accept responsibilities for care as well.

Figure 20.2 summarizes the ONS Patients' Bill of Rights for Quality Cancer Care.

Figure 20.2: ONS Position on Patient's Bill of Rights for Quality Care

- Education about cancer risks and lifestyle changes that affect the incidence of cancer should be available and accessible to all people.

- Cancer screening activities, tailored to a person's individual risk factors, that can lead to early detection of cancer should be covered by public and private health insurance plans.

- People must have timely access to appropriate treatment options for the management of specific cancers and cancer-related symptoms.

- People with cancer must have access to competent and qualified professional oncology care specialists.

- Public and private health insurance plans should cover supportive therapies that help manage the side effects of cancer and cancer treatment.

- People must have access to high-quality clinical trials.

- People need to have long-term follow-up by competent and qualified professional oncology care specialists.

- Palliative care to improve care provided at the end of life must be available and accessible to all people affected by cancer.

Adapted from the ONS Position on Patient's Bill of Rights for Quality Care. A copy of the complete position is available from the Oncology Nursing Society Customer Service Department (412) 921-7373, or for download from the ONS website at www.ons.org.

Self-Advocacy Strategies

It is important that every person assume responsibility for his or her own health. Just as we assume the responsibility to get routine maintenance and checkups for cars and other kinds of equipment important to our daily lives, we must give similar consideration to our bodies. Each person needs to be his own best advocate, which means taking the responsibility to know what is needed to preserve or regain optimal health, deciding on appropriate goals, and then taking action to achieve those goals.

Stories like Ron's, combined with the ONS Positions on Patients' Bill of Rights and Quality Cancer Care help outline suggestions for *self-advocacy*—taking control, having your needs met—that go a long way toward making sure the right things happen at the right time. These suggestions are highlighted in Figure 20.3.

Stages of Cancer-Related Advocacy

For most cancer survivors, advocacy is a critical, lifelong process. A growing number of cancer survivors take their advocacy skills to new levels. In fact, there is a recognized pathway of advocacy—referred to as the *advocacy continuum*—that starts as *personal advocacy*, broadens to *advocacy for others*

Figure 20.3: Self-Advocacy Strategies in Cancer Care

Before cancer

- Explore your personal risk factors for different kinds of cancer.

- Learn to recognize cancer's warning signs.

- Learn and follow recommended and regular schedules for cancer-related checkups.

- Know what preventive, screening, and management procedures and settings are and are not covered in your health insurance or HMO policy.

- If needed services are not covered in your existing health insurance policy, explore other options to help cover expenses.

- Create an "owner's manual" for your own body! Use a three-ring binder with a section or pocket for your personal follow-up schedule, each kind of report and forms of communication from doctors or treatment facilities, and other information you find of interest. Keep the records in chronological order. The Savard Health Record, distributed by Time Life Books, is a commercially produced version of this "owner's manual" idea, offering a ready-made system along with important advice to help survivors take charge of their health information.

- Learn to understand and speak the language of cancer.

- Demand copies of all laboratory and imaging tests that are part of routine checkups.

- Keep copies of all laboratory test and imaging study results. If you are asked to bring copies of results to a second health care provider's office, make sure you ask that they make their own copy. Keep your original.

- Read and review all test results. Learn what "normal" findings are, and compare normal results with those indicated on your own reports. If needed, ask the doctor or nurse to define terms used to describe unclear test results, to review with you all test reports, and to explain any test results that are not within normal limits.

- If any finding is abnormal, ask what the next step should be. Verify that this is the recommended protocol by reviewing additional resources such as relevant books and Internet sites and cancer-specific resources such as the National Cancer Institute and/or the American Cancer Society.

- Any abnormal finding warrants follow-up of some sort. Appropriate follow-up includes another appointment within a reasonable period of time to recheck the abnormal finding, additional laboratory or imaging studies, or biopsy.

When cancer (or a precancerous condition) is confirmed

- Institute a thorough information-seeking process: get information from trusted professional resources as well as peers or friends who have a similar diagnosis.

- Explore the staff resources, individual and organizational credentials, and competencies available at the cancer treatment center you consider using.

- Introduce yourself to the cancer treatment facility social worker. Social workers offer a wealth of information about community resources, financial assistance, peer and professional support groups, and more.

- Think through, identify, and make your needs known to members of the health care team.

- If you have questions that go unanswered, ask for a second (or third) opinion, or for a referral to another member of the cancer care team who can provide appropriate answers.

- Record conversations with members of the cancer care team so that you can listen to it again at a later time.
- Ask a family member or friend to accompany you for doctor's appointments to discuss plans for care and follow-up. A second set of ears never hurts.
- Get a full picture of what your treatment plan entails, including clear definitions of expected roles and responsibilities of each member of the cancer care team, with yourself as an important team player.
- Keep to the recommended guidelines for follow-up care after treatment, including the schedule for additional imaging, laboratory studies, and physical examinations.
- Ask the doctor, nurse, social worker, dietician, and pharmacist for their assistance in preparing your own "After-Cancer Wellness Plan." Include follow-up schedules, health-promoting behaviors such as smoking cessation, dietary changes, and exercise plans.
- Be persistent and assertive.

(including others in groups and organizations), and culminates in *public interest advocacy* efforts. Many cancer survivors get involved in advocacy efforts as a way to express gratitude for their survival. Others become advocates as a result of problems, dilemmas, oversights, or mistakes that occurred during their own or a loved one's cancer experience, in hopes of sparing others similar experiences.

Personal Advocacy Personal advocacy is a way of taking charge, through getting good information and asking the right questions. As personal advocacy evolves, survivors begin looking for other survivors with whom they can identify; together they look for ways to share their experience and wisdom even further. Survivors call this the "veteran helping the rookie" idea, the essence of the survivorship movement.

Advocacy for Others Successful self-advocates are often prepared to go on to advocate on behalf of others. Through the network of people who have faced similar problems, survivors learn how to address common specific issues and are ready to advocate for changes that affect survivorship. Many start advocating for others through relatively simple, everyday activities such as talking to a newly diagnosed friend or students in the health care professions, or speaking at community-based groups such as the Rotary Club, Lions Club, or church groups. Speaking out this way helps defy myths and stigmas about cancer. You're alive and living well!

Public Interest Advocacy Finally, many survivors become successful professional survivor advocates. They take their personal and group advocacy experiences and contribute to public interest advocacy in national and even international cancer survivorship movements. These advocacy efforts have the potential to change public policy. Examples of successful public interest advocacy include increased federal appropriations for cancer research to explore causes, cures, and effects of cancer; legislation to assure appropriate length of stay following some forms of cancer surgery; and legislation to provide funding for cancer-screening efforts. Cancer survivors now hold roles in meaningful cancer policy planning bodies such as the National Cancer Advisory Board, boards of directors of major universities and affiliated cancer care facilities, and governing boards of professional organizations such as the Oncology Nursing Society. The National Coalition for Cancer Survivorship, based in Silver Spring, Maryland, is the leading national cancer advocacy organization. The website for the National Coalition for Cancer Survivorship (NCCS) provides linkages to other national cancer advocacy groups. NCCS can also provide referrals to site-specific organizations. NCCS's toll-free telephone number is (888) 650-9127.

The Politics of Cancer

Cancer survivors have become increasingly visible and a recognized force in what is commonly referred to as *onco-politics*—the politics of cancer. During the last decade or so, three major issues that directly or indirectly affect cancer care and/or cancer survivors have come to the forefront. First, President Clinton's efforts to reform the American health care system provided the catalyst for a focus on how care is financed as well as where it occurs. A second major political drive focused on how little of our total national budget is expended on looking for answers to the questions "What causes cancer?" "How can cancer be prevented?" and "How can cancer be cured?" Last, there is growing recognition that different races and different cultures are affected in ways that indicate that the burden of cancer is unevenly distributed in the American population, with people in minority and underserved populations assuming more of the hardships imposed by the disease.

Health Care Reform

There are many things "right" about health care in America and other industrialized nations, particularly evidenced by the rise in numbers of cancer survivors. The May 15, 2000, issue of *USA Today* featured this front-page—"above the fold"—headline: "Cancer's decline continues: 28,000 fewer deaths." The report goes on to say that 55,000 fewer people will get cancer and 28,000 fewer will die of it in 2000 as compared to 1999. These numbers characterize a decade-long decline in the number of new cancers diagnosed and the number of cancer-related deaths in the U.S. Indeed, this is good news, and The National Center for Disease Prevention and Health Promotion heralds this news as a "turning point in the war against cancer." The decline is largely due to the drop in the numbers of smokers and the decline in lung cancers, but also relates to progress in prevention, early detection, and treatment. Another piece of good news for men: The cancer rate among men—who do have the highest cancer rates—dropped the most.

Amid the celebratory climate, it could be easy to forget or at least temporarily overlook other alarming news: the ever-increasing numbers of Americans without health care insurance or access to health care at all, the shocking costs associated with health care and cancer care in particular, the decreasing support for cancer research, and, perhaps most distressing, the lack of access to good cancer care and markedly less optimistic outcomes that characterize minority groups and other underserved populations.

On a broader scale, these issues have energized cancer-related advocacy groups in the U.S. and present unlimited opportunities for cancer survivors to apply newly developed advocacy skills.

Making Care Accessible

In the U.S., nearly forty-five million people have no health care insurance at all. At least another one million people become uninsured every year, and an unknown number have only limited coverage. Lack of insurance complicates cancer care. A person who is uninsured or underinsured may not find and use preventive care or take advantage of screening programs that find cancers when the chances for cure are highest; may not get timely cancer treatment; may forego help with emotional problems or distressing symptoms that accompany cancer; and may forego needed follow-up once treatment is completed.

From the self-advocacy perspective, people should be able to assess their own unique situations. A person might ask himself some simple questions related to the challenges of paying for cancer care. Key questions include:

- Is there someone in my life who can help me work through financial issues and/or insurance problems? A financial counselor, my company or insurance plan's benefits manager, an accountant, an attorney?

- What things will my insurance pay for? Will it pay for

    — my participation in a clinical trial?

    — inpatient services at the hospital I choose?

    — the doctor of my choice?

    — care and medicines I get in the ambulatory clinic or doctor's office?

    — the services of the home care nurse?

    — the services of or consultations with rehabilitation specialists such as a physiatrist (the M.D. with a specialty in rehabilitation), physical therapist, or occupational therapist?

    — supplies I need in the home, such as dressing supplies used postoperatively, a hospital bed, or other types of assistive devices?

    — medicines used to manage other symptoms such as nausea and vomiting or pain?

    — hospice care and needed supplies in my home and/or an inpatient facility?

    — follow-up visits with my oncologist for the period the oncologist says is necessary?

    — consultations with the oncology social worker, nutritional specialist, or oncology nurse?

    — consultations and/or long-term access to a mental health specialist—social worker, counselor, psychiatrist, or psychologist?

- Is there a cap—an upper spending limit—on what my insurance plan will pay for?

- Will I be able to continue on this insurance plan after my cancer treatment ends?

- If I move to another city or state, will I be able to continue with this insurance plan and will the costs remain the same?

- What is the approximate cost of care I can expect throughout my course of treatment and follow-up?

- What aspects of care am I prepared to pay for myself?

- What resources are there in my community to help cover or at least reduce costs or my own out-of-pocket expenses?

This kind of self-risk assessment can help identify issues and possible problems before they escalate into problems that threaten ongoing care or the maintenance of quality of life. Once potential problems are identified, appropriate actions can be taken.

Paying for Care

Over half of all Americans who have jobs get health insurance as an employment benefit. People with low-paying jobs—those who are considered *low-income*—may qualify for Medicaid, the insurance programs administered by each state. For Americans over sixty-five, the federal government provides the Medicare insurance program. That leaves many people in the middle—middle-income people and those who are self-employed—who need to pay for their own insurance, pay for the costs of care out of their own pocket, or look for other financial assistance to pay for care.

Table 20.1 provides a brief overview of a few of the health care financial assistance programs that are available.

Cancer Research

In the United States alone, over fifteen hundred people die every day from cancer. This number is the equivalent to the total passenger loads of at least three Boeing 747 jets crashing, killing all aboard, every day of the year.

For every $10 each of us pays in taxes, just *one penny* goes to fund cancer research. At the same time, health care costs for cancer exceed $107 billion annually. Only about 2 percent of these costs are invested back into research to find effective prevention, treatments, and cures for cancer. Three out of every four cancer research projects that are actually approved—meaning only that they are thought to have merit—go unfunded. Without research, there will be no advancement in the way cancer is managed. President Richard Nixon signed the National Cancer Act in 1971, declaring the War on Cancer. The number of cancer deaths each year exceeds *all* U.S. combat deaths in *all* of the wars in the twentieth century. This begs the question, "Are we really fighting a war?" Many believe a true war on cancer has never been mounted at all—there have only been minor skirmishes.

On September 26, 1998, the March to Conquer Cancer, spearheaded by the National Coalition for Cancer Survivorship, was held on the Mall in Washington, D.C. Over 350,000 people—cancer survivors, family members, nurses, doctors, and researchers—were there to demand *no more cancer*, and that a substantial increase in federal funding be made available for cancer research.

Table 20.1: Financial Assistance Programs

Program	Eligibility Criteria	Pays For	How to Access
Medicare	*65 years old or older *Entitled to Social Security, Widow's, or Railroad Retirement benefits *On kidney dialysis *Totally disabled and has collected Social Security for at least two years *Part B eligibility starts after a deductible amount has been reached	Part A pays for *inpatient hospital bills *treatment and rehabilitation in a skilled nursing facility *hospice care Part B pays for *doctors' services *outpatient hospital services including emergency room visits, outpatient surgery *laboratory services *some kinds of medical equipment	*Call the Social Security Administration: (800) 772-1213 *Talk to the social worker, hospital or clinic financial counselor
The Medicare Hospice Benefit	*Doctor's written statement that the patient is "terminally ill" *Informed consent of the patient *Care must be provided by a Medicare-certified hospice	*Team approach to care, including services of a dietician, physical therapist, occupational therapist, speech therapist *24-hour-a-day access to services *Home care *Home health aide assistance *Medical equipment and supplies *Prescription medicines for pain and other distressing symptoms *Bereavement care for family members	*Contact Medicare or ask for the assistance of a social worker, nurse, doctor. *Call a local hospice for admitting information *Contact the National Hospice Organization for the location of a nearby hospice program: (800) 658-8898 or www.nho.org
Medicaid	Specific eligibility criteria are defined by each state, but generally include: *low-income *elderly *blind *disabled *already receiving public assistance	Each state decides the type, amount, duration of services and how much it will pay; generally includes: *Inpatient hospital care *Outpatient hospital care *Nursing home care *Home health care *Care provided by doctors, midwives, nurse practitioners *Laboratory services	*Apply at local Medicaid state agency *Hospital social worker can assist with the application

Table 20.1: Financial Assistance Programs (Cont'd.)

Program	Eligibility Criteria	Pays For	How to Access
		*X-ray services *Screening services *Diagnosis and treatment for people under twenty-one years of age *May or may not pay for prescription drugs for low-income elderly and people who are disabled	
U.S. Veterans Administration	*Service in any of the U.S. Armed Services *Enrollment in the Uniform Benefits Package: qualifications including "service connection" to the current illness *Financial need	*Costs of care when enrolled in a clinical trial sponsored by the National Cancer Institute *Cancer treatment *Follow-up care *Burial costs	*The nearest VA Medical Center *VA social worker *VA benefits counselor *Veterans' benefit office *Department of Federal Benefits for Veterans and Dependents: (800) 827-1000
Hill-Burton funds	Hospitals that get Hill-Burton funding from the federal government (funding for construction of facilities) are required to offer some services to people who cannot pay for their care	Depends on funding available at the hospital; funding cycles start at the beginning of each year, and funds are made available on a first-come, first-served basis depending on eligibility criteria	*Hill-Burton toll-free number: (800) 638-0742
Viatical settlements (getting cash from life insurance policies before the policy holder dies)	*Made available by some insurance companies to persons whose life expectancy is short *Doctor's statement that the policy holder is "of sound mind"		*Not all life insurance policies offer the option of a viatical settlement; consult social worker, financial counselor, estate planner, or attorney for advice *State Insurance Commissioner or Insurance Department

Table 20.1: Financial Assistance Programs (Cont'd.)

Program	Eligibility Criteria	Pays For	How to Access
Prescription drug patient assistance programs	*Varies with each company's program; application will be made by the doctor or nurse who prescribes the medicine	*Full or partial provision of medicines prescribed by a doctor	*PhRMA: www.phrma.org *Call (or ask the social worker or nurse to call) the drug company's established Prescription Drug Patient Assistance Program
Private funding at community facilities and university medical centers	Privately established funds through local foundations often provide funds to help pay for specific kinds of care; for example, a teaching hospital might have a fund that helps pay for care provided in any of a number of specialty clinics	Varies	*Talk to the hospital or clinic social worker, nurse, or doctor about any special funding available in hospital-based foundations to help pay for cancer-care-related costs
Community funds	Many communities have nonprofit organizations established for the purpose of supporting health care services—many of them specific to cancer care	Varies according to the mission of the organization	*Hospital social workers, oncology nurses, or financial counselors generally have information about local assistive organizations

The federal government, still the largest source of monies for cancer research, has allocated increasing levels of funding to the National Cancer Institute. Prostate cancer research efforts, largely through the advocacy efforts of individual prostate cancer survivors and prostate cancer advocacy groups, have received substantial increases in funding.

Other funding issues concern academic medical centers, places where a great deal of research has traditionally been based, which are increasingly experiencing diminished funding from the local, state, and federal governments. In many of these institutions, the focus on cancer research is being cut back or even eliminated. Individual and public support for research is critical to the advancement of cancer care, and cancer survivors and their loved ones are compelling advocates for this cause. A simple phone call, letter, or in-person visit to a legislator or policy-maker can be enough to sway an opinion or a vote. Survivors or their loved ones who cannot act alone should consider joining other like-minded people: two voices are better than one. There is power in numbers. A favorite quotation says it all: *"Never doubt that a small group of committed citizens can change the world. Indeed, it is the only thing that ever has."*—Margaret Mead

The Unequal Burden of Cancer

The advances in cancer prevention, early detection, treatment, and supportive care are not equally available to all people in the United States. In late 1999, the U.S. Institute of Medicine (IOM) released its report, *The Unequal Burden of Cancer: An Assessment of NIH Research and Programs for Ethnic Minorities and the Medically Underserved*. This report highlights the fact that people—regardless of ethnic background—who are poor, lack insurance, or do not have access to high-quality cancer care have higher cancer rates *and* higher cancer-related death rates. Professional presentations offered at the 2000 meeting of the Intercultural Cancer Council reflect these findings:

- In cancers where the rates are similar for white Americans and African Americans, African Americans have higher mortality rates, pointing to differences in access to screening and treatment, quality of care, or compliance with care.

- There is "triple jeopardy": the combined negative effect of being poor, of a minority race, and elderly, since it is these individuals who are diagnosed at later stages of cancer and have the greatest chance of dying from cancer.

- African Americans are 15 percent more likely to develop cancer than whites and 34 percent more likely to die of cancer than whites.

- Hispanic men are less likely than white men of the same age to have a prostate exam.

- Men in certain racial groups are often confused about the meaning and value of cancer screening and the screening tests that are available.

- Men hold a more fatalistic view of cancer than women.

- African-American men with prostate cancer are more likely than white men to be diagnosed with advanced disease.

- African-American men are less likely to have radical prostatectomy as a treatment for prostate cancer and more likely to have orchiectomy, radiation, and hormonal therapy than white men with the same diagnosis.

- Smoking rates have declined more among African Americans aged eighteen to thirty-four than among similar-aged whites

- Smoking rates among Vietnamese American men is between two and three times the general rate of U.S. men.

- African Americans have been less willing than whites to participate in medical research studies.

Well, you get the gist. Getting the right cancer care to people in underserved, uninsured, and poor communities is a big, ongoing problem. Advocacy groups like the Intercultural Cancer Council (ICC), the Appalachia Leadership Initiative on Cancer, the Asian and Pacific Islander American Health Foundation, Native American Cancer Initiatives, and the National Rural Health Association are just a few of the many local and national groups focusing on cancer-related issues specific to these populations. For more information about the ICC, or to inquire about the existence of a specific population-based advocacy group, call ICC at (713) 798-4617. The Office of Minority Health Resource Center, a division of the National Institutes of Health, based in Washington, DC, is the largest U.S. resource and referral service on minority health.

What Does It All Mean?

Cancer is a personal and family dilemma and a huge public health issue. There are close to ten million cancer survivors in the U.S. alone, with nearly three thousand new survivors added to the roster every day. Personal advocacy is vital to living well beyond that initial diagnosis of cancer. Whether or not a cancer survivor is able and willing to work his way up the ladder to higher levels of advocacy is a personal decision. Advocacy at any level is a set of skills that can empower a person with cancer to maximize the quality of his own life *and* perhaps enhance the survival of others.

Bibliography

Chapter 1: About Cancer

American Cancer Society: Facts and Figures—2000. Atlanta, GA: American Cancer Society, 2000.

Braddock, C.H., Edwards, K.A., Hasenberg, N.M., Laidley, T.L., and Levinson, W. Informed decision making in outpatient practice: Time to get back to basics. *Journal of the American Medical Association* 282(24):2313–2320, 1999.

Clark, E.J., and Stovall, E.L. Advocacy: The cornerstone of cancer survivorship. *Cancer Practice* 4(5):239–244, 1996.

US TOO International, Inc. The Louis Harris Survey: Perspectives on prostate cancer treatments: Awareness, attitudes and relationships—A study of patients and urologists, 1995. www.ustoo.com/louis.html.

Chapter 4: Prostate Cancer

Abel, L.J., Blatt, H.J., Stipetich, R.L., Fuscardo, J.A., et al. Nursing management of patients receiving brachytherapy for early-stage prostate cancer. *Clinical Journal of Oncology Nursing* 3(1):7–15, 1999.

Cash, J.C., and Dattoli, M.J. Management of patients receiving transperineal Palladium-103 prostate implants. *Oncology Nursing Forum* 24(8):1361–1367, 1997.

Held-Warmkessel, J. Prostate Cancer. In Yarbro, C.H., Frogge, M.H., Goodman, M., and Groenwald, S.L., eds. *Cancer Nursing: Principles and Practice*, 5th Edition, 1427–1451, 2000.

Lewis, J., and Berger, E.R. *New Guidelines for Surviving Prostate Cancer*. Westbury, NY: Health Education Literary Publisher, 1997.

Chapter 7: Testicular Cancer

Bosl, G., and Motzer, R. Testicular Germ-Cell Cancer. *New England Journal of Medicine* 337(4):242–253,1997.

Henkel, J. Testicular cancer: Survival high with early treatment. *FDA Consumer Magazine*. January-February, 1996.

International Germ-Cell Cancer Collaborative Group: International Germ Cell Consensus Classification: A prognostic factor-based staging system for metastatic germ-cell cancers. *Journal of Clinical Oncology* 15(2):594–603, 1997.

Nichols, C., and the Indiana University Cancer Center, Testicular Cancer Resource Center Expert Interview. *The Testicular Cancer Resource Center*, Volume 1:22, March 23, 1999.

Smith, A. Cancer, Stress and the Search for Doogie Houser. *The Testicular Cancer Resource Center*, 1999.

Swanson, J., and Forrest, L. *Men's Reproductive Health*, Volume 3. New York: Springer Publishing Company, 1984.

Chapter 8: Penile Cancer

National Cancer Institute. Penile Cancer. In PDQ•Treatment•Health Professionals. http://cancernet.nci.nih.gov. Accessed August 9, 1999.

Chapter 9: Male Breast Cancer

Chapman, D.D., and Goodman, M. Breast Cancer. In Yarbro, C.H., Frogge, M.H., Goodman, M., and Groenwald, S.L.(eds). *Cancer Nursing: Principles and Practice*, 5th Edition. Boston: Jones and Bartlett Publishers, 994–1047, 2000.

Chrichlow, R.W. Carcinoma of the male breast. *Surgical Gynecology and Obstetrics* 134:1011–1019, 1972.

Donegan, W.L. Cancer of the breast in men. *CA—A Cancer Journal for Clinicians* 41:339–354, 1991.

Donnegan, W.L. Cancer of the male breast. In Donegan, W.L. and Spratt, J.S. *Cancer of the Breast*, 5th Edition. Philadelphia: W.B. Saunders, 765–777, 1995.

Evans, D.B., Crichlow, R.W. Carcinoma of the male breast and Kleinfelter's syndrome: Is there an association? *CA—A Cancer Journal for Clinicians* 37:246–251, 1987.

Kinne, D.W., Hakes, T.B. Male breast cancer. In Harris, J., Hellman, S., Henderson, I.C., Kinne, D.W. *Breast Diseases*. Philadelphia: J.B. Lippincott, 782–790, 1991.

Moore, M.P. Special therapeutic problems: Male breast cancer. In Harris, J., Lippman, M.E., Morrow, M., and Hellman, S. *Diseases of the Breast*. Philadelphia: Lippincott-Raven, 859–862, 1996.

Whooley, B.P., and Borgen, P.I. Male breast cancer. In Roses, D. *Breast Cancer*. New York: Churchill Livingstone, 613–622, 1999.

Chapter 11: An Overview of Cancer Treatment

Dodd, M.J. *Managing the Side Effects of Chemotherapy and Radiation Therapy: A Guide for Patients and Their Families*. 3rd Edition. San Francisco: Regents, University of California, UCSF Nursing Press, 1996.

Chapter 13: Radiation Therapy

Bruner, D.W., Bucholtz, J.D., Iwamoto, R., and Strohl, R., eds. *Manual for Radiation Oncology Nursing Practice and Education*. Pittsburgh: Oncology Nursing Press, 1998.

Kelly, L.D. Nursing assessment and patient management [in Radiation Therapy]. *Seminars in Oncology Nursing* 15(4):282–291, 1999.

Powell, L.L., ed. *Recycling Our Ideas: 10 Years of Practice Tips From the Oncology Nursing Forum (1982–1992)*. Pittsburgh: Oncology Nursing Press, 1993.

Preston, F.A. and Cunningham, R.S. *Clinical Guidelines for Symptom Management in Oncology: A Handbook for Advanced Practice Nurses*. New York: Clinical Insights Press, 1998.

Chapter 14: Systemic Therapy: Chemotherapy and Biotherapy

Fischer, D.S., Knobf, M.T., and Durivage, H.J. *The Cancer Chemotherapy Handbook*, 5th Edition. St. Louis: Mosby, 1997.

Fishman, M. and Mrozek-Orlowski, M., eds. *Cancer Chemotherapy Guidelines and Recommendations for Practice*. Pittsburgh: Oncology Nursing Press, 1999.

Gale, D., and Charette, J. *Oncology Nursing Care Plans*. El Paso: Skidmore-Roth Publishing, Inc., 1994.

Hahn, W.C., Counter, C.M., Lundberg, A.S., et al. Creation of human tumor cells with defined genetic elements. *Nature* 400:464–468, 1999.

Weitzman, J.B., and Yaniv, M. Rebuilding the road to cancer. *Nature* 400: 401–402, 1999.

Chapter 15: Clinical Trials

Giacalone, S.B. Cancer Clinical Trials. In Otto, S.E. (ed). *Oncology Nursing*, 3rd Edition. St. Louis: Mosby, 1997.

Oncology Nursing Society. Oncology Nursing Society position on cancer research and cancer clinical trials. *Oncology Nursing Forum* 25(6):973–974, 1997.

Chapter 16: Complementary and Alternative Therapies for Cancer

Astin, J.A. Why patients use alternative medicine: Results of a national study. *Journal of the American Medical Association* 279(19):1548–1553, 1998.

Blevins, S. Fighting Cancer and the FDA. *The Wall Street Journal*, June 2, 1997.

Booth, K. Are traditional evaluations right for alternative therapies? *Oncology Times*, April 8, 1998.

Cassileth, B., and Chapman, C. Alternative and complementary cancer therapies. *Cancer* 77(6):1026–1034, 1996.

Colt, G.H. See me, feel me, touch me, heal me. *Life Magazine*, September, 42–50, 1996.

Decker, G.M., ed. *An Introduction to Complementary and Alternative Therapies*. Pittsburgh: Oncology Nursing Press, Inc., 1999.

Eisenberg, D. Advising patients who seek alternative medical therapies. *Annals of Internal Medicine* 127:127–140, 1997.

Eisenberg, D., Davis, R.B., Ettner, S.L., Appel, M.S., et al. Trends in alternative medicine use in the United States, 1990–1997. *Journal of the American Medical Association* 280(18):1569–1575, 1998.

Foster, S. Battle weary: In the quest to cure cancer, we look to alternatives. *Herbs for Health*, May/June, 40–43, 1997.

Henkel, G. Talking points: What to say when patients are using alternative therapies. *Oncology Times*, April, 7–15, 1998.

Jonas, W. Alternative medicine: Learning from the past, examining the present, advancing to the future *Journal of the American Medical Association* 280(18):1616–1617, 1998.

Lane, W.I., and Comac, C. *Sharks Don't Get Cancer: How Shark Cartilage Could Save Your Life*. Garden City Park, NY: Avery Publishing Group Inc., 1993.

Montibrand, M. Past and present herbs used to treat cancer: Medicine, magic, or poison? *Oncology Nursing Forum* 26(1):49–60, 1999.

Montibrand, M. Decision tree model describing alternate health care choices made by oncology patients. *Cancer Nursing* 18(2):104–117, 1995.

Montibrand, M. Freedom of choice: an issue concerning alternate therapies chosen by patients with cancer. *Oncology Nursing Forum* 20(8):1195–1201, 1993.

Widman, L. Requests for medical advice from patients and families to health care providers who publish on the World Wide Web. *Archives of Internal Medicine* 157:209–212, 1997.

Wilt, T.J., Ishani, A., Stark, G., MacDonald, M.S., et al. Saw Palmetto extracts for treatment of benign prostatic hyperplasia: A systematic review. *Journal of the American Medical Association* 280:1604–1609, 1998.

Chapter 17: Taking Control of Cancer Pain

Patt, R.B. (With Contributors) *Cancer Pain*. Philadelphia: J.B. Lippincott Company, 1993.

Chapter 18: Cancer, Sexuality, and Sex

Barsevick, A.M., Much, J., and Sweeney, C. Psychosocial Responses to Cancer. In Yarbro, C.H., Frogge, M.H., Goodman, M., and Groenwald, S.L., eds. *Cancer Nursing: Principles and Practice*, 5th Edition. Boston: Jones and Bartlett Publishers, 1529–1549, 2000.

Masters, W.H., and Johnson, V.E. *Human Sexual Response*. New York: Lippincott Williams & Wilkens, 1966.

Chapter 19: End-of-Life and Palliative Care

Doyle, Hanks, and MacDonald. *The Oxford Textbook of Palliative Medicine*, 2nd Edition. New York: Oxford University Press, 1998.

Ferrell, R.R. *Suffering*. Sudbury, MA: Jones and Bartlett Publishers, 1996.

Field, M.J., and Cassel, C.K., eds. *Approaching Death: Improving Care at the End of Life*. Washington, D.C.: National Academy Press, 1997.

Houts, P.S., ed. *Home Care Guide for Advanced Cancer*. American College of Physcians, 1997.

Houts, P.S., and Bucher, J.A., eds. *Caregiving: A Step-By-Step Resource for Caring for the Person with Cancer at Home*. Atlanta, Georgia: American Cancer Society, 2000.

Kemp, C. *Terminal Illness: A Guide to Nursing Care*. Philadelphia: J.B. Lippincott Co., 1995.

Lynn, J., and Harrold, J., and The Center to Improve Care of the Dying. *Handbook for Mortals: Guidance for People Facing Serious Illness*. New York: Oxford University Press, 1999.

Chapter 20: Survivorship

Ferrell, B.R., and Dow, K.H. Quality of life among long-term cancer survivors. *Oncology* 11(4):565–576, 1997.

Ferrell, B.R., and Dow, K.H. Portraits of cancer survivorship: A glimpse through the lens of survivors' eyes. *Cancer Practice* 4(2):76–80, 1996.

Haylock, P.J., and Blackburn, K.M. Policy, politics and oncology nursing. In Yarbro, C.H., Frogge, M.H., Goodman, M., and Groenwald, S.L., eds. *Cancer Nursing: Principles and Practice*, 5th Edition. Boston: Jones and Bartlett Publishers, 1781–1800, 2000.

Haynes, M.A., and Smedley, B.D., eds. *The Unequal Burden of Cancer: An Assessment of NIH Research and Programs for Ethnic Minorities and the Medically Underserved*. Washington, D.C.: National Academy Press, 1999.

Leigh, S. Cancer survivorship: A consumer movement. *Seminars in Oncology* 21(6):783–786, 1994.

Resources

General Cancer Organizations

American Brain Tumor Association
2720 River Rd.
Des Plaines IL 60018
(847) 827-9910   Patient Line: (800) 886-2282

American Cancer Society (ACS)
1599 Clifton Rd. N.E.
Atlanta GA 30329
www.cancer.org   (800) ACS-2345 (227-2345)

The American Society of Clinical Oncologists (ASCO)
225 Reinekers Ln., Suite 650
Alexandria VA 22314
www.asco.org   (703) 299-1044

Canadian Cancer Society
565 W. 10th Ave.
Vancouver BC V5Z 4J4
Canada
www.bc.cancer.ca/ccs/   (604) 872-4400

Cancer Care, Inc.
275 7th Ave.
New York NY 10001   (212) 302-2400
www.cancercareinc.org   (800) 813-HOPE (813-4673)
Cancer Care, Inc. provides education, information, and referrals, and some direct financial assistance. There are national teleconferences for patients and families as well as health care professionals. The website offers a bookstore and helpful informational brochures.

The Leukemia & Lymphoma Society
600 Third Ave., 4th Floor
New York NY 10016   (800) 955-4LSA (955-4572)
www.leukemia.org   (212) 573-8484   (212) 856-9686, fax

The Leukemia Society gives callers the address and phone number of the nearest local chapter. Application for financial aid is made to the local chapter and must be made soon after diagnosis. Only bills incurred after application are eligible for reimbursement. This organization is also a very good resource for patient education brochures and booklets.

National Cancer Institute (NCI)
Cancer Information Service
Building 31, Room 10a24
9000 Rockville Pike
Bethesda MD 20892
www.nci.gov   (800) 4 CANCER (422-6237)

Oncology Nursing Society
501 Holiday Dr.
Pittsburg PA 15220
www.ons.org   (412) 921-7373

Specialized Organizations

Complementary and Alternative Therapy and Cancer

American Association of Acupuncture and Oriental Medicine
4101 Lake Boone Trail, Suite 201
Raleigh NC 27607   (919) 787-5181

The American Botanical Council
PO Box 144345
Austin TX 78714
www.herbalgram.org   (512) 926-4900

The American Dietetic Association
216 W. Jackson Blvd.
Chicago IL 60606   (800) 366-1655
www.eatright.org   (312) 899-0040

The American Holistic Health Association
PO Box 17400
Anaheim CA 90017   (714) 779-6152

The American Massage Therapy Association
820 Davis St.
Evanston IL 60201
www.amtamassage.org   (847) 864-0123

The American Society of Professional Hypnotherapists
PO Box 29
Boones Mill VA 24065   (703) 334-3035

The Better Business Bureau
The Council of Better Business Bureaus
4200 Wilson Blvd., Suite 800
Arlington VA 22203   (703) 276-0100

Commonweal Organization
PO Box 316
Bolinas CA 94924
www.commonweal.org   (415) 868-0970

The Food and Drug Administration (FDA)
HFI-40
Rockville MD 20857
www.fda.gov   (888) 463-6332

The National Center for Homeopathy
801 N. Fairfax St.
Alexandria VA 22314   (703) 548-7790
www.healthy.net/pan/pa/homeopathic/natcenhom/index.html

National Commission for the Certification of Acupuncturists
PO Box 97075
Washington DC 20090   (202) 232-1404

The Office of Cancer Complementary and Alternative Medicine
NCCAM at NIH
Bethesda MD 20892   (301) 496-1712
Clearinghouse #   (888) 644-6226
www.nccam.nih.gov

Incontinence

National Association for Continence (NAFC)
PO Box 8310
Spartanburg SC 29305
www.nafc.org   (864) 579-7900

Lung Cancer

The Alliance for Lung Cancer Advocacy, Support and Education (ALCASE)
1601 Lincoln Ave.
Vancouver WA 98660   (800) 298-2436
www.alcase.org   info@alcase.org

The American Lung Association
1740 Broadway
New York NY 10019
www.lungusa.org   (800) LUNG-USA (586-4872)

Ostomy

International Ostomy Association
15 Station Rd.
Reading
Berkshire RG1 1LG
United Kingdom   +44-1189-391-537

United Ostomy Association
19772 MacArthur Blvd., Suite 200
Irvine CA 92612-2405
www.uoa.org   (800) 826-0826

World Council of Enterostomal Therapists (WCET)
6 Ferrands Close
Hardin Bingley
W. Yorkshire BD16 1JA
United Kingdom   +44-1273-775-432

Wound, Ostomy and Continence Nurses Society (WOCN)
1550 South Coast Hwy., Suite 201
Laguna Beach CA 92651
www.wocn.org   (888) 224-WOCN (224-9626)

Pain

The American Alliance of Cancer Pain Initiatives
Resource Center of the AACPI
1300 University Avenue #4720
Madison WI 53706   (608) 262-0978

Mayday Pain Resource Center
City of Hope National Medical Center
1500 Duarte Rd.
Duarte CA 91010   (626) 359-8111, ext. 3829

Pediatric Service Organizations

Candlelighters Childhood Cancer Foundation
7910 Woodmont Ave., Suite 460
Bethesda MD 20814   (800) 366-CCCF (366-2223)
www.candlelighters.org   (301) 718-2686, fax

Candlelighters Childhood Cancer Foundation, Canada
55 Eglinton Ave. East, Suite 401
Toronto ON M4P 1G8
Canada   (800) 363-1062 (Canada only)
www.candlelighters.ca   (416) 489-9812, fax

Founded in 1970 by parents of children with cancer, Candlelighters now has over forty thousand members worldwide. Local chapters are available in larger cities. Its mission is to "educate, serve, and advocate for families of children with cancer, and the professionals who care for them." Free services include access to a library containing over 2800 articles related to childhood cancer, annual resource guide, computerized searches for protocols and treatment options, ability to match families with resources for help, newsletters, and various handbooks.

Childhood Cancer Ombudsman Program
12141 Pine Needle Ct.
Woodbridge VA 22192   (703) 492-0045
A free service provided by the Childhood Brain Tumor Foundation of Virginia to support children with cancer and their families who are experiencing difficulties gaining access to an appropriate education, medical care, coverage of the costs of health care, and meaningful employment.

Cancer Cured Kids
PO Box 189
Old Westbury NY 11568   (800) CCK-7525 (225-7525)
(516) 484-8160   (516) 484-8160, fax
Organization dedicated to the quality of life of kids who have survived cancer. It supplies information about educational and psychosocial needs of survivors.

Chai Lifeline/Camp Simcha
National Office
48 W. 25th St., 6th Fl.
New York NY 10010   (800) 343-2527
(212) 255-1160   (212) 255-1495, fax
National nonprofit Jewish organization provides free support service programs to children and their families in crisis. Sponsors the only kosher camp in North America for children with cancer.

The Compassionate Friends
National Office
PO Box 3696   (630) 990-0010
Oak Brook IL 60522-3696   (630) 990-0246, fax
www.jjt.com/~tcf_national/index.html
This organization offers understanding and friendship to bereaved parents and siblings. It sponsors local chapters that hold support meetings and makes personal contact with those experiencing the loss of a child. It also provides a catalog with a list of resources on adult and sibling grief.

Friends Network
PO Box 4545
Santa Barbara CA 93140
This organization distributes an activities newsletter printed in color, called *The Funletter*, to children with cancer.

Ronald McDonald House Coordinator
c/o Golin Communications, Inc.
500 North Michigan Ave.
Chicago IL 60614   (312) 836-7100
Ronald McDonald houses are close to hospitals in many major cities. The rates are extremely low and can be adjusted in cases of financial hardship. They provide an emotional haven for families facing similar situations.

Air Care Alliance
(800) 296-1217
www.angelflightfla.org/aircareall.org/acahome.html
A nationwide association of humanitarian flying organizations that flies patients to and from medical treatments.

Corporate Angel Network, Inc. (CAN)
Westchester County Airport, Bldg. 1
White Plains NY 10604   (914) 328-1313   (800) 328-4226
Provides use of available seats on corporate aircraft at no cost, to get to and from recognized cancer treatment centers. Child must travel with up to two adults. Also flies donors.

Mission Air Transportation Network
Proctor & Gamble Building
4711 Young St.
North York ON M2N 6K8
Canada   (416) 222-6335   (416) 222-6930
Arranges flights for Canadians in financial need using donated seats on corporate, commercial, or government aircraft.

Prostate Cancer

Association for the Cure of Cancer of the Prostate (CaP CURE)
www.capcure.org
CaP CURE identifies and supports prostate cancer research that will rapidly translate into treatments and cures. It encourages collaboration and reduced bureaucracy and speeds the process of discovery through encouraging partnerships among the advocacy community, government research institutions, and private industry. This organization has received considerable support from businessman Michael Milliken and retired General Norman Schwarzkopf, both prostate cancer survivors.

Man to Man
An American Cancer Society (ACS) program designed to educate and support men facing prostate cancer. The ACS offers a Facilitator Training Program that helps prepare interested men and women in planning and implementing a Man to Man program. Contact the local unit or state division of the ACS for further information.

National Prostate Cancer Coalition (NPPC)
1158 Fifteenth St., N.W.
Washington DC 20005
www.4npcc.org   (202) 463-9455

A grassroots advocacy organization dedicated to eliminating prostate cancer as a serious health concern for men and their families. NPCC's goals are to build a national grassroots movement that will press elected officials to increase federal funding for prostate cancer research and to make prostate cancer a national health priority.

US TOO International, Inc.
930 N. York Rd., Suite 50
Hinsdale IL 60521
www.ustoo.com   (630) 323-1002
Hotline: (800) 80-US TOO (808-7866)

An independent network of support group chapters for men with prostate cancer and their families. US TOO groups offer fellowship, peer counseling, education about treatment options, and discussion of medical alternatives without bias. A component of US TOO is the US TOO Partners Women's Support Network.

Sexuality and Sex

American Association of Sex Educators, Counselors and Therapists (AASECT)
PO Box 238
Mt. Vernon IA 52314
(Provides a free listing of certified sex educators and counselors in your state: Send a self-addressed, stamped, business-size envelope.)

Good Vibrations Catalogue
938 Howard St., Suite 101
San Francisco CA 94103   (800) 289-8243

Sinclair Intimacy Institute
Box 8865
Chapel Hill NC 27515

The Xandria Collection
874 Dubuque Ave.
South San Francisco CA 94080   (800) 848-2823

Survivorship

Intercultural Cancer Council
PMB-C
1720 Dryden
Houston TX 77030
www.icc.bcm.tmc.edu/   (713) 798-4617

National Coalition for Cancer Survivorship
1010 Wayne Ave.
Silver Spring MD 20910
www.cansearch.org   (301) 650-8868   (888) 650-9127

The Office of Minority Health Resource Center
PO Box 37337
Washington DC 20012
www.omhrc.gov   (800) 444-6472

Pharmaceutical Research and Manufacturers of America (PhRMA)
1100 15th St. N.W.
Washington DC 20005
www.phrma.org

The Uniform Benefits Package Enrollment Service Center
www.va.gov   (877) 222-VETS (222-8387)

Veterans Administration
Department of Federal Benefits for Veterans and Dependents
(800) 827-1000

Testicular Cancer

Centers of Excellence in the Treatment of Testicular Cancer

Indianapolis IN

Indiana University Medical Center   (317) 274-5000

Oncologists:

Lawrence Einhorn, M.D.
Department of Medicine   (317) 274-0920

Partick Loehrer, M.D.
Department of Medicine   (317) 274-0920

Bruce Roth, M.D.
Indiana Cancer Pavilion   (317) 274-3515

Steven Williams
Indiana University Cancer Center   (317) 278-0070

Urologists:

Richard Bihrle, M.D.
Department of Urology   (317) 630-7744

Richard Foster, M.D.
Department of Urology   (317) 274-3458

Portland OR

Oregon Health Sciences University

Bruce Lowe, M.D.
Associate Professor of Urology   (503) 474-7760

Craig Nichols, M.D.
Chairman Hematology/Oncology   (503) 494-8534

Boston MA

Dana-Farber Cancer Institute

Phil Kantoff, M.D.
Oncology, Harvard Medical School   (617) 632-3466

Marc Garnick, M.D.
Oncologist   (617) 732-3000

Jerome Richie, M.D.
Chief of Urology   (617) 566-3475

New York NY

Medical Oncology
   Dean Bajorin, M.D.   (212) 639-6708
   George Bosl, M.D.   (212) 639-8473
   Robert Motzer, M.D.   (212) 639-6667

Urology, Adult Surgery
   Harry Heer, M.D.   (212) 639-8264
   Joel Scheinfeld, M.D.   (212) 639-2592
   Pramod Sogani, M.D.   (212) 639-7704

Pediatric Surgery
   Michael Laquaglia, M.D.   (212) 639-7002
   Nicholas Saenz, M.D.   (212) 639-7929

Denver CO

University of Colorado Health Sciences Center

L. Michael Glodé, M.D.
Editor in Chief, ASCO OnLine   (303) 315-8825

Chicago IL

University of Chicago Hospitals

Nicholas Vogelzang, M.D. (773) 702-6743

Seattle WA

University of Washington School of Medicine
Paul Lange, M.D.   (206) 548-4294

San Francisco CA

University of California School of Medicine
Peter Carroll, M.D.   (415) 476-1611

Los Angeles CA

University of Southern California/Norris Comprehensive Cancer Center
Derek Raghavan, M.D.   (323) 865-3962
Donald Skinner, M.D.   (323) 764-3707

University of California, Los Angeles Medical Plaza
Daniel Lieber, M.D.   (310) 443-0466

Washington DC

Walter Reed Army Medical Center
David McLeod, M.D.   (202) 782-4118
Judd Moul, M.D.   (202) 780-4684

For Centers of Excellence outside of the United States and around the world, go to:
www.acor.org/diseases/TC/experts.html

General Internet Resources

CancerLynx
www.cancerlynx.com
Provides general information but also focuses on complementary therapies, and psychosocial needs of people facing cancer.

Physician Data Query (PDQ)
www.cancernet.nci.hih.gov
Provides links to PDQ and information about cancer treatment, screening, prevention, supportive care, and clinical trials. Also links to CANCERLIT, a bibliographic database.

www.cancernet.nci.nih.gov/prot/protsrch.shtml
Provides PDQ Clinical Trial Search Form, allowing searches for clinical trials to be done by the type of cancer, treatment, drug, and the sponsor of the trial.

Memorial Sloan Kettering Cancer Center
www.mskcc.org

National Cancer Institute Community Clinical Oncology Programs (CCOPs)
www.dcp.nic.nih.gov/CORB/

National Cancer Institute designated cancer centers
www.nci.nih.gov/cancercenters/

University of Pennsylvania Cancer Center-OncoLink
www.Oncolink.upenn.edu

U.S. Food and Drug Administration
www.fda.gov/fdac/search.html

Specific Internet Resources

Clinical Trials

Cancer Trials, National Cancer Institute
cancertrials.nci.nih.gov
Provides information to help understand clinical trials and how to find specific trials. Includes research news and links to other resources.

"Taking Part in Clinical Trials: What Cancer Patients Need to Know"
cancertrials.nci.nih.gov/NCI_CANCER_TRIALS/zones/Booklet

Complementary and Alternative Therapies

Ask Dr. Weil Integrative Medicine
cgi.pathfinder.com/drweil

Innovations in Cancer Therapy
www.bu.edu/cohis/cancer/innovtx.htm/

Monica Miller's site for insurance reform for alternatives
www.healthlobby.com/welcome.html/

National Center for Homeopathy
www.healthy.net/nch/

Office of Alternative Medicine website
altmed.od.nih.gov/

The University of Texas Center for Alternative Medicine Research website
chprd.sph.uth.tmc.edu/utcam/

End of Life and Palliative Care

American Academy of Hospice and Palliative Care
www.aahpm.org

Americans for Better Care of the Dying
www.abcd-caring.com

Center to Improve the Care of the Dying
www.gwu.edu/~cicd

Choice in Dying
www.choices.org

Growth House
www.growthhouse.org

Last Acts Campaign
www.lastacts.org

National Hospice Association
www.nho.org

Fertility

Internet Health Resources-Fertility Clinics
www.ihr.com/infertility/provider/index.html

Lung Cancer

Alliance for Lung Cancer Advocacy, Support, and Education (ALCASE)
www.alcase.org
info@alcase.org

Pain

Wisconsin Cancer Pain Initiative
www.wisc.edu/wcpi/

Prostate Cancer

Brachytherapy
www.rattler.cameron.edu/seedpods

Medscape
www.medscape.com/urology

National Coalition of Cancer Centers—Prostate Cancer Treatment Guidelines
www.nccn.org/patient_guidelines/prostate_cancer

The Prostate Cancer Info Link
www.comed.com/prostate

Prostate Cancer Support Groups
www.mediconsult.com

Prostate Pointers
www.rattler.cameron.edu/prostate

Texas Department of Health
www.tdh.state.tx.us/osp/PROSTATE/HTM

Sexuality and Sex

Good Vibrations
www.goodvibes.com
(For sexual materials, including lubricants, condoms, videotapes, books, vibrators, sex toys, and educational materials)

Sinclair Intimacy Institute
www.bettersex.com

Testicular Cancer

Mayo Clinic Health Oasis
www.mayohealth.org/mayo/9511/htm.testica.htm

Testicular Cancer Resource Center
www.acor.org/diseases/TC

Virginia Urology Clinic
www.uro.com/tcancer.htm

General Print and Other Media Resources

American Cancer Society: Facts and Figures—2000. Atlanta, GA: American Cancer Society, 2000.

Cancer Care, Inc. *A Helping Hand Resource Guide*. New York: Cancer Care, Inc.

Dollinger, M., Rosenbaum, E.H., and Cable, G. *Everyone's Guide to Cancer Therapy*, 3rd Revised Edition. Kansas City, KS: Somerville House Books, Ltd., Andrews McMeel Publishing, 1998.

Gullo, S.M., and Glass, E., eds. *Silver Linings: The Other Side of Cancer*. Pittsburgh PA: The Oncology Nursing Press, 1997.

Harpham, W.S. *Diagnosis: Cancer—Your Guide Through the First Few Months*. New York: W.W. Norton Co., 1998.

Harpham, W.S. *When a Parent Has Cancer: A Guide to Caring for Your Children*. New York: Harper Collins, 1997.

Harpham, W.S. *Becky and the Worry Cup*. (Accompanies *When A Parent Has Cancer*) New York: Harper Collins, 1997.

Hoffman, B., ed. *A Cancer Survivor's Almanac: Charting Your Journey*. Minneapolis, MN: Chronimed Publishing, 1996.

Houts, P.S., ed. *Home Care Guide for Cancer: How to Care for Family and Friends at Home*. Philadelphia: American College of Physicians, 1994.

Luggen, A.S., and Meiner, S.E., eds. *Handbook for the Care of the Older Adult with Cancer*. Pittsburgh: Oncology Nursing Press, Inc., 2000.

Wilkes, G.M. *Cancer and HIV Clinical Nutrition: Pocket Guide*, 2nd edition. Boston: Jones and Bartlett, 1999.

Specialized Print and Other Media Resources

Chemotherapy and Biotherapy

Dollinger, M.M., Rosenbaum, E.H., and Cable, G. *Everyone's Guide to Cancer Therapy*, 3rd Revised Edition. Kansas City, KS: Somerville House Books Limited, Andrews McMeel Publishing, 1998.

McKay, J. and Hirano, N. *Chemotherapy and Radiation Therapy Survival Guide*. Oakland, CA: New Harbinger Publications, 1998.

National Cancer Institute. *Understanding the Immune System*. National Cancer Institute, NIH Publication No. 93–529.

U.S. Department of Health and Human Services. *Chemotherapy and You: A Guide to Self-Help During Treatment*. National Institutes of Health, NIH Publication No. 88–1136.

Clinical Trials

National Cancer Institute. *What Are Clinical Trials All About? A Booklet for Patients with Cancer*. National Institutes of Health, National Cancer Institute, 1997.

Complementary and Alternative Therapy and Cancer

Cassidy, C.M. Healing Herbs, *Prevention Health Specials*, p. 1–93, 1996.

Cassileth, B. *The Alternative Medicine Handbook: The Complete Reference Guide to Alternative and Complementary Therapies*. New York: W.W. Norton, 1998.

Diamond, W.J., Cowden, W.L., and Goldberg B. *An Alternative Medicine: The Definitive Guide To Cancer*. Puyallup, WA: Future Medicine Publishing, Inc., 1994.

Jacobs, J. *The Encyclopedia of Alternative Medicine*. London: Carlton Books Ltd., 1996.

Jacobs, J. *A Guide to Alternative Medicine CD Rom*. Cambridge, MA: The Learning Company, 1996.

Lerner, M. *Choices in Healing: Integrating the Best of Conventional and Complementary Medicine*. Cambridge, MA: MIT Press, 1996.

Marti, J.E. *The Alternative Health & Medicine Encyclopedia*. Detroit, MI: Visible Ink Press, 1995.

Simone, C.B. *Cancer and Nutrition: A Ten Point Plan to Reduce Your Risk of Getting Cancer*. Garden City Park, NY: Avery Publishing Group, Inc., 1992.

Weil, A. *Spontaneous Healing*. New York: The Ballantine Publishing Group, 1995.

Weil, A. *Natural Health, Natural Medicine*. New York: Houghton, Mifflin & Company, 1994.

Zwicky, J.F., Hafner, A.W., Barrett, S., and Jarvis, W.T. *Reader's Guide to Alternative Health Methods*. Milwaukee, WI: American Medical Association, 1993.

End-of-Life and Palliative Care

Furman, J. and McNabb, D. *The Dying Time: Practical Wisdom for the Dying and Their Caregivers*. New York: Random House, Inc.1997.

Lynn, J., Harrold, J. and The Center to Improve Care of the Dying. *Handbook for Mortals: Guidance for People Facing Serious Illness*. New York: Oxford University Press, 1999.

McFarlane, R. and Bashe, P. *The Complete Bedside Companion: No-Nonsense Advice on Caring for the Seriously Ill*. New York: Simon and Schuster, 1998. (Hardback) (Paperback available from Fireside Publishers, 1999.)

Sankar, A. *Dying At Home: A Family Guide for Caregiving*. Baltimore, MD: Johns Hopkins Press, 1999.

Lung Cancer

ALCASE: *The Lung Cancer Manual*. Vancouver, WA: Alliance for Lung Cancer Advocacy, Support, and Education.

Ruckdeschel, J.C. *Myths and Facts About Lung Cancer—What You Need to Know*. Melville, NY: PRR, 1999.

Pain

Agency for Health Care Policy and Research. *Managing Cancer Pain: Patient Guide*. 1994. (Call 1-800-4-CANCER for a free copy.)

American Cancer Society. *Get Relief from Cancer Pain*. Atlanta, GA: American Cancer Society, 1994.

Coluzzi, P., Volker B., and Miaskowski, C. *Comprehensive Pain Management in Terminal Illness*. Sacramento, CA: California State Hospice Association, 1996.

Haylock, P.J., and Curtis, C. *Cancer Doesn't Have to Hurt*. Alameda, CA: Hunter House Publishers, 1997.

Pediatric Cancer

Adams, D. and Deveau, E. *Coping with Childhood Cancer: Where Do We Go From Here?* Toronto, ON: Kinbridge Publications, 1993.

American Brain Tumor Association. *Alex's Journey: The Story of a Child with a Brain Tumor*. Des Plaines, IL: American Brain Tumor Association, 1999. (Video available from the American Brain Tumor Association.)

Baker, L. *You and Leukemia: A Day at a Time*. Phildadelphia, PA: W.B. Saunders Co., 1988.

Bearison, D.J. *They Never Want to Tell You: Children Talk About Cancer*. Cambridge: Harvard University Press, 1991.

Bombeck, E. *I Want to Grow Hair, I Want to Grow Up, I Want to Go to Boise*. New York: Harper & Row Publishers, 1989.

Gill, K.A. *Teenage Cancer Journey*. Pittsburgh, PA: Oncology Nursing Press, 1999.

Keene, N. *Childhood Leukemia: A Guide for Families, Friends, and Caregivers*. Sebastopol, CA: O'Reilly, 1997.

Lozowski-Sullivan, S. *Know Before You Go: The Childhood Cancer Journey*. Bethesda, MD: The Candlelighters Childhood Cancer Foundation, 1998.

O'Toole, D. *Aarvy Aardvark Finds Hope*. Burnsville, NC: Mountain Rainbow Publications, 1997.

Shultz, C. *Why Charlie Brown Why?* New York: Topper Books, 1990. (Video available through the American Cancer Society.)

Prostate Cancer

National Comprehensive Cancer Network and the American Cancer Society. Prostate Cancer: Treatment Guidelines for Patients: Version I. *INTOUCH Magazine*. August/September 1999, pp. 74–103. Available at the website (www.nccn.org) or by calling the toll-free telephone numbers (800) ACS-2345 or (888) 909-NCCN (909-6226).

Radiation Therapy

National Cancer Institute. *Radiation Therapy and You: A Guide to Self-Help During Cancer Treatment.* National Institutes of Health, NIH Publication No. 99-2227.

Sexuality, Sex, and Cancer

Comfort, A. *The New Joy of Sex*. New York: Crown Publishers, Inc., 1993.

Danielou, A. (translator). *The Complete Kama Sutra*. Rochester, VT: Part Street Press, 1994.

Fox, S.I. *Human Physiology*, 2nd edition. Dubuque, IA: Wm. C. Brown Publishers, 1987.

Klein, M. and Robbins, R. *Let Me Count the Ways: Discovering Great Sex Without Intercourse*. New York: Jeremy P. Tarcher/Putnam, 1998.

Locker, S. *The Complete Idiot's Guide to Amazing Sex*. New York: Macmillan Publishing USA, 1999.

Schover, L.R. *Sexuality and Fertility After Cancer*. New York: John Wiley & Sons, 1997.

Wilmoth, M.D. Sexuality. In Burke, C.C. (ed). *Psychosocial Dimensions of Oncology Nursing Care*. Pittsburgh, PA: Oncology Nursing Press, Inc., 1998.

Zilbergeld, B. *The New Male Sexuality*. New York: Bantam Books, 1992.

Survivorship

Calder, K.J. and Pollitz, K. *What Cancer Survivors Need to Know About Health Insurance*. Silver Spring, MD: National Coalition for Cancer Survivorship, 1998.

Clark, E.J., ed. *Teamwork: The Cancer Patient's Guide to Talking with Your Doctor*. Silver Spring, MD: National Coalition for Cancer Survivorship, 3rd printing, 1998.

Herzlinger, R. *Market Driven Health Care: Who Wins, Who Loses in the Transformation of America's Largest Service Industry*. Reading, MA: Perseus Books, 1997.

Nash, D.B., Manfredi, M.P., Bozarth, B., and Howell, S. *Connecting with the New Healthcare Consumer: Defining Your Strategy*. New York: McGraw-Hill, 2000.

National Coalition for Cancer Survivorship. *The Cancer Survival Toolbox* (audio-tapes). Silver Spring, MD: National Coalition for Cancer Survivorship, 1998. Available in English, Spanish, and (print version only) Chinese. Also available at the NCCS website (www.cansearch.org).

National Coalition for Cancer Survivorship. *Finding Ways to Pay for Care: The Cancer Survival Toolbox* (audiotape). Silver Spring, MD: National Coalition for Cancer Survivorship, 1999. Also available at the NCCS website (www.cansearch.org).

National Coalition for Cancer Survivorship. *Topics for Older Persons: The Cancer Survival Toolbox* (audiotape). Silver Spring, MD: National Coalition for Cancer Survivorship, 1999. Also available at the NCCS website (www.cansearch.org).

National Coalition for Cancer Survivorship. *Caring for the Caregiver: The Cancer Survival Toolbox* (audiotape). Silver Spring, MD: National Coalition for Cancer Survivorship, 2000. Also available at the NCCS website (www.cansearch.org).

Spingarn, N.D. *The New Cancer Survivors: Living with Grace, Fighting with Spirit.* Baltimore, MD: Johns Hopkins Press, 1999.

Walsh-Burke, K. and Marcusen, C. Self-advocacy training for cancer survivors: The Cancer Survival Toolbox. *Cancer Practice* 7(6):297-301, 1999.

Index

A

acetaminophen, 254
Actinomycin-D, 202
Actiq, 255
acupressure, 227
acupuncture, 226–227
adenocarcinomas, 60; colorectal cancer, 102–103; lung cancer, 87
adenomatous polyposis coli, 103–104
adenosis, 60
adjuvant therapy, 157
Adrenocortical agents, 196
advance directives, 282
advanced oncology certified nurses, 43
aflatoxin, 17
African American men, and breast cancer, 137; and prostate cancer, 55, 56
age, and breast cancer, 137; and colorectal cancer, 102; and prostate cancer, 55, 56; mortality rates, 315–316
Aging with Dignity, 283
AIDS, 269
alcohol, and cancer treatment, 45
alkaloids, plant, 195
alkylating agents, 195, 199
Alliance for Lung Cancer Advocacy, Support, and Education, 324
aloe vera, 237
alopecia (hair loss), 189, 202
alpha-fetoprotein, 124

alternative therapies, 220–246; definition of, 221–223; risks of, 222–223
American Association of Acupuncture and Oriental Medicine, 323
American Association of Sex Educators, Counselors and Therapists, 328
American Botanical Council, 323
American Brain Tumor Association, 322
American Cancer Society, 39, 47, 322
American Dietetic Association, 323
American Holistic Health Association, 323
American Lung Association, 324
American Massage Therapy Association, 323
American Medical Dictionary, 37
American Society of Clinical Oncologists, 37, 322
American Society of Professional Hypnotherapists, 323
American Urologic Association System, 63
Aminoglutethamide, 196
amygdalin, 241
anal sex, 276, 277
anaphase, 10
anaplasia, 30
anchorage-dependent growth, 11
androgens, 196
anemia, 192
anesthesia, 169–171

aniline dyes, 13
anorexia, 190
antiandrogen, 196
antiangiogenesis drugs, 99, 207
antibiotics, 199
antibody-mediated drugs, 99
antiestrogens, 196
antimetabolites, 195, 199
antineoplastins, 231–232
antioxidants, 85
antitumor antibiotics, 195
anxiety, 206
Appalachia Leadership Initiative on
    Cancer, 316
Armstrong, Lance, 118
aromatic amines, 13
arsenic, 17, 193; and lung cancer, 85
art therapy, 229
asbestos, 1, 14, 17; and lung cancer, 85
Asian and Pacific Islander American
    Health Foundation, 316
Asparaginase, 196
aspirin, 18, 205; protection against co-
    lorectal cancer, 105
Association for the Cure of Cancer of
    the Prostate, 328
Association of Community Cancer
    Centers, 42
Association of Oncology Social
    Workers, 281
astragalus, 235
astrocytoma, 31
atypical adenomatous hyperplasia, 60
Australia, euthanasia, 289
ayurvedic medicine, 238–239
Azacytadine, 195

B

bacterial carcinogenesis, 15
barium enema, 106, 107, 110
BASE Camp Children's Cancer
    Foundation, 153
bedsores, interventions, 287
benign cells, 29, 30
benign prostatic hyperplasia, 55
benzene, 17
benzodiazepines, 206

Better Business Bureau, 323
bicalutamide, 79
biologic response modifier, 204
biopsy, 28–29; lung cancer, 87;
    prostate, 60, 62
biotherapy, 193, 203–208; mechanism
    of, 204–205; research, 207–208;
    side effects, 205–207
bladder cancer, 13; chemotherapy treat-
    ment, 195
bladder irritation, 191
Blenoxane, 127
bleomycin sulfate, 127
Bleomycin, 195, 200
bloating, 190
blood tests, 62
blood transfusions, 167
blood, in sputum, 95
B-Mode acquisition and targeting, 183
bone marrow depression, 192; symp-
    toms of, 199
bone marrow transplant, 128
bone marrow, cancer of, 142–144
bone scan, 60, 62
bone tumors, 147–148
botanical medicine, 234
brachytherapy, 66, 72–77, 183–184;
    care after, 74–77; side effects, 74
brain tumors, 145–146; chemotherapy
    treatment, 195, 196
BRCA genes, 14, 137
breast cancer, male, 14, 136–141; and
    diet, 16–17; chemotherapy, 195,
    196; diagnosis, 139; incidence,
    137; prognosis, 140; risk factors,
    137; treatment, 139–140
breast enlargement, 79
breath, shortness of, 95
bronchodilators, 95
bronchoscopy, 27, 88
buckthorn, 235
Burzynski, Stanislaw, 231
Buschke-Lowenstein condition, 132
Busulfan, 195, 199, 200

C

cachexia, 233–234

cadmium, and lung cancer, 85
Canadian Cancer Society, 322
Cancer Care, Inc., 322
Cancer Cured Kids, 326
Cancer Information Service, 48
cancer of unknown origin, 31
cancer suppressor genes, 13, 14
cancer (see also specific cancers), causes of, 12–15; definition, 8–12; diagnosing, 23–33; environmental exposure, 1; occurrence of, 1, 9; staging, 32–33
cancers, secondary, lung cancer, 98
Candlelighters Childhood Cancer Foundation, 325
Carboplatin, 195, 199, 200, 204
carcinoembryonic antigen level, 26, 109
carcinogens, 12–13; familial, 14; physical, 14
carcinogenesis, 12–15
carcinoid lung cancer, 87
carcinomas, 30; infiltrating ductal, 139
cardiac side effects, 206
caregivers, cancer, 34–49
Carmustine (BCNU), 195, 200
castration, 78
catheters, 70, 73
celecoxib, 254
cell cycle, 9–11
cell-cycle-specific and nonspecific drugs, 194, 195
cells, cancerous, 10–12
cell traits, 31
cell types, prostate cancer, 60
Centers of Excellence in the Treatment of Testicular Cancer, 329
central nervous system lymphoma, 269
central nervous system tumors, 148–149
cervical cancer, and penile cancer, 131
cesium-137, 184
Chai Lifeline/Camp Simcha, 326
chaparral, 236
chat rooms, 46
chemical carcinogenesis, 13
chemoprevention, 18
chemotherapy, 193–208; combination,

194, 197; failure, 197–198; mechanism of, 194–198; side effects, 186, 198–203; single agent, 194
chemotherapy, and breast cancer, 140; and colorectal cancer, 112; and leukemia, 143; and lymphoma, 145; and lung cancer, 92; and prostate cancer, 66, 80; and testicular cancer, 126, 127–128
childhood cancer, 141–153
Childhood Cancer Ombudsman Program, 326
children, and family member's cancer treatment, 45
Chinese medicine, 226–227
Chlorambucil, 195, 199
Chlorodeoxyadenosine (2-CdA), 199
chloroform, 17
choline magnesium trisalicyclate, 254
Chopra, Deepak, 238–239
chromium, and lung cancer, 85
circumcision and penile cancer, 131
cisplatin, 118, 127, 128, 193, 195, 199, 200, 202, 203
clinical trials, 42, 209–219; participating in, 212–218; types of, 210–212
coal, and lung cancer, 85
cobalt-60, 184
cocaine, crack, and lung cancer, 85
codeine, 95
colchine, 193
colectomy, 111–113
colon cancer, 18; and diet, 16–17
colon, 101–102
colonoscopy, 27, 106, 107, 108
colorectal cancer, 100–117; diagnosis, 108–111; recurrence, 115; risk factors, 102–105; screening, 106–108; staging, 110–111; survivorship, 116–117; symptoms, 108–109; treatment, 111–115
colostomy, 112, 114–115; and sex, 273
combined precision irradiation, 72
Commonweal, 240, 324
communication, 35, 40; and health needs, 2; prostate cancer, 53
Community Clinical Oncology Programs, 212, 218

community funds, for treatment, 314
Compassionate Friends, 326
complementary therapies, 220–246; definition of, 221–223; diet therapies, 224–226; vitamin therapy, 225
Comprehensive Cancer Centers, 41–42
Comprehensive Community Oncology Programs, 42
computerized axial tomographic (CT) scans, 27
condoms, 278
conformal radiation therapy, 182
confusion, interventions, 286
conjunctivitis, 189
connective tissue, 30
contact inhibition, 11
Corporate Angel Network, Inc., 327
costs, end-of-life care, 294–295; of treatment, 215–216
cough, interventions, 286; treatment, 94–95
CPT-11 (Irinotecan), 199
Crohn's disease, 104
cryosurgery, 66, 71
cryotherapy, 150
cryptorchidism, 120, 138
CT scan, 60, 62, 110; and lung cancer detection, 86, 87
Cyclophosphamide, 195, 200, 202
cystitis, 191
cystoscopy, 60
cystourethroscopy, 73
Cytarabine, 195, 199, 200, 203
Cytosine arabinoside, 201
cytotoxic drugs, 194

D

Dacarbazine, 195, 200
Dactinomycin, 195, 199, 201
daughter cells, 10
Daunorubicin, 195, 199, 200, 202
DDT, 17
delirium, interventions, 286
dementia, interventions, 286
Demoral, 205
depression, 206

detection, lung cancer, 86; penis cancer, 131–132; prostate cancer, 56–58; testicular cancer, 121–123
Dexamethasone, 196
diagnosis, breast cancer, 139; colorectal cancer, 108–111; lung cancer, 87–90; penis cancer, 132–133; prostate cancer, 59–64; testicular cancer, 123–125
diarrhea, 191
diet and cancer prevention, 16–17; and colorectal cancer, 105
diet therapies, 224–226
dietary additives, 16
diethylstilbestrol (DES), 79, 121
differentiation, 12
digestive system, 101–102
digital rectal examination (DRE), 54, 59, 60, 61, 106, 107
Dilaudid, 255
dioxin, 13
Directory of Medical Specialists, 37
DNA ploidy analysis, 62
Docetaxel, 203
doctor, choosing, 36–40
Dolophine, 255
doubling time, 9
Doxorubicin, 195, 199, 200, 201, 202
Dromostanolone, 196
Duke's staging system, 110
Duragesic, 255
dysplasia, 30
dyspnea, 95; interventions, 286

E

ear inflammation, 189
echinacea, 235
ejaculation, dry, 71; pain, 59; problems with, 268
emphysema, 95
end-of-life care, 279–295; euthanasia, 285, 289–290; maintaining control, 280–290; palliative care, 290–295
enemas, 233, 242
epididymis, 119
Epirubicin (4,Epidoxorubicin), 199

epithelial tissue, 30
Epogen, 204
Epstein-Barr virus, 15
erectile dysfunction, 265–268; and
    prostate cancer treatment, 71, 77
erythema, 185
Erythroplasia of Queyrat, 132
esophagitis, 189
essiac, 237
estrogens, 196
Etoposide, 127, 196, 199, 201, 202,
    203
euthanasia, 285, 289–290
Exceptional Cancer Patients, 240
external beam radiation therapy, 66,
    71–72, 81, 180–183
eye inflammation, 189

F

family history, and colorectal cancer,
    104–105
family, and cancer treatment, 44
fat, dietary, 13
fatigue, and radiation therapy, 186;
    chemotherapy side effect, 201
fecal occult blood test, 106, 107
Fentanyl, 255
fertility, 263–265
fiber, dietary, 13
fibrosis, 191; radiation, 97
financial assistance, sources, 312–314
finasteride, 18, 56
Five Wishes, 284
flow cytometry, 31
Floxuridine, 199, 201
Fludarabine, 195
flu-like syndrome, 205
Fluorouracil (5-FU), 112, 195, 199,
    201, 202
Food and Drug Administration, 213,
    323; clinical trials, 213
formaldehyde, 17
fractions, radiation therapy, 179, 181
friends, and cancer treatment, 44

G

gap phase, 10
gastrointestinal cancers, chemotherapy
    treatment, 195
gastroscopy, 27
generation time, 9
genetic counseling, 20–21
genetic testing, 20
genital warts, 278. *See also* human
    papillomavirus
Gerson Therapy, 241–242
ginseng, 236
Gleason score, 60, 67
glioblastoma, 31
gold-198l, 184
gonadotropin releasing hormone, 196
Good Vibrations, 328
goserelin, 79
gynecomastia, 79, 137, 138, 139

H

hair loss, 189, 202; treating, 97, 202
Halotestin, 196
Hamilton, Scott, 118
head and neck cancers, chemotherapy
    treatment, 195
headaches, 205
health care reform, 308–309
health insurance, 294–295
health philosophies, 234–239
Helicobacter pylori, 15
hematopoietic growth factors, 199,
    204–205
hemoptysis, 95; interventions, 287
hepatitis, 278; hepatitis B, 15
herbal therapies, 234
hereditary nonpolyposis colorectal can-
    cer, 104–105
hernia, inguinal, 120
herpes, 278
Hill-Burton funds, 313
histological traits, 29
HIV, 278
Hodgkin's disease (lymphoma),
    144–145
homeopathy, 234, 238

hormonal therapy, prostate cancer, 66, 78–80
hormones, 275
hospice care, 290–295
hospitals, and intimacy, 271–272; receiving treatment in, 161–162
Hoxey Therapy, 242
human chorionic gonadotropin, 124
human papillomavirus, 15, 131, 269
hydrazine sulfate, 233–234
hydrocele, 120
Hydrocortisone, 196
Hydromorphone, 255
Hydroxyurea, 196
hypercholesteremia, 138
hyperestrogenism, 137
hyperplasia, 30
hyperprolactinemia, 138
hyperthermia, 188
hypertrophy, 30
hypnotherapy, 230
hypothalamus injury, 138

I

ibuprofen, 254
Idarubicin, 199, 201, 202
Ifex, 127
ifosfamide, 127, 195, 199, 202
imagery, mental, 229
imaging techniques, 26–28
immortality, cancer cell, 11
immune system deficiencies, 15, 275
Immuno-Augmentative Therapy, 241
impotence, 71, 77
infertility, and breast cancer, 138
inflammatory bowel disease, 104
infections, 192
information sources, 48
informed consent, 166, 214
initiating event, 13
insomnia, 206
intensity-modulated radiation therapy, 182
intensive care unit, 173–174
Intercultural Cancer Council, 316, 328
Interleukin-2, 206
International Ostomy Association, 325

Internet, and cancer information, 46, 48, 331–334
interstitial radioactive seed implants, 66, 72–77
intravenous pyelogram, 124
iodine, radioactive, 72
iodine-125, 184
ionization, 14
iridium-192, 184
Irinotecan, 113
iscador (mistletoe), 237
itching, interventions, 287

J

Jewish men, and breast cancer, 137
joint pain, 205
journaling, 229

K

Kadian, 255
Kaposi's sarcoma, 269
Kelly's Nutritional-Metabolic Therapy, 242
ketoprofen, 254
kidney tumors, 149
Kleinfelter's Syndrome, 137

L

laboratory tests, 26
lactate dehydrogenase, 124
large cell lung cancer, 87
Leatrile, 241
Leucovorin, 112
leukemia, 31; acute lymphocytic, 142–144; and boys, 141; chemotherapy treatment, 195, 196; virus, 15
The Leukemia & Lymphoma Society, 322
Leukine, 205
leukocoria, 150
Leukoplakia, 132
Leuprolide (Lupron), 79, 196

Levamisole, 112

libido, 272–273

Lisa Madonia Memorial Fund, 153

lithotomy, 72–73

Live Cell Therapy, 242–243

liver cancer, 15

living will, 282

Lomustine, 195, 200

lung cancer, 84–99; causes, 84–85; detection, 86; diagnosis, 87–90; prevention, 85; recurrence, 98; research, 98–99; side effects, treatment, 94; staging, 89–90; survivorship, 97–98; symptom management, 94–97; symptoms, 86; treatment, 90–94, 195; types of, 86–87

luteinizing hormone, 78

lymph nodes, 59

lymphoma, 15, 31, 144–145; and boys, 141; Burkitt's, 15; chemotherapy treatment, 195, 196; T-cell, 15

M

macrobiotic diet, 224

magnetic resonance imaging (MRI) scans, 27

Make a Wish Foundation of America, 153

malignant cells, 30

mammography, 139

Man to Man, 328

marijuana, and lung cancer, 85

massage, 227–228

Mayday Pain Resource Center, 325

mediastinoscopy, 88

Medicaid, 37, 294, 312–313

medical history, patient's, 24

Medical Miranda, 67

Medi-Cal, 37

Medicare Hospice Benefit, 312

Medicare, 37, 294, 312

meditation, 230

Medroxyprogesterone (Depo-Provera), 196

medulloblastoma, and boys, 141, 145–146

Megestrol (Megace), 196

melanoma, 14, 17, 31; chemotherapy treatment, 195

Melphalan, 200

memory loss, 98

mental health professionals, 43

mentors, 46–47

Mercaptopurine, 195

mesodermal germ layer, 142

mesothelioma (lung cancer), 14, 87

metaphase, 10

metastasis, cells, 11; lung cancer, 87; sites of, 32

Methadone, 255

Methadose, 255

Methotrexate, 195, 199, 202, 203

mind-body approaches, 228–231

Mission Air Transportation Network, 327

Mithramycin, 195, 202

Mitomycin, 195, 199, 201

mitosis, 9, 10

Mitotane, 196

Mitxantrone (Novantrone), 199

mixed cell lung cancer, 87

Modified Astler-Coller staging system, 110

monoclonal antibodies, 204

morphine, 205, 255

mouth infections, interventions, 287

MRI scan, 60, 62; and lung cancer detection, 87

MSContin, 255

MSIR, 255

multi-drug resistance, 197

mumps, 120

muscular tissue, 30

music therapy, 229

mustard gas, 193

myeloma, 31; chemotherapy treatment, 195; multiple, 277

N

naproxin, 254

nasopharyngeal carcinoma, 15

National Association for Continence, 324

National Cancer Institute, 39, 41, 48; Cancer Information Service, 323; and clinical trials, 212

National Center for Homeopathy, 324

National Coalition for Cancer Survivorship, 329

National Commission for the Certification of Acupuncturists, 324

National Prostate Cancer Coalition, 328

Native American Cancer Initiatives, 316

nausea, 190; chemotherapy side effect, 200; interventions, 287

neoadjuvant hormone blockade, 68, 79

neoadjuvant therapy, 157

neoplasia, 29

nerve sparing surgery, 266

nervous tissue, cancers of, 30, 31

Netherlands, euthanasia, 289

Neupogen, 205

neuroblastoma, 142, 148–149; chemotherapy treatment, 196

neuroectodermal tissue, 142

neuroendocrine tumor, 110

nickel, and lung cancer, 85

Nitrogen mustard, 200

Nitrosureas, 200

non-Hodgkin's lymphoma, 144–145, 269

non-seminoma tumors, 125, 126

non-small-cell lung cancer, 87; staging, 89, 90, 91; surviving, 89; treatment, 93–94

nonsteroidal anti-inflammatory drugs (NSAIDs), 105, 205, 254

Novocain, 170

nuclear scans, 27

nurses, 3–4, 43

nutritional supplements, 224–225

O

obesity, 13, 18

Occupational Safety and Health Administration, 85

Office of Alternative Medicine, 221

Office of Cancer Complementary and Alternative Medicine, 221, 323

Office of Minority Health Resource Center, 316, 329

OMS Concentrate, 255

oncogenes, 13

oncologists, 38

Oncology Nursing Society, 21, 323; clinical trials position, 210; position on end-of-life care, 281

open lung biopsy, 89

opiods, 254

oral sex, 276

Oramorph SR, 255

orchiectomy, 66, 78; inguinal, 124

organic foods, 224

osteogenesis imperfecta, 147

osteosarcoma, 147–148

otitis media, 189

ovarian cancer, 14

Oxycodone, 255

Oxygen Therapy, 243

P

Paclitaxel (Taxol), 199, 203

Paget's disease, 132, 147

pain control, 205, 248–258; assessment, 252–253; barriers to, 249–252; management, 253–258; medications, 253, 286; nondrug approaches, 255–256, 286; postoperative, 175–176

pain, lung cancer, 95, 97; neuropathic, pain, 248–249; nociceptive, 248

palladium, 184

Palladone, 255

palliative care, 157, 290–295

pancreatic cancer, chemotherapy treatment, 195

parallel biochemical defense system, 232

paralysis, interventions, 286

parent cell, 9

pathology reports, understanding, 29–30

patients' rights, 67

Patient Self-Determination Act, 282

Patients' Bill of Rights for Quality Cancer Care, 162, 304–305
pau d'arco, 237
Pauling, Linus, 225
pediatric cancers, 141–153; chemotherapy treatment, 195, 196
pelvic exenteration, 114
pelvic lymphadenectomy, 66
penectomy, 134
penile cancer, 15, 130–141, 277; detection, 131–132; diagnosis, 132–133; prevention, 131–132; risk factors, 130–131; staging, 133–134; survivorship, 135; treatment, 134–135
penile implant, 267
Percocet, 255
Percodan, 255
perineal urethrostomy, 135
peripheral stem cell therapy, 128
PET scans, and lung cancer detection, 87
Pharmaceutical Research and Manufacturers of America, 329
pharmacologic therapies, 231–234
photocoagulation, 150
physical activity, 18
Physician Data Query, 42, 48
physicians, and cancer treatment, 162–163
placental alkaline phosphatase, 124
Plant Alkaloids, 199
platelets, low, 276
Platinol, 118, 127, 128
Plicamycin, 201
pneumonitis, 191
podophyllotoxins, 195
politics, 308–316; accessibility to health care, 309–311, 315–316; costs of care, 311, 312–314; health care reform, 308–309; research, 311
pollutants, 17–18
polychlorinated biphenyls, 17
polycyclic aromatic hydrocarbons, 17; and lung cancer, 85
polypectomy, 113
polyps, colorectal, 102–103

postoperative surgical unit, 174–175
power of attorney, 282–283
Prednisone, 196
preputial sac, 131
prescription drug assistance programs, 314
prevention, 15–18; lung cancer, 85; penis cancer, 131–132; prostate cancer, 55–56
Procarbazine, 196, 203
Procrit, 204
ProctoScinct, 82
Progestational agents, 196
prognosis, breast cancer, 140
prolonging life, 285
prophase, 10
prophylactic cranial radiation, 92
Prostate Cancer Prevention Trial, 56
prostate cancer, 15, 18, 38, 47, 52–83, 196; detection, 56–58; diagnosis, 59–64; follow-up, 80–81; issues and concerns, 52–54; prevention, 55–56; recurrence, 81; research, 82–83; risk factors, 55; screening, 53–54; staging, 63–64; symptoms, 58–59; treatment, 65–80
prostate carcinoma cells, 31
prostate, healthy, 54–55
prostate-specific antigen (PSA) testing, 24, 26, 57–58, 60, 61, 65, 80
prostate-specific membrane antigen (PSMA), 58
prostatic acid phosphatase (PAP) test, 62
prostatic intraepithelial neoplasia, 60
prostatitis, 57
prosthesis, penile, 267, 274
psychoneuroimmunology, 229
psychosis, 206

R

race, and cancer, 120, 315, 316
radiation, as carcinogen, 17, and breast cancer; 138; and lung cancer, 85
radiation recall reaction, 186
radiation therapy, and breast cancer, ' 140; and leukemia, 144; and lung

cancer, 92; and lymphoma, 145; and penis cancer, 134; and testicular cancer, 126, 127

radiation therapy, description of, 178–179; research in, 188; risk factors, 186; side effects, 184–188, 189–192; techniques, 180–184; uses of, 178–192

radical peritoneal lymph node dissection, 126

radical prostatectomy, 66, 69–71, 81

radiologists, 27

radiopharmaceutical application, 77

radium-226, 184

Radner, Gilda, 239

radon, 14, 18, and lung cancer, 85

rectal cancer, 277

rectum, 101–102

recurrence, prostate cancer, 81

red blood cell counts, 275

religion and healing, 231

research, lung cancer, 98–99; prostate cancer, 82–83; systemic therapy, 207

retinoblastoma, 142, 150–151

retinoids, 225

rhabdomyosarcoma, 146–147

risk analysis, 18–19

risk factors, 16–17; breast cancer, 137; colorectal cancer, 102–105; penis cancer, 130–131; prostate cancer, 55; testicular cancer, 120–121

rofecoxib, 254

Ronald McDonald House, 327

rosemary, 236

Roxanol, 255

Roxicodone Intensol, 255

S

salvage therapy, 81, 157

sarcoma (see specific cancers), 30; chemotherapy treatment, 195

saw palmetto, 235

schedule dependent drugs, 194

schistosomiasis, 137

scirrhous tumour, 110

screening, colorectal cancer, 106–108; prostate cancer, 53–54

scrotum, 119

second opinions, 41–42

seed implants, 66, 72–77

seizures, interventions, 286

selenium, 85

seminomas, 125, 126

sexuality and cancer, 260–278; changes, 272; fertility, 263–265; intimacy, 269–272; sexual response, 262–263

sexually transmitted diseases, 277–278; and penile cancer, 131

shark cartilage, 232–233

side effects, lung cancer treatment, 94

Siegel, Bernie, 240

sigmoidoscopy, 106, 107

Sinclair Intimacy Institute, 328

skin cancer, 17–18; basal cell, 14; chemotherapy treatment, 195; squamous cell, 14

skin care, during radiation therapy, 187

small-cell lung cancer, 87; staging, 89; surviving, 89; treatment, 92–93

smegma, 131

smoking, 1, 16, and asbestos exposure, 14; and lung cancer, 84–85; quitting, 85

sonogram, 123

sores, digestive system, 200

speculated lesions, 139

sperm banking, 263–264

sperm count, 265

spiritual approaches, 230–231

sputum, interventions, 287

squamous cell carcinoma, 60; lung cancer, 87; penis cancer, 132

staging, colorectal cancer, 110–111; lung cancer, 89–90; penis cancer, 133–134; prostate cancer, 63–64; testicular cancer, 124–125

Starlight Foundation, 153

stereotactic radiosurgery, 182–183

stomach cancer, 15; chemotherapy treatment, 195

Streptozotocin, 195, 200

Strontium 89, 77

suicide, assisted, 285, 289–290

Sunshine Foundation, 153
superior vena cava syndrome, 96
support groups, 46–47
Suramin, 196
surgery, 68–69; and breast cancer, 140; and colorectal cancer, 111–113; and lung cancer, 92, 93; and penile cancer, 134; and testicular cancer, 124, 126
surgery, after, 171–176; care at home, 176–177; complications, 166–167; preparation for, 165–170; testing before, 166; use of, 164–177
survivor support, post-surgery, 176–177
survivorship skills, advocacy, 304–308; communication, 301; decision making, 302; finding information, 300–301; negotiation, 303–304; problem solving, 303
survivorship, 3, 4–5, 35, 296–316; colorectal cancer, 116–117; lung cancer, 97–98; needs of survivors, 297–298; penis cancer, 135; skills, 299–307; testicular cancer, 128–129
swelling, face, 95
symptom management, 284; lung cancer, 94–97; prostate cancer, 66
symptoms, 24; colorectal cancer, 108–109; lung cancer, 86; prostate cancer, 58–59; testicular cancer, 122–123
systemic therapies. *See also* chemotherapy, biotherapy

T

tags, mucosal, 103
tai chi, 227
Tamoxifen, 196
Taxol, 196, 202
Taxotere, 82, 196, 199
tea, 236
telehealth technology, 41
telophase, 10
Teniposide, 196, 199, 203
testes, structure and function, 119–120
testicular cancer, 118–129; chemother- apy treatment, 195, 196; detection, 121–123; diagnosis, 123–125; risk factors, 120–121; staging, 124–125; survivorship, 128–129; symptoms, 122–123; treatment, 125–128
testicular implants, 129
testicular leukemia, 143–144
testicular self-exam (TSE), 119
testosterone, 54, 78, 119, 196
tests, for cancer, 24, 26–31
thalidomide, 82, 208
Thioguanine, 195, 201, 203
Thiotepa, 199
thoracotomy, 89
tissue diagnosis, 28–29
TNM system, 32
tobacco, 13, 16; and cancer treatment, 45; and lung cancer, 84–85
Topotecan, 196, 199
total androgen ablation, 79
transillumination, 123
transitional cell carcinoma, 60
transrectal ultrascan, 60, 61
transsexuals, and breast cancer, 138
transurethral resection of the prostate (TURP), 69
treatment team, forming, 36–40
treatment, breast cancer, 139–140; colorectal cancer, 111–115; lung cancer, 90–94; penis cancer, 134–135; prostate cancer, 65–80; stopping, 290; testicular cancer, 125–128
treatments, cancer, 156–163; deciding on, 158–160; goals, 156–157; hospitals and, 160–162; sequence of, 157–158
TSE, 121–122
tumor boards, 41
tumors, 29; germ-cell, 124; grades of, 31, 60
Tylox, 255
tyrosine kinase inhibitors, 99

U

U.S. Office of Technology Assessment, 221

U.S. Veteran's Administration, 57, 295, 313, 329
ulcerative colitis, 104
ultrasound scans, 27, 123
ultrasound-guided percutaneous cryosurgery, 66
ultraviolet radiation, 14, 18; prostate cancer, 55
United Ostomy Association, 325
urinary tract cancers, 38
urination, difficulty with, 59
urine, blood in, 59
US TOO International, Inc., 47, 53, 67, 328

V

vegetarian diet, 224
Velban, 127
Vepesid, 127
Viagra, 267
viatical settlements, 313
vinblastine sulfate, 127, 195, 201, 203
vinca, 195
Vincristine, 195, 203
Vindesine, 195, 203
Vinorelbine, 203
vinyl chloride, 17; and lung cancer, 85
Vioxx, 254
viral carcinogenesis, 15
vitamin A, 85, 225
vitamin B17, 241
vitamin C, 85, 225
vitamin D, 225, 226
vitamin E, 225
vitamin therapy, 225–226
vomiting, 190

W

Ward, Mathew, 118
watchful waiting, prostate cancer, 65–66
Weil, Andrew, 240
Wellness Community, 239–240
Wellspring Center, 240
white blood cell counts, 275, 276–277
Wilms' tumor, 142, 149; chemotherapy treatment, 195
wish organizations, 152–154
World Council of Enterostomal Therapists, 325
Wound, Ostomy and Continence Nurses Society, 325

X

Xandria Collection, 328
xerostomia, 189
X-ray tests, 27; and lung cancer detection, 86, 87
X-rays, as carcinogens, 18

Y

Y-Me National Breast Cancer Organization, 140

WOMEN'S CANCERS: How to Prevent Them, How to Treat Them, How to Beat Them *by* Kerry A. McGinn, R.N., N.P., and Pamela J. Haylock, R.N., M.A.

This award-winning guide offers information, ideas, and support for treating and surviving cancer—from lung and colon cancer to the malignancies that exclusively affect women: breast, cervical, ovarian, uterine, and vaginal cancer, as well as rarer forms of reproductive cancers.

The authors clearly and sensitively address the issues that surround a cancer diagnosis, from finding the right physician to psychological factors. They discuss risk factors, complementary therapies, and how to cope with all aspects of chemotherapy, including nausea and hair loss.

The second edition covers the latest screening guidelines and diagnostic tests, the discovery of the breast cancer gene, and how changes in health care and insurance industries affect cancer treatment. Also included is a new chapter on lung cancer, the leading cause of death from cancer in women.

512 pages ... 68 illus. ... 2nd edition ... Paperback $19.95 ... Hardcover $29.95

CANCER — INCREASING YOUR ODDS FOR SURVIVAL: A Resource Guide for Integrating Mainstream, Alternative and Complementary Therapies *by* David Bognar, with a Preface by O. Carl Simonton, Ph.D.

Based on the four-part television series hosted by Walter Cronkite.

This book describes all the current conventional, alternative, and complementary treatments for cancer. Each listing covers the treatment and its success rates and gives contact information for experts, organizations, and support groups, and book, video, and Internet resource listings. Full-length interviews with leaders in the field of healing, including Joan Borysenko, Stephen Levine, and Bernie Siegel, cover the powerful effect the mind has on the body and the therapies that strengthen the connection between spiritual healing and issues of death and dying.

352 pages ... Paperback $15.95 ... Hard Cover $25.95

CANCER DOESN'T HAVE TO HURT: How to Conquer the Pain Caused by Cancer and Cancer Treatment
by Pamela J. Haylock, R.N., M.A., and Carol P. Curtiss, R.N., OCN

People with cancer suffer needlessly because of the belief that cancer and pain go hand-in-hand. Haylock and Curtiss show that not only can cancer pain be relieved, but patients who have less pain do better.

Readers learn how to describe their pain in specific terms that doctors understand, as well as how to read prescriptions, administer medications, and adjust dosages if necessary. Also included are non-drug methods of pain relief that patients and caregivers can implement on their own, including massage, exercise, visual imagery, and music therapy.

192 pages ... 12 illus. ... Paperback... $14.95 ... Hardcover... $24.95

To order or for our FREE catalog call (800) 266-5592

THE FEISTY WOMAN'S BREAST CANCER BOOK *by* Elaine Ratner.

Weaving her own story with information about treatment choices, Elaine Ratner has written a book that challenges many popular assumptions. Among her leading concerns: the paternalistic attitude of the medical establishment toward women patients, why thousands of women already cured by surgery routinely accept invasive therapies that don't really help them, and the ways our culture shapes women's attitudes toward their bodies and affects their health care decisions.

"I heartily endorse [Ms. Ratner's] emphasis on the importance of learning all you can about treatment options and not allowing doctors to make all the decisions for you." — Jane Brody, *New York Times*

"There are times when a woman needs a wise and level-headed friend, someone kind, savvy, and caring... [This] book...is just such a friend..." — Rachel Naomi Remen, M.D., author of *Kitchen Table Wisdom*

288 pages ... Paperback.... $14.95 ... Hardcover... $24.95

LYMPHEDEMA: A Breast Cancer Patient's Guide to Prevention and Healing *by* Jeannie Burt & Gwen White, P.T.; Foreword by Judith R. Casley-Smith, M.D.

Thirty percent of all breast cancer survivors in the U.S. may get lymphedema after surgery or radiation. This book emphasizes active self-help—more than 50 illustrations explain treatment procedures, bandaging techniques, and exercises to make treatment more effective. Chapters cover garments, pumps, diet, the effects of environmental chemicals, and the benefits of relaxation. Personal stories highlight practical issues and factors in success.

"Finally, here is a superbly informative and useful book about lymphedema.... Reading (it) is emotionally satisfying, as well as empowering." — National Lymphedema Network Newsletter

224 pages... 50 illus... Paperback... $12.95... Hardcover... $22.95

RECOVERING FROM BREAST SURGERY: Exercises to Strengthen Your Body and Relieve Pain *by* Diana Stumm, P.T.

Until now, no book has specifically addressed how to eliminate the pain and loss of mobility that follows a mastectomy or other breast surgery. Physical therapist Diana Stumm has worked with women recovering from breast surgery for more than 30 years. In this book, she discusses the best exercises for mastectomy, lumpectomy, radiation, reconstruction, and lymphedema. Clear drawings illustrate a program of specific stretches, massage techniques, and general exercises that form the crucial steps to a full and pain-free recovery.

"[Diana Stumm's] knowledge of breast cancer management is unsurpassed in the world of physical therapy." — Francis A. Marzoni, Jr., M.D.

128 pages ... 25 illus. ... Paperback ... $11.95

All prices and availability subject to change